ADVANCES IN
Pediatrics

Editor-in-Chief
Michael S. Kappy, MD, PhD

Professor, Department of Pediatrics
University of Colorado Health Sciences Center
The Children's Hospital, Denver, Colorado

PHILADELPHIA   LONDON   TORONTO   MONTREAL   SYDNEY   TOKYO

ADVANCES IN
Pediatrics

VOLUMES 1 THROUGH 55 (OUT OF PRINT)

VOLUME 56

Vice President, Continuity Publishing: Kimberly Murphy
Editor: Carla Holloway

Reprints: For copies of 100 or more of articles in this publication, please contact the Commercial Reprints Department, Elsevier Inc., 360 Park Avenue South, New York, NY 10010-1710. Tel: (212) 633-3812; Fax: (212) 462-1935; E-mail: reprints@elsevier.com.

Printed and bound in the United Kingdom
Transferred to Digital Print 2011

Editorial Office:
Elsevier
1600 John F. Kennedy Blvd,
Suite 1800
Philadelphia, PA 19103-2899

International Standard Serial Number: 0065-3101
International Standard Book Number: 13: 978-0-323-06822-2

ADVANCES IN
Pediatrics

Editor-in-Chief

MICHAEL S. KAPPY, MD, PhD, Professor, Department of Pediatrics, University of Colorado Health Sciences Center, The Children's Hospital, Denver, Colorado

Associate Editors

LEWIS A. BARNESS, MD, DSci(hc), DPH(hc), Distinguished University Professor Emeritus, Department of Pediatrics, University of South Florida College of Medicine, Tampa, Florida

LESLIE L. BARTON, MD, Professor Emerita, Department of Pediatrics, Steele Memorial Children's Research Center, University of Arizona, Tucson, Arizona

CAROL D. BERKOWITZ, MD, Executive Vice Chair, Department of Pediatrics, Harbor-UCLA Medical Center; Professor of Clinical Pediatrics, David Geffen School of Medicine at UCLA, Torrance, California

ENID GILBERT-BARNESS, AO, MD, MBBS, FRCPA, FRCPath, DSci(hc), MD(hc), Professor, Departments of Pathology and Cell Biology, Pediatrics, and Obstetrics and Gynecology, University of South Florida College of Medicine, Tampa General Hospital, Tampa, Florida

MORITZ ZIEGLER, MD, Chief, Pediatric Surgery, The Children's Hospital, Denver, Colorado

ADVANCES IN
Pediatrics

CONTRIBUTORS

MARK BALLOW, MD, Professor of Pediatrics, Division of Allergy, Immunology and Pediatric Rheumatology, Women and Children's Hospital of Buffalo, State University of New York at Buffalo School of Medicine and Biomedical Sciences, New York, New York

CAROL D. BERKOWITZ, MD, Executive Vice Chair, Department of Pediatrics, Harbor-UCLA Medical Center; Professor of Clinical Pediatrics, David Geffen School of Medicine at UCLA, Los Angeles, California

STEPHEN BERMAN, MD, Professor and Chair, General Academic Pediatrics; Department of Pediatrics Attending, The Children's Hospital, University of Colorado, Aurora, Colorado

ARTURO BRITO, MD, MPH, Chief Medical Officer, Children's Health Fund; Associate Clinical Professor, Department of Pediatrics, Columbia University College of Physicians and Surgeons, New York, New York

GLADYS CAMPA, LMHC, Department of Pediatrics, University of Miami Miller School of Medicine, Miami, Florida

DARA CANNATA, MD, Division of Endocrinology, Diabetes and Bone Diseases, The Samuel Bronfman Department of Medicine, Mount Sinai School of Medicine, New York, New York

ANAI CUADRA, PhD, Assistant Professor of Clinical Pediatrics, Department of Pediatrics, University of Miami Miller School of Medicine, Miami, Florida

MELISSA K. EGGE, MD, Fellow, Department of Pediatrics, Harbor-UCLA Medical Center, Torrance, California

KAM-LUN ELLIS HON, MD (CUHK), FAAP, FCCM, Department of Paediatrics, Prince of Wales Hospital, The Chinese University of Hong Kong, Shatin, Hong Kong

YVONNE FIERZ, MD, Division of Endocrinology, Diabetes and Bone Diseases, The Samuel Bronfman Department of Medicine, Mount Sinai School of Medicine, New York, New York

ALAN W. FLAKE, MD, Center for Fetal Diagnosis and Treatment, Children's Hospital of Philadelphia; Professor of Surgery and Obstetrics and Gynecology, Department of Surgery, University of Pennsylvania School of Medicine, Philadelphia, Pennsylvania; Ruth and Tristram C. Colket, Jr Endowed Chair in Pediatric Surgery, Director, Children's Center for Fetal Research, Children's Hospital of Philadelphia; Director, Pediatric Surgery Fellowship Training Program, Children's Hospital of Philadelphia, Philadelphia, Pennsylvania

JOHN M. FREEMAN, MD, Professor, Neurology and Pediatrics (Emeritus), Johns Hopkins Medical Institutions, Baltimore, Maryland

CHARLES GABBERT, MD, Division of Gastroenterology, Hepatology, and Nutrition, Department of Pediatrics, University of California, San Diego School of Medicine, San Diego; Department of Medicine, University of California, San Diego School of Medicine, La Jolla, California

NATALIE GARCIA, MD, Department of Medicine, University of California, San Diego School of Medicine, La Jolla, California

ROY GRANT, MA, Senior Director, Applied Research, Children's Health Fund, New York, New York

BENJAMIN L. JOHNSON, MEd, Liver Imaging Group, Department of Radiology, University of California, San Diego School of Medicine, San Diego, California

SHARON JOSEPH, MD, Children's Hospital at Montefiore Medical Center, Bronx; Assistant Clinical Professor, Department of Pediatrics, Albert Einstein College of Medicine, New York, New York

SHERYL KENT, PhD, Department of Anesthesiology, University of Colorado Denver; Chronic Pain Consultative Service, The Children's Hospital, Aurora, Colorado

ADRIAN J. KHAW, MD, Assistant Professor of Clinical Pediatrics, Department of Pediatrics, University of Miami Miller School of Medicine, Miami, Florida

KRISTIN D. KISTLER, PhD, Division of Gastroenterology, Hepatology, and Nutrition, Department of Pediatrics, University of California, San Diego School of Medicine, San Diego, California

ERIC H. KOSSOFF, MD, Associate Professor, Neurology and Pediatrics, Johns Hopkins Medical Institutions, Baltimore, Maryland

HEATHER LEHMAN, MD, Assistant Professor of Pediatrics, Division of Allergy, Immunology and Pediatric Rheumatology, Women and Children's Hospital of Buffalo, State University of New York at Buffalo School of Medicine and Biomedical Sciences, New York, New York

DEREK LEROITH, MD, PhD, Division of Endocrinology, Diabetes and Bone Diseases, The Samuel Bronfman Department of Medicine, Mount Sinai School of Medicine, New York, New York

ALEXANDER K.C. LEUNG, MBBS, FRCPC, FRCP(UK&Irel), FRCPCH, FAAP, Department of Paediatrics, The Alberta Children's Hospital, The University of Calgary, Calgary, Alberta, Canada

SARAH M. LINDBÄCK, MD, MPH, Division of Gastroenterology, Hepatology, and Nutrition, Department of Pediatrics, University of California, San Diego School of Medicine, San Diego, California

LYNN LORIAUX, MD, PhD, Professor and Chair, Department of Medicine, Oregon Health and Science University, Portland, Oregon

JULIA LYNCH, MD, Director, Military Infectious Disease Research Program, US Army, Medical Research and Material Command (US Army, MRMC), Fort Detrick, Massachusetts

PATRICK MAHAR, MD, Assistant Professor, Department of Pediatrics, Emergency Medicine Attending, The Children's Hospital, University of Colorado, Aurora, Colorado

MARILYN J. MANCO-JOHNSON, MD, Department of Pediatrics, Hemophilia and Thrombosis Center, The Children's Hospital, University of Colorado Denver, Aurora, Colorado

NIZAR F. MARAQA, MD, Assistant Professor, Pediatric Infectious Diseases and Immunology, University of Florida College of Medicine-Jacksonville, Jacksonville, Florida

GAIL L. NEUENKIRCHEN, MS, RN, CPNP, Department of Anesthesiology, University of Colorado Denver; Chronic Pain Consultative Service, The Children's Hospital, Aurora, Colorado

SOLA OLAMIKAN, MD, Chronic Pain Consultative Service, The Children's Hospital, Aurora, Colorado

ALINA OLTEANU, MD, PhD, Head, Section of Community Pediatrics and Global Health, Department of Pediatrics, Tulane University School of Medicine, New Orleans, Louisiana

JORDAN S. ORANGE, MD, PhD, Division of Immunology, Children's Hospital of Philadelphia, University of Pennsylvania School of Medicine, Philadelphia, Pennsylvania

PERRIE E. PARDEE, BS, Division of Gastroenterology, Hepatology, and Nutrition, Department of Pediatrics, University of California, San Diego School of Medicine, San Diego, California

DAVID A. PARTRICK, MD, Associate Professor of Surgery, University of Colorado School of Medicine, Department of Pediatric Surgery, Director of Surgical Endoscopy, The Children's Hospital, University of Colorado, Aurora, Colorado

IAN M. PAUL, MD, MSc, Associate Professor, Departments of Pediatrics and Public Health Sciences, The Milton S. Hershey Medical Center, Penn State College of Medicine, Hershey, Pennsylvania

MOBEEN H. RATHORE, MD, CPE, Professor and Associate Chairman, Chief, Pediatric Infectious Diseases and Immunology; Wolfson Children's Hospital, University of Florida College of Medicine-Jacksonville, Jacksonville, Florida

ARLETA REWERS, MD, PhD, Associate Professor, Emergency Medicine, Department of Pediatrics, School of Medicine, University of Colorado Denver, Aurora, Colorado

LOURDES RIGUAL-LYNCH, PhD, Children's Hospital at Montefiore Medical Center, Bronx; Department of Pediatrics, Albert Einstein College of Medicine, New York, New York

JOHN A. SANDOVAL, MD, Assistant Member, St Jude Children's Research Hospital, Department of Surgery, Memphis, Tennessee

JEFFREY B. SCHWIMMER, MD, Division of Gastroenterology, Hepatology, and Nutrition, Department of Pediatrics; Liver Imaging Group, Department of Radiology, University of California, San Diego School of Medicine; Department of Gastroenterology, Rady Children's Hospital San Diego, San Diego, California

ALAN SHAPIRO, MD, Children's Hospital at Montefiore Medical Center, Bronx; Department of Pediatrics, Albert Einstein College of Medicine, New York, New York

ZIAD M. SHEHAB, MD, Professor of Pediatrics and Pathology, Head, Section of Infectious Diseases, Department of Pediatrics, Arizona Health Sciences Center, Tucson, Arizona

CLAUDE B. SIRLIN, MD, Liver Imaging Group, Department of Radiology, University of California, San Diego School of Medicine, San Diego, California

ROBIN SLOVER, MD, Associate Professor, Department of Anesthesiology, University of Colorado Denver; Interim Director, Chronic Pain Consultative Service, The Children's Hospital, Aurora, Colorado

EMMANUIL SMORODINSKY, MD, Department of Medicine, University of California, San Diego School of Medicine, La Jolla; Liver Imaging Group, Department of Radiology, University of California, San Diego School of Medicine, San Diego, California

E. RICHARD STIEHM, MD, Division of Immunology/Allergy/Rheumatology, Mattel Children's Hospital, UCLA School of Medicine University of California, Los Angeles, California

ERIC THAM, MD, Assistant Professor, Department of Pediatrics, Emergency Medicine Attending, The Children's Hospital, University of Colorado, Aurora, Colorado

ARCHANA VIJAYAKUMAR, BS, Division of Endocrinology, Diabetes and Bone Diseases, The Samuel Bronfman Department of Medicine, Mount Sinai School of Medicine, New York, New York

MIHO WATANABE, MD, Center for Fetal Diagnosis and Treatment, Children's Hospital of Philadelphia; Department of Surgery, University of Pennsylvania School of Medicine; Fetal Surgery Research Fellow, Children's Center for Fetal Research, Children's Hospital of Philadelphia, Philadelphia, Pennsylvania

JOE WATHEN, MD, Assistant Professor, Department of Pediatric, Emergency Medicine Attending, The Children's Hospital, University of Colorado, Aurora, Colorado

CONTENTS

VOLUME 57 • 2010

Childhood Accidents: Injuries and Poisoning
By Kam-Lun Ellis Hon and Alexander K.C. Leung

Controversies in the Evaluation of Young Children with Fractures
By Melissa K. Egge and Carol D. Berkowitz

Pediatric Nonalcoholic Fatty Liver Disease: A Comprehensive Review

By Sarah M. Lindbäck, Charles Gabbert, Benjamin L. Johnson, Emmanuil Smorodinsky, Claude B. Sirlin, Natalie Garcia, Perrie E. Pardee, Kristin D. Kistler, and Jeffrey B. Schwimmer

Chronic Pediatric Pain

By Robin Slover, Gail L. Neuenkirchen, Sola Olamikan,
and Sheryl Kent

Advances in Pediatric Pharmacology, Therapeutics, and Toxicology

By Ian M. Paul

Therapeutic Use of Immunoglobulins

By E. Richard Stiehm, Jordan S. Orange, Mark Ballow,
and Heather Lehman

Pediatric Outpatient Parenteral Antimicrobial Therapy: An Update

By Nizar F. Maraqa and Mobeen H. Rathore

Current Controversies in Treatment and Prevention of Diabetic Ketoacidosis

By Arleta Rewers

Coccidioidomycosis

By Ziad M. Shehab

Advances in the Care and Treatment of Children with Hemophilia

By Marilyn J. Manco-Johnson

Bridging Mental Health and Medical Care in Underserved Pediatric Populations: Three Integrative Models

By Arturo Brito, Adrian J. Khaw, Gladys Campa, Anai Cuadra, Sharon Joseph, Lourdes Rigual-Lynch, Alina Olteanu, Alan Shapiro, and Roy Grant

Ketosis and the Ketogenic Diet, 2010: Advances in Treating Epilepsy and Other Disorders

By John M. Freeman and Eric H. Kossoff

The GH/IGF-1 Axis in Growth and Development: New Insights Derived from Animal Models

Dara Cannata, Archana Vijayakumar, Yvonne Fierz, and Derek LeRoith

Fetal Surgery: Progress and Perspectives

By Miho Watanabe and Alan W. Flake

Advances in the Surgical Management of Gastroesophageal Reflux

By John A. Sandoval and David A. Partrick

Advances in Pediatrics 57 (2010) xxv–xxvi

ADVANCES IN PEDIATRICS

Introduction

Michael S. Kappy, MD, PhD, FAAP

The Editors welcome Carol Berkowitz, MD to our Board. Dr Berkowitz is Executive Vice Chair in the Department of Pediatrics, David Geffen School of Medicine at UCLA. She is a distinguished pediatrician who has published extensively on matters of child behavior and child abuse, including articles in this Journal. We welcome her input in selecting future articles in her area of interest, based on her vast experience.

This year's "Foundations of Pediatrics" feature, contributed by Dr Lynn Loriaux, Chair of the Department of Medicine at the University of Oregon Health Sciences University, honors Fuller Albright, MD, whose contributions to our understanding of metabolic and endocrine disorders are legendary.

The article by Lynch et al describes of how disasters affect children and how we can participate in their care, a particularly timely topic considering recent events in Haiti, Mexico, China, and other parts of the world.

Advances in our medical treatment of childhood disorders are presented in articles by Freeman and Kosoff, Maraqa and Rathore, Paul, Shehab, Slover, Stiehm et al, and Rewers, whose recent contributions to our understanding of the pathogenesis and treatment of diabetic ketoacidosis represent a significant advance.

General advances in the diagnosis and treatment of childhood disorders are contributed by Egge and Berkowitz (child abuse), Manco-Johnson (hemophilia), and Brito et al, a continuing feature from the Children's Health Fund regarding the provision of mental health and medical care to underserved children. Schwimmer provides an update on non-alcoholic fatty liver disease in children, an increasing medical problem in children associated with obesity and a probable prelude to Type 2 diabetes.

Advances in fetal surgery, a burgeoning field, are well-documented by Watanabe and Flake, and Sandoval and Partrick present advances in the surgical treatment of gastroesophageal reflux. Cannata et al revise our understanding of the growth hormone/IGF-I axis in its latest iteration.

0065-3101/10/$ – see front matter
doi:10.1016/j.yapd.2010.09.006

As always, the editors welcome your suggestions for future articles, and these can be sent to: kappy.michael@tchden.org.

Michael S. Kappy, MD, PhD, FAAP
University of Colorado Health Sciences Center
The Children's Hospital
13123 East 16th Avenue
B-265 Aurora, CO 80045, USA

E-mail address: kappy.michael@tchden.org

Advances in Pediatrics 57 (2010) 1–6

ADVANCES IN PEDIATRICS

Foundations of Pediatrics: Fuller Albright, MD (1900–1969)

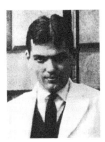

Fuller Albright, MD

Lynn Loriaux, MD, PhD

Department of Medicine, Oregon Health and Science University, Portland, OR, USA

F uller Albright was born in Buffalo, New York, on Jan. 12, 1900. His father, John Joseph Albright, was a man of property, making his fortune in coal, steel, and automobiles. John's first wife, Harriet, died in 1895. He was left with three motherless children, Raymond, Ruth, and Langdon. To remedy this situation, he wrote to the president of Smith College inquiring if there might not be a recent graduate who might like the job of governess to the children. Susan Fuller accepted the job. She rapidly became one of the family, and she and John were married 2 years later. Together they had five children. Fuller, after his mother's maiden name, was the middle child and the second of two boys.

John Albright founded the Nichols School for boys and the Franklin School for girls, and all of his eight children were educated in these two institutions. Fuller was a good student with a strong interest in sports. He was the captain of the football team. He went to Harvard College when he was 17. Eighteen months later, he joined the Army and was sent to the Officer Candidate School in Plattsburg, New York. It was during this year that he likely fell victim to the influenza pandemic. He recovered, but almost certainly had Von Economo encephalitis, which revisited him many years later in the form of postencephalitic Parkinson disease.

The end of World War I found Albright an instructor in the Student Army Corps at Princeton University. Despite having attended only 18 months of

E-mail address: loriauxl@ohsu.edu

0065-3101/10/$ – see front matter
doi:10.1016/j.yapd.2010.08.010

college, he applied to Harvard Medical School, and was accepted. He was elected to Alpha Omega Alpha in 1923, and graduated in 1924. He took a 2-year internship at the Massachusetts General Hospital.

Fuller and a cointern, Read Ellsworth, became fast friends during this time. Read was from Coos Bay, Oregon, at that time the timber capital of the western United States. His family was a wealthy one. Read graduated from Reed College in Portland, Oregon. He was handsome, outgoing, musically talented, and could tell a good joke. Fuller was quiet, reserved, serious, and tone deaf. Together they made a famous team. They both developed an interest in endocrinology. Fuller followed this interest as a fellow with Joseph Aub, a leading endocrinologist at the Massachusetts General Hospital. Ellsworth returned to Johns Hopkins to work with John Eager Howard. Albright joined Ellsworth at Hopkins for a year in 1927. Thus began a fertile collaboration on the physiology and pathophysiology of disorders of calcium metabolism that endured until Ellsworth's death from tuberculosis in 1937.

Albright left Hopkins in 1928 to spend a year with Jacob Erdheim, the famed Viennese pathologist. Erdheim had shown that parathyroidectomy prevents calcification of the teeth in rats, an important insight into the regulation of calcium homeostasis. Albright described Erdheim as follows:

> "Was ist die Ursacke dafür." (What is the cause of this?) These words meet our ears as we approach. They are spoken by the head gardener for the tree, the fruit of which can save lives. The appearance of the head gardener is so arresting that, for the moment, we turn our full attention to him. He has a huge frame. Although he is not excessively tall, his hips are as high as an average man's chest. The hands are large and deft. His eyes smile from behind gold-rimmed spectacles as he expostulates in a somewhat high-pitched voice, "Manche Leute sehen sehr gut aber sie schauen nicht an" (many people see well but neglect to look) [1].

This was probably Albright's first introduction to the syndrome of hypogonadotropic hypogonadism.

Albright returned to the Massachusetts General Hospital in 1929. He established the Biological Laboratory in order to offer the Ascheim-Zondek pregnancy test to the hospital clinical services. More tests followed, and the name was changed to the Endocrine Laboratory. It was this laboratory that, in time, became the core of the world famous Endocrine Unit of the Massachusetts Hospital.

In 1930, Albright met Claire Birge of Greenwich, Connecticut, and they were married 2 years later. Their first child, a boy, was named Birge, his mother's maiden name. As a wedding present, Fuller's father gave them a house in Brookline. Serge Koussevitsky was their next door neighbor.

At the annual Atlantic City meetings of 1936, John Eager Howard noted the beginnings of a "pill rolling" tremor in Albright's right hand. The Parkinson disease advanced rapidly. By 1940, Albright could no longer write. By 1945, his speech was so impaired that he could be understood only by family and a few close associates. By 1950, Albright was sure that the disease was affecting his thought processes. Sometimes, he said, it could take him an entire evening to write a single paragraph. He resolved to do something about it.

A young neurosurgeon at the Mayo Clinic, Irving Cooper, had developed an operation that helped many patients and Parkinson disease [2]. It was called chemopallidectomy. The operation was called chemopallidectomy, because Cooper believed that the cannula tip was in the body of the globus pallidus. Subsequent postmortem studies showed that the successful operations ablated the posterior portion of the ventrolateral nucleus of the thalamus. A burr hole was drilled, and a cannula was advanced into the center of the globus pallidus. A balloon at the tip of the cannula was inflated, and if the tremor and rigidity responded positively, a small amount of ethanol was introduced through the cannula, killing the adjacent neurons. Every 2 or 3 days, another dose was given until maximum benefit was achieved in terms of a reduction in rigidity, tremor, or both. Cooper had recently moved from the Mayo Clinic to St Barnabas Hospital in New York City. The surgery was performed in June of 1956. The early results were favorable. Albright was free of tremor and rigidity on the left side. He could write better, and could perform useful acts with his left hand. The family, in a state of euphoria, returned to Boston. Only his son Read remained behind in order to accompany his father home. The cannula was removed on the seventh postoperative day at about noon. At 3 p.m., Albright was found in bed, akinetic and mute. He lived in this state for another 13 years.

This was a devastating outcome for both patient and surgeon. Cooper wrote in his book "The Vital Probe:"

> "During the next two decades, on a least one hundred occasions, when my name was mentioned during an introduction at a dinner party or at a medical conference or at an airport or in a hotel lobby, the mention of my name was followed by the comment, 'Oh you're the man who operated on Fuller Albright.' On two occasions, when I was introduced at a dinner party, one of the doctors rose, stating he would not stay in the same room with the man who had destroyed Fuller Albright. It is a marvelous thing to behold a teacher of medicine held in such affection and respect that the surgeon considered to be his enemy could not be tolerated by some in the same room. It was a painful, irreversibly traumatic experience for me, a young surgeon, continuing even when I was no longer young" [2].

Albright was moved back to Boston into the Lemuel Shattuck Hospital and then to Massachusetts General Hospital. It was in this time that a young psychiatrist, Paul McHugh, was the resident neurologist for a medical team responsible for 25 permanently disabled patients suffering from advanced neuropsychiatric disorders. They rounded on Fuller Albright daily. Dr McHugh would comment, on each occasion, that they should be careful about what they said because it was possible that the patient could hear and perhaps understand them. One day, an aggressive intern asked Dr McHugh to demonstrate to them that that Albright could hear and understand. McHugh turned to the patient and said, "Dr Albright, what is the serum calcium in pseudo-pseudohypoparathyroidism?" Fuller Albright turned his head slightly and said, "just about normal" [3].

> "A full and complete sentence had emerged from a man who none of us had ever heard speak before. His answer was correct—as he should know, having discovered and named the condition I asked him about. Subsequently, in all the months we cared for him, he would never utter another word. But what a difference that moment had made to all of us. We matured that day not only in matters of the mind but in matters of the heart. Somehow, deep inside that body and damaged brain, he was there—and our job was to help him. If we had ever had misgivings before, we would never again doubt the value of caring for people like him. And we didn't give a fig that his EEG was grossly abnormal" [3].

Over the years, others were convinced that Fuller Albright could understand discussions with him, but as far as I know, he never spoke again. He died of pneumonia in 1969 in the Massachusetts General Hospital.

These years of progressive disability coincided with Albright's most fertile period of translational research. This was in an era before the "least publishable" unit. A paper was written when something substantive could be reported. His curriculum vitae contained 118-peer reviewed papers (appendix). One can see the first American description of hyper- and hypoparathyroidism [4,5], the first description of pseudo hypoparathyroidism [6] and pseudo-pseudo hypoparathyroidism [7] One can see the first descriptions of Klinefelter syndrome [8], the McCune Albright syndrome [9], the Forbes Albright syndrome [10], renal tubular acidosis [11], Vitamin D-resistant rickets [12], the first convincing explanation of the pathophysiology of congenital adrenal hyperplasia [13], the second substantive paper on Turner syndrome [14], the best paper on Cushing syndrome ever written [15], and the first description of the polyendocrine deficiency syndrome [16]. The list goes on.

How did he do this? First, he was blessed with the gift of inductive reasoning. He was homozygous for this trait. Second, he saw patients every day, and spent time in the laboratory every day. He never lost touch with the patient and depended upon his patients to teach him about their illness and to reveal fruitful questions for investigation. He was a bedside-to-bench translational investigator. He insisted that problems chosen for study be generated by real illness in real patients.

In 1944, Albright gave the presidential address at the annual meeting of the American Society of Clinical Investigation [17]. In this address, he set forth a list of suggestions for success. Among them are these:

> "This rider of two horses, however, must remember that there are two horses: He must avoid the danger, on one side, that he as a clinician, be swamped with patients and the other equal danger or the other side that he, as an investigator, be sequestered entirely from the bedside."
> "Any theory is better than none at all."

"Hypotheses are subject to change without notice."
"The man, not the project, should be endowed."
"Whatever else you do, no not become a professor of medicine or the head of a department."

The research world can be divided into basic and applied, and into bench and clinical. Applied clinical research is, basically, the clinical trial. Applied bench research might be thought of as the process that leads to new "cosmetics," or perfume. An example of basic bench research might be understanding how oxygen binds to hemoglobin. An example of basic clinical research might be the untangling of the pathophysiology of premature thelarche.

Albright was a pure basic clinical investigator. There was no profit tied to his work; it was a gift to the world of medicine. For a long time, academic heroes were almost all modeled on Albright's example. The RO-1, the institutional review board, and the cost of doing clinical research have changed all that. A young physician aspiring to a life in translational research faces a very tough uphill struggle, and that struggle is for funding. If this young aspirant's time is truly split between patients and laboratory, the probability of ongoing funding is attenuated. To survive and pay the mortgage, the young proto-scientist will probably give up the laboratory and see patients all of the time or, he will give up patients and enter the laboratory forever. The issue is how to fund the "rider of two horses." Nobody has found the answer to this; only the intramural National Institutes of Health (NIH) do it well. The NIH, however, has not been successful in replicating the model in the non-NIH scientific community. This is where the problem lies. This is where focus needs to be if basic clinical scientists are to continue. Some say that their era is past. Maybe so, but it is hard for me to imagine medicine without them. In that world, scholarship will become the substitute for discovery. Is that what is wanted? As Willy Loman's wife says, "attention must be paid."

References
[1] Albright F, Ellsworth R. Uncharted seas. Portland (OR): Kalmia Press; 1990.
[2] Cooper I. The vital probe. Toronto: George J. McLeod; 1981.
[3] McHugh P. The mind has mountains. Baltimore (MD): The Johns Hopkins University Press; 2006.
[4] Bauer W, Aub JC, Albright F. Studies of calcium and phosphorus metabolism: V. A study of the bone trabeculae as a readily available reserve supply of calcium. J Exp Med 1929;49(1):145.
[5] Albright F. Hyperparathyroidism: its diagnosis and exclusion. N Engl J Med 1933;209(10): 475.
[6] Albright F, Burnett CH, Smith PH, et al. Pseudohypoparathyroidism—an example of seabright's bantam syndrome. Endocrinology 1942;30(6):922.
[7] Albright F, Forbes AP. Pseudo-pseudohypoparathyroidism. Trans Assoc Am Physicians 1952;65:337.
[8] Klinefelter HE Jr, Reifenstein EC Jr, Albright F. Syndrome characterized by gynecomastia, aspermatogenesis without a-leydigism, and increased excretion of follicle-stimulating hormone. J Clin Endocrinol 1942;2:615.

[9] Albright F, Butler AM, Hampton AO, et al. Syndrome characterized by osteitis fibrosa disseminata, areas of pigmentation and endocrine dysfunction, with precocious puberty in females. N Engl J Med 1937;216(17):727.

[10] Forbes AP, Hanneman PH, Griswold GC, et al. Syndrome characterized by galactorrhea, amenorrhea and low urinary FSH: comparison with acromegaly and normal lactation. J Clin Endocrinol Metab 1954;14:265.

[11] Dawson J, Dempsey B, Bartter FC, et al. Evidence for the presence of an amphoteric electrolyte in the urine of patients with renal tubular acidosis. Metabolism 1953;2(3):225.

[12] Albright F, Butler AM, Bloomberg E. Rickets resistant to vitamin D therapy. Am J Dis Child 1937;54:529.

[13] Bartter FC, Albright F, Forbes AP, et al. The effects of adrenocortocostropic hormone and cortisone in the adrenogenital syndrome associated with congenital adrenal hyperplasia: an attempt to explain and correct its disordered hormonal pattern. J Clin Invest 1951;20:237.

[14] Albright F, Smith PM, Fraser R. A syndrome characterized by primary ovarian insufficiency and decreased stature. Report of 11 cases with a digression on hormonal control of auxiliary and pubic hair. Am J Med Sci 1942;204(5):625.

[15] Albright F. Cushing's syndrome, its pathological physiology, its relationship to the adrenogenital syndrome, and its connection with the problem of the reaction of the body to injorious agents (alarm reastion of selye). Harvey Lect 1942–43;38:123.

[16] Sutphin A, Albright F, McCune DJ. Five cases (three in siblings) of idiopathic hypoparathyroidism associated with moniliasis. J Clin Endocrinol 1943;3(12):625.

[17] Albright F. Some of the do's and don'ts in clinical investigation. J Clin Invest 1944;23:921.

Advances in Pediatrics 57 (2010) 7–31

ADVANCES IN PEDIATRICS

Disasters and Their Effects on Children

Julia Lynch, MD[a], Joe Wathen, MD[b], Eric Tham, MD[b],
Patrick Mahar, MD[b], Stephen Berman, MD[c],*

[a]Military Infectious Disease Research Program, US Army, Medical Research and Material
Command (US Army, MRMC), 504 Scott Street, Fort Detrick, MA 21702, USA
[b]Department of Pediatrics, Emergency Medicine, University of Colorado, The Children's Hospital,
13123 East 16th Avenue, B251, Aurora, CO 80045, USA
[c]Department of Pediatrics, General Academic Pediatrics, The Children's Hospital,
University of Colorado, Aurora, CO, USA

The recent magnitude 7.0 M_w earthquake in Haiti on January 12, 2010, created one of the most severe humanitarian disasters in modern recorded times. According to the most recent estimates, 222,570 people died during the earthquake, with an additional 600,000 injured, and more than 1 million being internally displaced persons [1]. Some statistical models estimated that 110,000 of the injured were children [2]. These estimates rival the 230,000 who perished during the Asian tsunami of 2004. Although the destruction of the Asian tsunami occurred in more than 14 countries, the deaths and destruction of the January earthquake were centered on the tiny island of Hispaniola in the country of Haiti with the epicenter in Leogane, which is 25 km from the capital of Port-au-Prince.

Although there was an overwhelming desire by physicians and other health professionals to respond to this tragedy, many of the immediate responders were poorly prepared to perform medical procedures without the support of modern facilities [3]. This included having to perform many amputations without the use of anesthesia or sedation in the immediate aftermath of the earthquake. In this article, we review disaster definitions, classifications, and measures of severity; describe the phases of a disaster; review the 10 World Health Organization emergency relief measures; discuss the role of international relief organizations; and present key issues that medical volunteers faced in Haiti. The key message of this article is to understand that although it is not possible to predict disasters of this magnitude, planning and preparation can help mitigate some of the morbidity and mortality that occur in the aftermath of such disasters. This message has been clearly stated by Benjamin Franklin: "Failing to plan is planning to fail."

*Corresponding author. E-mail address: Berman.Stephen@tchden.org

0065-3101/10/$ – see front matter
doi:10.1016/j.yapd.2010.09.005

DEFINITIONS

The World Health Organization and the Pan American Health Organization (WHO/PAHO) define a disaster as an event that most often occurs suddenly and unexpectedly, resulting in loss of life, harm to the health of the population, destruction of community property, and damage to the environment. The disaster disrupts the normal pattern of life, causing suffering and an overwhelming sense of helplessness and hopelessness. The impact on the socioeconomic structure of a region and environment often requires outside assistance and intervention. Although there are many definitions for disaster, there are 3 common factors. First, there is an event or phenomenon that impacts a population or an environment. Second, a vulnerable condition or characteristic allows the event to have a more serious impact. For example, the large number of collapsed buildings, including schools and hospitals, caused by earthquakes were related to substandard building practices in both China and Haiti. The damage from the 2009 earthquake in Tokyo and the 2010 earthquake in Chile had far less loss of life in large part because of the high quality of construction. Identifying these factors has practical implications for communities' preparedness and provides a basis for prevention. Third, local resources are inadequate to cope with the problems created by the phenomenon or event.

Disasters affect communities in multiple ways. Their impact on the health care infrastructure is multifactorial. They can cause an unexpected number of deaths. In addition, the large number of wounded and sick often exceeds the local community's health care delivery capacity. The community's capacity to care for those affected is often reduced because professionals, clinics, and hospitals have been affected or destroyed. This will have long-term consequences leading to increased morbidity and mortality. Before the January 12 earthquake in Haiti, there were only 11 hospitals in Port-au-Prince. The earthquake damaged or destroyed at least 8 of these hospitals. The remaining health facilities were quickly overwhelmed by large numbers of survivors requiring a wide range of care, particularly for trauma injuries. To help with immediate health care needs, field hospitals were established by a variety of groups (Fig. 1). The 2010 earthquake in Haiti demonstrates how a disaster becomes much more devastating when the preexisting medical system is already inadequate and poorly functional. This makes integrating and organizing outside assistance more fragmented and chaotic.

The disaster can have adverse effects on the environment that will increase the risk for infectious transmissible diseases and environmental hazards. This will affect morbidity, premature death, and future quality of life. There can be shortages of food, with severe nutritional consequences. All these conditions lead to a sense of hopelessness and inability to think that the future will be better. This means that people no longer visualize their future by making plans such as finishing school, getting married, and working. This "foreshortened future" affects the psychological and social behavior of the community.

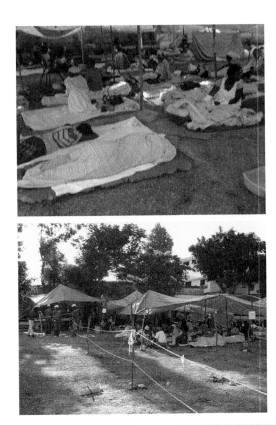

Fig. 1. Field hospital Haiti 2010. These are pictures taken by the team that went to Haiti from TCH. This was their field hospital.

CLASSIFICATION OF DISASTERS

Disasters can be divided into those caused by natural forces and those caused by humans, as shown in Box 1.

Natural forces include earthquakes, tsunamis, volcanic eruptions, hurricanes, fires, tornados, and extreme weather conditions. They can be classified as rapid-onset disasters such as earthquakes or tsunamis, and those with progressive onset, such as droughts that lead to famine. Natural events, usually sudden, can have tremendous effects. For instance, in December 2004, more than 230,000 people died in southern Asia as a result of a tsunami, and in February 2010, more than 220,000 people died following an earthquake in Haiti. Although similar types of disasters have predictable patterns of disruption, as shown in Table 1, the degree of severity and type of response is affected by local features.

Disasters caused by humans are those in which major direct causes are identifiable intentional or nonintentional human actions. They can be subdivided into 3 main categories: technological disasters, terrorism, and complex humanitarian emergencies.

Box 1: Types of disasters

Natural disasters

- Hurricanes or cyclones
- Tornadoes
- Floods
- Avalanches and mud slides
- Tsunamis
- Hailstorms
- Droughts
- Forest fires
- Earthquakes
- Epidemics

Human-provoked disasters

Technological/industrial disasters

- Leaks of hazardous materials
- Accidental explosions
- Bridge or road collapses, or vehicle
- Collisions
- Power cuts

Terrorism/International violence

- Bombs or explosions
- Release of chemical materials
- Release of biologic agents
- Release of radioactive agents
- Multiple or massive shootings
- Mutinies
- Intentional fires

Complex emergencies

- Conflicts or wars
- Genocide

Technological disasters are most often industrial events resulting from unregulated industrialization and inadequate safety standards. Examples include the radioactive leak in the Chernobyl nuclear station in Ukraine (1986) and the toxic gas leak in a Bhopal factory in India (1984). Both of these disasters were associated with many deaths as well as long-term health effects in the affected population. The threat of terrorism has also increased owing to the

Table 1
Frequent effects of disasters

Disaster type / Effect	Complex emergency	Earthquake	Strong winds	Floods	Gradual floods	Mud slides	Volcanic eruptions
Immediate deaths	Numerous	Numerous	Few	Numerous	Few	Numerous	Numerous
Severe lesions	Numerous	Numerous	Moderate	Few	Few	Few	Few
Increased risk for transmissible diseases	This risk applies to ALL significant disasters, and increases with overcrowding and deterioration of sanitary conditions						
Damage to health centers	Moderate; can be severe if health centers are military targets	Severe	Severe	Severe but localized	Severe (only for equipment)	Severe but localized	Severe
Damage to water supply	Severe	Severe	Slight	Severe	Slight	Severe but localized	Severe
Food shortage	Severe	May result from economic and logistic factors		Frequent	Frequent	Not frequent	Not frequent
Significant population displacements	Frequent	Frequent; increased likelihood in severely damaged urban areas	Not frequent	Frequent			

spread of technologies involving nuclear, biologic, and chemical agents as well as the use of explosives and firearms. Explosive or blast events are the most common type of terrorist event causing morbidity and mortality. The term complex humanitarian emergency describes the situation resulting from either an international or civil war. War often results in a staggering loss of civilian lives. There is a disruption of the basic societal infrastructure, including food distribution, water, electricity, sanitation, and health care. In addition, the ability to carry out an emergency relief response is hindered by a lack of security as well as political instability.

Both natural disasters and complex emergencies can force many people to leave their homes. The specific job of the office of the United Nations High Commissioner for Refugees (UNHCR) is to register and assist displaced populations and individuals. This office recognizes 2 categories of affected people: refugees and internally displaced persons (IDP).

Refugees flee their countries because of war, violence, famine, or well-founded fear of persecution for political, ethnical, religious, or nationality reasons. A person recognized as a refugee is entitled to certain protections under the terms of international humanitarian laws. IDPs leave their homes for similar reasons but do not cross the boundaries of their countries. These individuals do not receive the same kind of legal protection, so helping them can be much more difficult. The current worldwide number of IDPs can be monitored by accessing information available at http://www.internal-displacement.org.

PHASES OF DISASTERS

Because relief interventions in emergencies evolve as a continuum, it is useful to prioritize activities and resources according to 4 phases: planning, response, recovery, and mitigation/prevention. Planning comprises all the activities and actions taken before a disaster. Base the planning on the analysis of the community's or organization's risk for exposure to specific types of disasters. Plans should take into account the frequency of occurrence of each type of disaster, the anticipated magnitude of effect, the likelihood that there will be an advanced warning, characteristics of the populations most likely to be affected, the amount and types of resources available within the community or organizational structure, and the ability to function independently without additional outside resources for periods of time.

The response phase includes all activities and actions taken during and immediately after a disaster. This includes notification of the organizations involved in disaster response, setting up of initial communication networks, initial search and rescue, disposal of the dead, damage assessment, evacuation, sheltering, and other multiple activities. The response phase is characterized by initial chaos, high crude mortality rate (CMR), and hopefully, rapid assessments of the situation by specialized response teams. The response phase is often complicated by the lack of functional communications and central organization. The response phase lasts until the initial casualties have been either rescued or acknowledged as lost, and enough resources have been made available to allow the population to assess damages and begin planning restoration and recovery. This phase can last hours to weeks. During the first few days following a disaster, local communities must usually rely on their own resources and disaster plans.

The recovery phase is the period in which the affected organization or community works toward reestablishing self-sufficiency. This is the period of new community planning, rebuilding, and reestablishment of government and public service infrastructure. The health status of the affected population begins to return to predisaster conditions and the outside support services are gradually withdrawn.

During the mitigation and prevention phase, all aspects of emergency management are scrutinized for "lessons learned," and the lessons are then applied in an effort to prevent the recurrence of the disaster itself or to lessen the effects of subsequent events. Mitigation includes preventive and precautionary measures such as changing building codes and practices, redesigning public utilities and services, reviewing mandatory evacuation practices and warning policies, and educating members of the community. Mitigation and planning are continuous processes, as lessons learned from a previous disaster are included in planning for the next one.

SEVERITY OF A DISASTER

As was demonstrated in Haiti, the more fragile the pre-event health status of the affected population and inadequate the predisaster infrastructure, the more severe the disaster. Disaster severity will, therefore, vary according to its magnitude and the vulnerability of the population. When assessing the outcome of a disaster, public health officers describe its severity by the number of human lives lost using the CMR. CMR is usually defined as the number of deaths per 10,000 inhabitants per day. In developing nations, the reference CMR value varies from 0.4 to 0.7 deaths per 10,000 people per day. A CMR above 1 death per 10,000 people per day is considered a humanitarian emergency. To assess the progression of a disaster and the effectiveness of relief interventions, measure the CMR over several appropriate time intervals. For example, during the month following the massive movement of Rwandan refugees to Eastern Zaire, the CMR in that region was 40 to 60 times above the

Table 2 Crude mortality rate: baseline and after humanitarian disaster				
Date	Origin	Host country	CMR crisis	CMR baseline
1991	Somalia	Ethiopia	4.7	0.6
1991	Iraq	Turkey/Iraq	4.2	0.2
1994	Rwanda	Zaire	34.0	0.6

Data from Toole MJ. Mass population displacement—a global public health challenge. Infect Dis Clin North Am 1995:9(2):353–66.

corresponding reference value. The CMR is usually highest during the initial phase of a disaster (Table 2).

The immediate mortality in any type of disaster is not higher in a specific age range; instead, it usually reflects the age distribution of the overall population. However, later the mortality rate is disproportionately higher among the youngest and oldest people. Fig. 2 shows this phenomenon related to a refugee crisis in Northern Iraq in 1991. Although children aged 0 to 5 years accounted for only 18% of the total refugee population, they accounted for 64% of the overall refugee mortality rate.

The most vulnerable groups include children, especially those displaced from their families; women who are pregnant, lactating, or live without their spouse; individuals living in households headed only by women; disabled individuals; and the elderly. In addition to disproportionately high mortality rates, children displaced from their family are at high risk for a number of adverse consequences, including rape, torture, robbery, and exploitation in child labor,

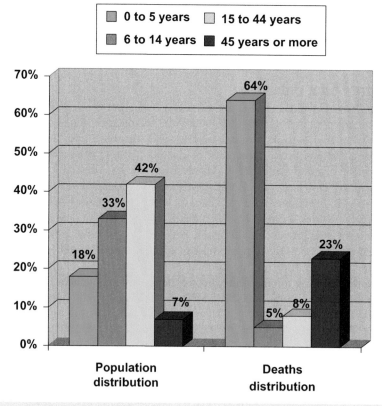

Fig. 2. Mortality rate per age group: refugee crisis Northern Iraq (1991). (*Data from* Toole MJ. Mass population displacement—a global public health challenge. Infect Dis Clin North Am 1995;9(2):353–66.)

child trafficking, and child soldiering. Additionally, because of certain physical and physiologic characteristics, infants and children are more vulnerable to the release of toxic substances and the overcrowding associated with the displacement of large populations. Consequently, in all disaster response planning, it is critical to attempt to reunite children with their families as soon as possible and pay special attention to reducing their vulnerability.

Trauma is often the leading cause of mortality from the immediate impact of a disaster. After the initial impact phase, there are 5 leading medical problems that have consistently been found to be the major causes of mortality in postwar or post–natural disaster settings: diarrhea and dehydration, measles, malaria, respiratory infections, and malnutrition. Unique features in each disaster (eg, climate, topography, preexisting social structure, and physical conditions) affect the proportion of deaths associated with each of these, as well as other causes. Fig. 3 shows the number of natural and complex disasters in the world between 1985 and 1995. Malnutrition, although not identified as a significant immediate cause of death, is the most important factor correlated to the high mortality rates attributable to transmissible diseases. A study including 41 displaced populations (Fig. 4) showed a clear correlation between the CMR (ie, death from all causes) and the prevalence of malnutrition.

ESSENTIAL EMERGENCY RELIEF MEASURES
At a World Health Organization conference, international relief experts identified 10 essential emergency relief measures to consider when responding to a disaster. Each of these measures is described in the following sections. These interventions are not intended to be implemented in strict order; rather, priority for each intervention should be suited to the particular needs relating to each individual emergency situation. The immediate goal for any intervention in humanitarian emergencies is to reduce the number of deaths. Although

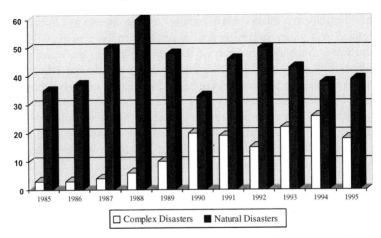

Fig. 3. Number of natural and complex disasters worldwide, 1985–1995.

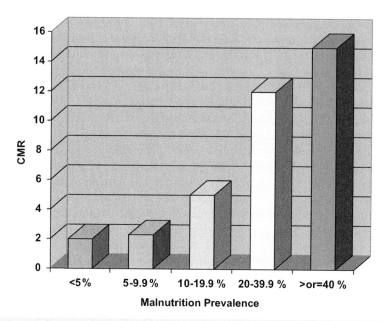

Fig. 4. Effects of malnutrition on mortality rates during disasters. Malnutrition = <80% weight/height WHO reference population; CMR = crude mortality rate (deaths per 1,000 individuals/month) in relation to malnutrition prevalence.

both conflict and natural disasters can result in immediate deaths, there are many preventable deaths that occur in later phases of a disaster over a longer time period. Interventions that are based on speculations rather than on accurate information obtained in the place of the disaster are likely to waste time and valuable resources, ultimately increasing the suffering of the affected population. Unpredicted effects may require urgent attention. For example, compromise of a water supply system is unlikely to be a predicted effect of a storm-related mudslide. However, if the regional system for water pumping or purification is in the mudslide zone, the shortage of safe water becomes the key issue that must be addressed to prevent disease and excessive mortality in the affected population. Resources need to match both the need and the time frame to be useful. For example, trauma is likely to be the major cause of death immediately after an earthquake. If trauma surgery teams and field hospitals arrive a week after the earthquake, most of the trauma-related deaths will already have occurred and very little benefit will be obtained from this high-cost resource.

Do a Rapid Assessment of the Emergency Situation and the Affected Population

An assessment should accurately define what is needed, so that limited resources will be efficiently used to minimize morbidity and mortality as well as reduce the likelihood of additional problems/complications during subsequent phases of response.

National level
Assessments are typically done by expert teams focused on promptly defining the event magnitude, the environmental conditions and infrastructure damage, the major health and nutrition needs of the affected population, and the local response capacity.

Community level
In the immediate aftermath of a disaster, the initial response will primarily come from local resources. Communities must be prepared to do a local assessment of disaster impact. Health care professionals should be prepared to assess the health issues in their community, and understand how information will be shared with higher levels of authority, to contribute to regional or national assessments.

Assessments need to be an ongoing process so that the quality and specificity of data will improve during the rescue and recovery phases. This is especially important whenever any major change occurs, such as an aftershock earthquake. Information gathered through these assessments should be used by the resource managers to determine the allocation of resources in any large-scale disaster.

Provide Adequate Shelter and Clothing
Shelter and clothing is essential as exposure to the climatic conditions in disaster situations can increase caloric requirements and lead to death.

Community level
Find short-term shelters for all homeless individuals, particularly focusing on vulnerable populations. Shelters should be appropriate for the climate and focus on providing a safe environment from subsequent events related to the disaster. After an earthquake, shelters should be established in locations that would not have potential for further damage from collapsing buildings or falling debris from anticipated aftershocks. During times of flooding, it is important that shelter for the displaced individuals is located in an area that is not at risk of rising floodwaters. Displaced victims will not use these shelters if they do not feel safe. Keep individuals within their communities and family networks as much as possible. In general, it is recommended to direct resources to rebuilding within the community, rather than building large camps or temporary settlements outside the disaster area. Schools are often used as emergency shelters following a disaster; however, it is important for children to return to as normal a routine as possible as early as possible. This means that schools should be reopened as soon as possible and teachers should be trained to understand stress reactions and recognize when additional help is needed.

Provide Adequate Nutrition
Large-scale bulk food requirements are typically calculated based on a minimum of 2000 kcal per person per day.

Community level

Communities must plan to distribute food equitably and include vulnerable groups. As global food resources improve, establish targeted supplemental and therapeutic feeding programs for malnourished individuals.

Provide Elementary Sanitation and Clean Water

The estimated minimum requirement for water is 3 to 5 L per person per day of clean water.

Community level

Reestablish supplies of clean water and effective sanitation and waste disposal services as soon as possible. Consider how to address the needs of vulnerable groups related to access, safety, and security in the planning process.

Set Up Diarrhea Control Program

An increase in diarrheal disease is a predictable outcome of disasters because of infrastructure and health care services disruption.

Community level

Rapidly implement community-based education on appropriate household sanitation measures, diarrhea prevention, and household case management, particularly for young children with diarrhea. Health care centers should anticipate the needs for additional cases of dehydration, using appropriate low-cost strategies (oral rehydration solution/oral rehydration therapy [ORS/ORT]) and recognize possible cases of cholera and dysentery.

Immunize Against Measles and Provide Vitamin A Supplements

Measles has been a major source of mortality among crowded, displaced populations in which malnutrition is prevalent. Therefore, measles immunization is the only vaccine that is routinely considered for use as a preventive measure immediately following a disaster. Because vitamin A deficiency is common and contributes to measles-related mortality, consider mass distribution of vitamin A for vulnerable populations.

National level

National and international agencies must work together to determine if measles immunization or vitamin A distribution is necessary following a particular event. If necessary for all or part of the affected population, national authorities should establish the central logistics (eg, cold chain, personnel, materials) to manage a mass immunization/distribution campaign.

Community level

Health officers must immediately assess the available cold chain as part of its health care assessment. Health care professionals must monitor for cases of measles and develop a plan for mass immunization and/or mass distribution of vitamin A to the vulnerable groups in their community.

Reestablish and Improve Primary Medical Care

Immediate casualties (rescue phase) of a sudden impact disaster are likely to include a limited number of trauma victims. In most disasters in fragile communities, the larger number of disaster-related deaths (ie, deaths above the baseline CMR) will be a result of preventable causes of mortality in the weeks and months following the impact. These casualties can largely be prevented by community health education and access to appropriate primary care.

Community level
Health professionals should know the emergency transport and response systems in their community. Health care interventions during the rescue phase should include minimizing loss of life caused by the direct impact of the event (eg, trauma, drowning). After the rescue phase, health care resources should be focused on reestablishing and improving the access and quality of primary care, particularly for the most vulnerable groups.

Set Up Disease Surveillance and Health Information Systems

Effective health information and disease surveillance systems are necessary to monitor effectiveness of health interventions and reassign priorities.

National level
Health authorities should use available information to define initial priorities in the use of limited resources. They should develop specific surveillance guidelines for each disaster to track relevant disease/mortality trends.

Community level
Every health care delivery setting should immediately implement a simple but effective health information collection system based on established WHO, PAHO, or governmental guidelines. Health care professionals should know how to share this information regularly with regional and/or federal health authorities.

Organize Human Resources

The initial shock of an event can make it difficult for a disaster-affected population to effectively respond in a quick and organized fashion. Having a predefined emergency plan with clearly identified leaders can help the local community to cope until more external resources arrive.

Community level
Have an emergency plan and predefined community leaders for the following:

- Conducting rescue operations
- Conducting assessments (eg, health services, transportation, food, sanitation/ water systems)
- Organization of food and water distribution, and the sanitary program
- Health services management
- Corpses and gravesite management

- Identification of unaccompanied minors and other extremely vulnerable individuals (eg, elderly or persons with a disability) and plans for caring for these individuals.

Coordinate Activities

National level

In a large-scale disaster there will be many national and international agencies attempting to assess, develop plans, and establish priorities for funding at national and regional levels. Most effective relief efforts require effective collaboration among many agencies, each bringing their own expertise and experience. However, all of these agencies will ultimately depend on accurate assessments from the affected communities to make appropriate decisions.

Community level

Develop local emergency plans that link into regional and national plans and agencies. Understand the mechanisms for communicating information (eg, assessments, surveillance data) during disasters. Build relationships with key individuals within and outside the community before a disaster occurs.

INTERNATIONAL RELIEF ORGANIZATIONS

When local resources are insufficient, assistance from multiple national or perhaps multinational organizations will be needed. Each involved organization has its own institutional structure and culture, in addition to other features, such as capacity for response, technical and logistic resources, and thematic or regional approach.

Several international agencies may have activities in the country before the event. In response to the disaster, these agencies may retarget their resources in the country to emergency relief. Effective coordination and cooperation among involved organizations are essential but very difficult to achieve in the chaotic situation of a massive emergency. There are 2 major types of organizations that can get involved in assistance when a disaster occurs: governmental and nongovernmental organizations (NGOs).

GOVERNMENTAL ORGANIZATIONS

National Ministries

These are agencies at the national ministry level that have authority for disaster planning and response. Nations should establish a health disaster coordinator within the Ministry of Health (MoH). The health disaster coordinator not only coordinates health-related relief efforts in the event of a disaster, but also continuously updates emergency plans and conducts preparedness training for health care professionals.

The Pan American Health Organization

PAHO is an international public health agency serving as the Regional Office for the Americas of WHO. It provides health policy guidance and technical assistance in disaster planning and response. More information is available at www.paho.org.

World Health Organization

WHO provides technical advice and develops health policies relating to disasters. More information is available at www.who.int.

SUMA

SUMA (Humanitarian Supply Administration System, developed by PAHO) facilitates the reception, inventory, and rapid distribution of essential humanitarian supplies and equipment. In the event of a disaster, PAHO can send SUMA-trained staff to the affected country to assist in managing the inflow of supplies.

United Nations

The UN is a multinational organization that functions mainly through its subagencies, which are independently funded. More information is available at: www.un.org.

The Office of the United Nations High Commissioner for Refugees

The Office of the United Nations High Commissioner for Refugees (UNHCR) is mainly responsible for providing needed food, supplies, and other material, but it also plays a central role in protecting and advocating for displaced populations. More information is available at www.unhcr.org.

World Food Program

The World Food Program (WFP) coordinates the delivery of food to regions in need around the world. More information available at www.wfp.org.

United Nations International Children's Emergency Fund

The United Nations International Children's Emergency Fund (UNICEF) was created by the UN General Assembly to advocate and protect children's rights, to help fulfill their basic needs, and to provide opportunities for maximizing the development of their potential. When an emergency occurs, UNICEF focuses on ensuring that basic needs of women and children are fulfilled and on protecting their basic rights. More information is available at www.unicef.org.

Office for the Coordination of Humanitarian Affairs

In 1998, the Office for the Coordination of Humanitarian Affairs (OCHA) was established by the reorganization of the UN Department of Humanitarian Affairs (DHA). Its mission was expanded to include the coordination of humanitarian response, policy development, and advocacy. OCHA's tasks are done through the Inter Agency Permanent Committee that includes multiple participating organizations, such as UN agencies, funds, and programs, the Red Cross, and NGOs. More information is available at http://ochaonline.un.org.

Foreign Organizations That Provide Help in Case of Disaster

Table 3 identifies some of the governmental agencies of developed countries that provide funding and technical help to countries affected by humanitarian emergencies.

Table 3	
Foreign agencies for disaster assistance	
US Agency for International Development - Office for Foreign Disaster Assistance (OFDA)	http://www.usaid.gov/our_work/humanitarian_assistance/disaster_assistance/
Canadian International Development Agency (CIDA)	www.acdi-cida.gc.ca
European Commission Humanitarian Organization (ECHO)	http://ec.europa.eu/echo/about/actors/specialised_agencies_en.htm
United Kingdom Department for International Development (DFID)	www.dfid.gov.uk
Japan International Cooperation Agency (JICA)	http://www.jica.go.jp/worldmap/english.html

PAHO and WHO have developed guidelines to assist disaster-affected countries in managing donor offers from various agencies, according to the 1999 PAHO publication *Humanitarian Assistance in Disaster Situations: A Guide for Effective Aid.*

Military Help

Both local and foreign military can be mobilized to assist in the response to natural disasters or complex emergencies. Certain unique features make military organizations useful in a disaster.

Advantages

> *Speed:* Few organizations are capable of implementing a large logistic response as rapidly as the military.
> *Security:* The military can secure a specified environment, population, and material.
> *Transportation:* Their fleet of planes and helicopters, as well as land and naval equipment, enable them to transport resources readily.
> *Logistics:* They have experience in maintaining supply lines in problematic environments and situations.
> *Command, control, and communication:* They have a well-defined and responsive organizational structure.
> *Self-sufficiency in the field:* When military arrive to the region where the event has occurred, they are capable of fulfilling the needs of their own personnel.
> *Specialized units:* They often have specifically trained and equipped units. These include engineers who can provide technical assistance and preventive medicine teams capable of rapidly performing epidemiologic evaluations and surveillance, outbreak investigations, vector control, and water purification and treatment.
> *Field hospitals and capacity for medical evacuation:* Hospitals can be helpful in certain circumstances. See the WHO-PAHO guidelines for the use of field hospitals in sudden-impact disasters (as mentioned above).

Shortcomings

Despite all the advantages mentioned previously, the use of the military can have significant shortcomings and limitations in some situations.

Medical care: Field hospitals are designed for the care of soldiers wounded in combat (ie, for the care of wounds suffered by healthy adults). During a disaster, primary care and preventive interventions for women and children are major needs.

Logistics: Supplies available in the military response system may not be appropriate for a disaster in terms of prevailing diseases or types of food.

Political objectives: The military are an asset of governments; in addition, certain humanitarian objectives can be subordinated to other political or strategic goals. The presence of the army in certain scenarios can cause tension in certain groups of the population and compromise relief workers who, for their own safety and function, wish to be considered neutral.

Cost: Military activities are expensive.

NONGOVERNMENTAL ORGANIZATIONS

NGOs are nonprofit organizations working on a full-time basis in assistance for appropriate development. Thousands of NGOs, both international and national, are functioning throughout the world. Most NGOs are small agencies focusing on very specific development projects (eg, providing education, working tools, or training in sustainable development). Only a few of them have the resources required for supporting activities targeted to promote development and to respond to disasters in multiple countries or regions. Although NGOs may receive contributions from individuals, most of their funds come from the governments of industrialized countries. These governments distribute their money for assisting projects through contracts with NGOs. Unlike the International Committee of the Red Cross (ICRC), some NGOs maintain a "right to interfere." This means they can operate across borders without written approval of their hosts. Although usually looking for the neutrality of the ICRC, some NGOs may be more willing to report any perceived injustice. They perform well in emergencies within their area of specialty (eg, water provision, food distribution), but most cannot achieve self-sufficiency in an emergency setting and rely on UN, military, or other agencies for security, transportation to remote sites, communication, support of logistics, or medical care for their own personnel. NGOs have an enhanced ability to provide person-to-person assistance because they are likely to have a predisaster relationship with the affected communities and understand the local culture and public health issues. They can also shift easily from disaster relief to development, and are willing to make a long-term commitment to community development and rebuilding.

International Committee of the Red Cross

The ICRC is a hybrid agency: neither private nor controlled by a government. A number of its characteristics are unique; its mission is defined by the international humanitarian law passed by the 1949 Geneva Convention and the two 1977 protocols. The ICRC gets involved mainly when civil disturbances are present; it has the right and duty to intervene across borders when national or international conflicts break out, regardless of whether a "state of war" has been declared. The ICRC brokers relief assistance during war, assures legal protection for victims, and monitors the way Prisoners of War are managed. Also, the ICRC plays a critical role in reuniting families. The ICRC strives to preserve its neutrality, which is essential for its mission and enables its members to work unarmed in war regions under the control of any of the involved parties. The ICRC provides a complete account of its activities to all the parties involved in the conflict. It will refuse to participate in any activity that can be seen as showing favoritism. This may include transportation in vehicles belonging to one of the parties or joining efforts with groups that have their own interests. The ICRC is usually self-sufficient and can use its own resources for air lifts, communication, and logistics. It will participate only if all parties involved in the conflict sign an agreement recognizing and showing respect for its neutrality and mission. The ICRC is related to but independent from the Red Cross and the Red Crescent Societies national agencies. These organizations provide assistance primarily to victims of disasters or wars within their own nations. They have a similar commitment with neutrality, provision of assistance based only on the need, and independence from national governments.

Coordinating the activities of all these organizations poses a tremendous challenge. Following a natural disaster the host nation's government/agencies and military are likely to have operational command. Most nations now have defined governmental authorities responsible for global disaster planning and response, as well as coordinators for individual sectors such as health. External agencies or governments play a supportive role in providing technical assistance and resources.

In complex emergencies related to a conflict, the armed forces or government authorities will have the command of operations, including the coordination of humanitarian help. The coordination in this scenario can be particularly difficult if the hostile groups are stationed nearby and try to block assistance of civilians. In this context, humanitarian help can be used as a political and strategic instrument.

MEDICAL VOLUNTEERING

Following a disaster, many pediatricians and other health professionals volunteer for a limited time. During the initial response phase, the greatest pediatric needs include air transport teams, surgical teams (a surgeon, operating room [OR] nurse, anesthesiologist, and critical care pediatrician), as well as pediatricians with training and experience in emergency medicine and critical care. Volunteers may have to be self-sufficient for a period of time in terms of food, water, and shelter. Volunteers should work through an established NGO or governmental agency rather than simply "show up" to help.

Volunteers should be prepared to respond quickly, as the quicker the response teams can provide appropriate care, the more effective they can be at saving lives and limiting morbidity. Part of preparation is anticipating the types of injuries that will be seen with different types of disasters. When sending a response team into a disaster during the acute response phase, it is important to have the personnel with the ability to treat the most likely injuries seen with the specific type of disaster. In a major earthquake like the one in Haiti in January 2010, one would expect most of the casualties to be secondary to traumatic injuries related to collapsed buildings. Therefore, a team should be prepared to have personnel and supplies that can be used to treat crush injuries and a large number of open wounds, along with a variety of orthopedic injuries. In a disaster involving an explosion (large industrial accident or terrorist attack), the pattern of injuries would include many of the same traumatic injuries as seen in an earthquake, but would also include a large number of burns and blast injuries such as blast lung. Personnel required in this type of disaster should include those with training in caring for burns as well as experience with other traumatic injuries.

In the first days following the Haiti earthquake, there were a large number of complex orthopedic injuries that required emergent treatment. These included open fractures, traumatic amputations, and crush injuries. The treatment of these injuries included fracture reductions, wound debridement, and amputations. Thus, it was essential to have personnel with the training to perform the needed procedures. Personnel with training in emergency medicine, general surgery, and orthopedics are best suited to be part of the initial response team when a large number of traumatic injuries are expected.

Supplies that were essential in caring for these patients included plaster splinting/casting supplies, wound dressing supplies, and medications for pain control and sedation. When caring for open wounds, the ability to appropriately irrigate and clean wounds can greatly reduce subsequent secondary infections of these wounds. Response teams should come prepared with supplies that would be able to provide pressure irrigation of wounds with either clean water or saline, antibiotic ointments, and large supplies of wound dressings. A large number of the orthopedic injuries can be treated with casting or splinting. Plaster casting material is far superior in this setting because casts made of fiberglass cannot be easily removed without a cast saw, whereas patients/families can be instructed to remove a plaster cast by soaking it in water. Adequate sedation for painful procedures such as amputations and fracture reductions can be safely obtained using either ketamine intravascularly or intramuscularly. Ketamine is the ideal sedative in this situation, as the safety profile is such that it can be used when minimal monitoring equipment is available because it causes minimal respiratory or cardiovascular effects. Procedural sedation with ketamine is a basic skill set of pediatric emergency medicine–trained physicians and can provide adequate sedation and analgesia for most of the procedures that will be needed during the response phase.

Box 2 provides a list of pediatric equipment that, if possible, should be brought in. An article in the *New England Journal of Medicine* by the Israeli mobile hospital reviews the ethical dilemmas encountered in Haiti when the need for care far exceeded the capacity [4].

Among the recommended equipment, elements for proper airway management in children are crucial. A major challenge of any disaster response is gathering, organizing, and moving supplies to the affected area. Resource

Box 2: Recommended equipment to bring for pediatric emergencies in disaster situations

Airway Management/Breathing
- Tongue blades
- Suctioning machine (portable, battery powered)
- Suction catheters: Yankauer, 8, 10, 14F
- Simple face masks: infant, child, adult
- Pediatric and adult masks for assisted ventilation
- Self-inflating bag with 250-mL, 500-mL, and 1000-mL reservoir
- Optional for intubation
- Laryngoscope handle with batteries (extra batteries AA, laryngoscope bulbs)
  Miler blades: 0, 1, 2, 3 Macintosh blades 2, 3
  Endotracheal tubes, uncuffed: 3.0, 3.5, 4.0, 4.5, 5.0, 6.0; cuffed: 7.0, 8.0
  Laryngeal mask airways
  Stylets: small, large
  Easycap (ETCO2 analyzer), 2 sizes
  Adhesive tape to secure endotracheal tube (ETT)

Circulation/intravascular access or fluid management
- IV catheters: 18-, 20-, 22-, 24-gauge
- Butterfly needles: 23-gauge
- Intraosseous needles: 15- or 18-gauge, or Eazy IO device
- Boards, tape, tourniquet IV
- Pediatric drip chambers and tubing
- 5% dextrose in normal saline and half normal saline
- Isotonic fluids (normal saline or lactated Ringer's solution)
- Medications: epinephrine, atropine, sodium bicarbonate, calcium chloride, lidocaine, D25, D10

Miscellaneous
- Broselow tape
- Nasogastric tubes: 8, 10, 14F
- Splints and gauze padding
- Rolling carts with supplies such as abundant blankets
- Warm water source and portable showers for decontamination
- Thermal control (radiant cradle, lamps)
- Geiger counter (if suspicion of radioactive contamination)
- Personal protective equipment (PPE)
- Pain\Sedation medications: ketamine, morphine, ketoralac

- Other potential medications: albuterol, keflex, ancef, Ceftriaxone, Diazepam
- Surgical equipment for amputations, incision and drainage of wounds, laceration repairs
- Headlamps with replacement batteries
- Scissors
- Plaster for casting, not fiberglass (hard to remove)

Monitoring equipment
- Sphygmomanometer/Blood pressure cuffs: premature, infant, child, adult
- Portable monitor/defibrillator (with settings <10)
- Pediatric defibrillation paddles
- Pediatric electrocardiogram (ECG) skin electrode contacts (peel and stick)
- Pulse oxymeter with reusable (older children) and nonreusable (small children) sensors
- Device to check serum glucose and strips to check urine for glucose, blood, etc.

management within the hospital and other facilities or agencies may prove to be a decisive factor in whether a mass casualty event can be handled.

Communication in a disaster situation is essential among disaster relief team members as well as with coordinating groups and logistical support personnel in home countries. Modern technology has provided many different types of communication devices, which have different advantages and disadvantages. Radios are useful for short-range communications when a disaster relief team is separated. However, they are limited by range and will not allow communication with the other teams or organizations that are a long distance away. Satellite phones are ideal for communication with the team as well as with the home country. They provide a reliable method of communication when telephone services are not working or there is no infrastructure, because they rely on orbiting satellites to transmit data. However, they are a scarce resource as well as an expensive resource. The main drawback for many portable satellite phones is that the phone's antenna needs an unobstructed view of the sky. Cellular phones are an ideal method for communication. Voice calls can be made to team members as well as to coordinate in the home country. E-mail and SMS texting are other methods of communicating through the cellular network. Haiti was the first disaster where social media was widely used. For example, our team from The Children's Hospital was able to arrange the evacuation of a patient via a Blackhawk helicopter to the USNS *Comfort* through SMS texting and electronic mail alone. With the availability of smart phones such as the RIM Blackberry and the Apple I-phone, access to the mobile Internet has allowed the use of the Internet for communication using electronic e-mail or other social media. Because the voice cellular circuits in Haiti were congested during the day, we communicated with team members as well as the United States almost exclusively via SMS text messaging and e-mail through our smart phones.

However, cellular technology is dependent on a cellular infrastructure and network that has survived a disaster. Another disadvantage of cellular phones is that different countries have different cellular standards that are not compatible with each other. For example, although the countries of Haiti and the Dominican Republic are on the same island of Hispaniola, each country has a different cellular standard. Haiti uses the GSM (Global System for Mobile Communications) standard, and the Dominican Republic uses the CDMA (Code Division Multiple Access) standard. We encountered relief workers from the Dominican Republic who could not communicate in Haiti because they did not have the right equipment for Haiti.

The availability of the Internet through various means including satellite links and data over cellular networks has allowed for many novel methods of communication over the Internet. There are traditional methods such as electronic mail. Web blogs also allow relief workers as well as those affected by the disaster to reach out to the world. Other social media tools such as Facebook and the microblogging service Twitter allow almost instantaneous updates from the field. Haitians and relief workers were able to keep their families and loved ones up to date using social media tools such as Facebook and Twitter.

One of the most novel uses of social media was the adoption of the Ushahidi technology to Haiti (http://haiti.ushahidi.com/main). Ushahidi was originally developed for people to report ethnic violence in Kenya so it could be tracked. Using an instance of Ushahidi developed specifically for Haiti, Haitians could send a Creole text message on their cellular phones to the Ushahidi phone number asking for help. The message would be translated to English by translators, mapped, and assigned to a relief organization such as the US military, the United Nations, or other NGOs to complete the task (http://haitirewired. wired.com/profiles/blogs/ushahidi-amp-the-unprecedented).

Mental Health Considerations

Disaster response providers, especially those coming from developed countries to disasters occurring in developing counties, are often thrust into a high-stress situation with exposure to situations they may have never experienced before. The degree of destruction and death will likely be much greater than what the health care providers are accustomed to dealing with in their daily lives. The emotional impact of large-scale destruction, suffering, and death will elicit different responses in different people, but all volunteer providers should recognize how their experiences can affect their well-being both emotionally and physically. The emotional stress experienced by disaster response providers has been well documented after events such as 9/11 and Hurricane Katrina [5–8]. The affect of stress is amplified by the long hours of intense work experienced during the response to a disaster. Environmental conditions (such as extreme heat/cold/rain/flooding), lack of sleep, and inadequate nutrition impair

Table 4
Common stress reactions

Behavioral	Physical	Psychological/Emotional	Thinking	Social
• Increase or decrease in activity level	• Gastrointestinal problems	• Feeling heroic, euphoric, or invulnerable	• Memory problems	• Isolation
• Substance use or abuse (alcohol or drugs)	• Headaches, other aches and pains	• Denial	• Disorientation and confusion	• Blaming
• Difficulty communicating or listening	• Visual disturbances	• Anxiety or fear	• Slow thought processes; lack of concentration	• Difficulty in giving or accepting support or help
• Irritability, outbursts of anger, frequent arguments	• Weight loss or gain	• Depression	• Difficulty setting priorities or making decisions	• Inability to experience pleasure or have fun
• Inability to rest or relax	• Sweating or chills	• Guilt	• Loss of objectivity	
• Decline in job performance; absenteeism	• Tremors or muscle twitching	• Apathy		
• Frequent crying	• Being easily startled	• Grief		
• Hypervigilance or excessive worry	• Chronic fatigue or sleep disturbances			
• Avoidance of activities or places that trigger memories	• Immune system disorders			
• Becoming accident prone				

Adapted from The US Department of Health and Human Services, Substance Abuse and Mental Health Services Administration (SAMHSA), and Center for Mental Health Services (CMHS). Available at: http://mentalhealth.samhsa.gov/publications/allpubs/SMA-4113/default.asp. Accessed September 2, 2010.

a provider's ability to deal with the stressful situation. Crisis response workers and managers, including first responders, public health workers, construction workers, transportation workers, utilities workers, and other volunteers, are repeatedly exposed to extraordinarily stressful events. This places them at higher than normal risk for developing stress reactions [9].

It is important for all disaster response providers to recognize the potential emotional stress they will be entering before arriving on scene. Stress prevention and management needs to be considered and addressed from the start of the deployment to prevent problems. By anticipating stressors and individuals' responses to these stressors, the response team and individuals can potentially prevent a crisis within the team of care providers. The US Department of Health and Human Services, Substance Abuse and Mental Health Services Administration (SAMHSA), and Center for Mental Health Services (CMHS) have published a guide focusing on general principles of stress management and offers simple, practical strategies that can be incorporated into the daily routine of managers and workers. It also provides a concise orientation to the signs and symptoms of stress. This can be found online at http://mentalhealth.samhsa.gov/publications/allpubs/SMA-4113/default.asp.

Although most people are resilient, the stress response becomes problematic when it does not or cannot turn off; that is, when symptoms last too long or interfere with daily life. Table 4 provides a list of the common stress reactions.

SUMMARY

Disasters are, to a great extent, beyond our control and inevitable; however, we can be better prepared for the consequences and thus reduce the degree of human suffering. As Vernon Law [10] has said, "Experience is a hard teacher. She gives the test first and the lessons afterwards." Knowledge and understanding are needed for more effective preparation and planning. Pediatricians have a special role in the planning and preparation process to ensure that the needs of children are adequately considered in this process. Pediatric volunteers should be prepared for their experiences from the standpoint of training, available materials and resources, and mental health considerations.

Acknowledgments

This article has been adapted from the American Academy of Pediatrics manual on disaster training for developing countries entitled "Pediatrics in Disasters."

References

[1] ReliefWeb. Haiti: Earthquake Situation Report #25. Available at: http://www.reliefweb.int/rw/rwb.nsf/db900sid/EGUA-836R39?OpenDocument&;RSS20&RSS20=FS. Accessed March 2010.

[2] Available at: http://www.google.com/hostednews/afp/article/ALeqM5hOiPk5G7TMLiYsBbZ1ajaBMS_lWg. Accessed March 2010.

[3] Sontag D. Doctors haunted by Haitians they couldn't help. New York Times. February 12, 2010. Available at: http://www.nytimes.com/2010/02/13/world/americas/13doctors.html?hp. Accessed March 2010.

[4] Merin O, Ash N, Levy G, et al. The Israeli Field Hospital in Haiti—ethical dilemmas in early disaster response. N Engl J Med 2010;362(11):e38.

[5] Levenson RL Jr, Acosta JK. Observations from ground zero at the World Trade Center in New York City, part I. Int J Emerg Ment Health 2001;3(4):241–4.

[6] Centers for Disease Control and Prevention (CDC). Mental health status of World Trade Center rescue and recovery workers and volunteers—New York City, July 2002-August 2004. MMWR Morb Mortal Wkly Rep 2004;53(35):812–5.

[7] Bills CB, Levy NA, Sharma V, et al. Mental health of workers and volunteers responding to events of 9/11: review of the literature. Mt Sinai J Med 2008;75(2):115–27.

[8] Palm KM, Polusny MA, Follette VM. Vicarious traumatization: potential hazards and interventions for disaster and trauma workers. Prehospital Disaster Med 2004;19(1):73–8.

[9] Pan American Health Organization. Stress management in disasters. Washington, DC: Pan American Health Organization; 2001.

[10] Nathan, David H. The McFarland Baseball Quotations Dictionary. McFarland & Company; 2000. ISBN 9780786408887.

Advances in Pediatrics 57 (2010) 33–62

ADVANCES IN PEDIATRICS

Childhood Accidents: Injuries and Poisoning

Kam-Lun Ellis Hon, MD (CUHK)[a,*],
Alexander K.C. Leung, MBBS, FRCPC,
FRCP(UK&Irel), FRCPCH[b]

[a]Department of Paediatrics, Prince of Wales Hospital, The Chinese University of Hong Kong,
6/F, Clinical Sciences Building, Shatin, Hong Kong
[b]Department of Paediatrics, The Alberta Children's Hospital, The University of Calgary,
#200, 233-16th Avenue, NW, Calgary, Alberta, Canada T2M 5H5

A ccidents, injuries, and poisonings are important, but potentially avoidable, causes of mortality and morbidity in children. Injury is not synonymous with accident and is regarded by some as understandable, predictable, and preventable. Nevertheless, an injury may also be the consequence of an accident. Conversely, it may be a sequela of a harmful or abusive act. In the literature, the term nonaccidental injury (NAI) is often equivalent to child abuse. NAI carries medicolegal consequences and must be used with caution. Injury is the leading cause of death and disability in children and adolescents.

EPIDEMIOLOGY
International Differences
Epidemiologic data on accidents, injuries and poisoning are available in many industrialized nations, and many factors have been studied in predicting outcome and guiding national policy on injury prevention [1–11]. The causes of injury are heterogeneous and vary from city to city. Nevertheless, road traffic accident (RTA) is the leading cause of death for all age groups after the first year of life [1,5,9]. There are fundamental differences in mortality and morbidity between indoor and outdoor injuries. Injuries are the leading cause of childhood mortality and morbidity in most industrialized countries, especially for children after the first year of life [1,4,9,10,12]. In the United Kingdom, there have been dramatic decreases in childhood mortality for injuries in recent years [1]. In Canada during the period 1979 to 2002, there were also dramatic decreases in childhood mortality for total injuries and unintentional injuries as well as various degrees of reduction for many causes of

*Corresponding author. E-mail address: ehon@cuhk.edu.hk

0065-3101/10/$ – see front matter
doi:10.1016/j.yapd.2009.08.010

injury [4]. The investigators reported that motor vehicle–related injuries were the most common causes of injury deaths, accounting for an average of 36.4% of total injury deaths, followed by suffocation (14.3%), drowning (13.5%), and burning (11.1%); however, suffocation was the leading cause of injury mortality for infants [4]. In the United States, injuries are the leading cause of mortality from early childhood until middle adulthood, which include motor vehicle crashes, submersion injury, homicide, suicide, and fires [9]. Preventable childhood injuries account for nearly half of all deaths in individuals aged 1 to 19 years, and unintentional injury resulted in the death of 20,000 children, adolescents, and young adults in 2002. From 1950 to 1993, the overall annual death rate for children aged less than 15 years in the United States declined substantially, primarily reflecting decreases in deaths associated with unintentional injuries, pneumonia, influenza, cancer, and congenital anomalies [13]. However, during the same period, childhood homicide rates tripled, and suicide rates quadrupled. In 1994, among children aged 1 to 4 years, homicide was the fourth leading cause of death; among children aged 5 to 14 years, homicide was the third leading cause of death, and suicide was the sixth [13]. In this study, the investigators also compared patterns and the effect of violent deaths among children in the United States and other industrialized countries. They analyzed data on childhood homicide, suicide, and firearm-related death in the United States and 25 other industrialized countries for the most recent year for which data were available in each country. The analysis indicated that the United States had the highest rates of childhood homicide, suicide, and firearm-related death among industrialized countries [13]. Elsewhere, Kibel and colleagues [6] examined trends in major causes of injury mortality and the proportion of total deaths attributable to injuries from 1968 to 1985 for white, colored, and Asian children less than 15 years old in South Africa. No clear trends in overall mortalities were observed. There were marked fluctuations in injury mortalities from year to year. The effect of injury as a cause of death increased relative to a decrease in other diseases, notably gastroenteritis and malnutrition, in children less than 5 years old. Patterns varied considerably between age, sex, and population groups. The investigators concluded that road and burn death rates decreased, whereas drowning and assault rates increased [6]. In Singapore, drowning, falls from height, rollover falls from beds, slamming door injuries, the low use of child car restraints, bicycle injuries, and playground falls were highlighted as areas of concern [10].

Injury from a motor vehicle collision is the leading cause of death in children [2,9]. The victims are often unrestrained or inappropriately restrained [14]. In a motor vehicle collision, children are more likely to die in a pickup truck than in any other type of automobile. Rehabilitation costs and long-term consequences of motor vehicle injuries are substantial [15]. There are likely to be significant international differences in injury epidemiology, so the statistical data cannot be extrapolated from city to city. For instance, in Hong Kong most people travel on public transport. Pickup trunks are rarely used for transport of children, and most of the severe RTA victims are pedestrians.

An estimated 23,000 children sustained head injuries (excluding the face) while bicycling in 1998 in the United States [16,17]. Two-thirds of bicycle-related deaths were due to traumatic brain injury (TBI) [9]. Wearing a bicycle helmet reduces the risk of brain injury in a crash by 74% to 85% [17–19]. Approximately 1 fatal head injury could be prevented every day, and 1 nonfatal head injury every 4 seconds, if every rider wore a helmet [20]. Only about 50% of children in the United States between 5 and 14 years old own a helmet, and only 25% of them always wear it while bicycling [21].

Falls of all kinds represent an important cause of child injury and death. In the United States, approximately 140 deaths from falls occur annually in children younger than 15 years [22]. Three million children require emergency department care for fall-related injuries [22]. Although falls are the most common cause of injury in childhood, they are usually nonfatal. Nevertheless, fatalities attributable to falls do occur in children aged 15 years or younger.

Fires and burns combined are the third most common cause of unintentional childhood injury death, after motor vehicle collisions and falls. The highest death rates in residential injuries are attributable to fires. Each year in the United States, approximately 1000 children aged 15 years and younger die in residential fires [23–26]. Children younger than 5 years are found to be twice as likely to die in a residential fire than the rest of the population [26,27].

In Hong Kong, the injury statistics are different from those of many other countries [12]. Firearm, drowning, near-drowning, fire, electrical burn, and bicycle injuries are uncommon. A male predominance is observed in several studies in indoor and outdoor injuries [12]. A consistent excess of males in pediatric emergency department attendances and hospital admissions have been observed [12,28]. Although male vulnerability to illness has long been recognized, the consistency and magnitude of these gender differentials in admissions are impressive. More vigorous exploration of the underlying mechanisms responsible for this phenomenon is warranted so that preventive measures can be more appropriately targeted.

There are significant differences between indoor and outdoor accidents in that victims of indoor accidents are generally younger, with scalds, poisoning, and foreign-body aspiration predominant, whereas RTAs are the principal category in outdoor accidents [9,10,12,29]. As a risk factor, premorbid neurodevelopmental conditions, such as mental retardation, seizures, or cerebral palsy, are often present in indoor accidents. Scalds by hot fluids are the most common category of injury involving young children and are associated with long hospital stay. Outdoor injuries generally occur in healthy children. Nevertheless, both groups are associated with significant morbidity. Morbidity following major injuries is often high. Most children require cardiopulmonary or neurologic/neurosurgical supports in the pediatric intensive care unit (PICU). The determining factor for mortality or poor neurodevelopmental outcomes is the presence of central nervous system (CNS) involvement. Pediatric TBI caused by various mechanisms, such as falls, motor vehicle collisions, child abuse, and gunshot wounds, affects children of all ages. From 1989 to 1998,

84,792 children died as a result of TBI in the United States, with a male/female ratio of 2.5:1 [30,31]. Although TBI is one of the leading causes of acquired disability and death in infants and children, little research has been done on TBI compared with research efforts directed at other pediatric diseases such as cancer.

Firearm-related deaths account for the highest percentage of injury death in individuals aged 10 to 19 years in the United States [32]. Between 1962 and1993, the total number of firearm-related deaths increased by 137%, from 16,720 in 1962 to 39,595 in 1993. Suicide and homicide were responsible for most firearm fatalities [33,34]. In 2002, 2893 firearm-related deaths occurred in the United States in individuals 20 years or younger [34]. In the study by Eber and colleagues [34] from 1993 to 2000, an estimated 22,661 (95% confidence interval [CI]: 16,668–28,654) or 4.9 per 100,000 (95% CI: 3.6–6.2) children 14 years old or younger with nonfatal firearm injuries were treated in United States hospital emergency departments. Assaults accounted for 41.5% of nonfatal firearm injuries, and unintentional injuries accounted for 43.1%. Approximately 4 of 5 children who sustained a nonfatal, unintentional firearm injury were shot by themselves or by a friend, a relative, or another person known to them. During this period, 5542, or 1.20 per 100,000 (95% CI: 1.17, 1.23) children 14 years old or younger died of firearm injuries; 1 of every 5 children who were wounded by a firearm gunshot died of that injury. Most firearm deaths were violence related, with homicides and suicides constituting 54.7% and 21.9% of these deaths, respectively. For children 14 years old or younger, the burden of morbidity and mortality associated with firearm injuries falls disproportionately on boys, blacks, and children 10 to 14 years old. Fatal and nonfatal injury rates declined by more than 50% during the study period [34].

Sports- and gymnastic-related injuries are prevalent in many Western nations. In 2002, the number of cheerleading participants increased 18% in the United States [35–37]. This increase in participation, along with new cheerleading styles, has increased the number of gymnastic-related injuries by 110% [38]. An estimated 7.5 injuries occur per 1000 participants aged 6 to 17 years. Approximately 4.8 million children aged 5 to 14 years play baseball or softball. In 1995, an estimated 162,000 children visited the emergency department after a baseball- or softball-related injury [36,39]. The peak age for injury in these sports was 12 years. Approximately 43% of injuries were from a ball-chest impact; 24% were from a ball-head impact; 15% were from a bat impact; 10% were from a ball-neck, ball-ear, or ball-throat impact; and 8% were unknown. Approximately 50,000 emergency department visits per year are attributable to skateboard injuries, and approximately 9400 emergency department visits due to nonmotorized scooter–related injury were reported between January and August 2000 [37]. Emergency departments treat more than 200,000 children aged 14 years and younger each year for playground-related injuries [40,41]. Inline skating has become popular and many children younger than 18 years participate [42]. Injuries include wrist injuries and fractures.

Fatalities are rare and almost always associated with a motor vehicle collision. In 1999, approximately 8800 children younger than 15 months went to the emergency department because of injuries related to infant walkers in the United States [43,44]. In 1996, approximately 83,400 injuries in the United States were caused by trampoline use; 66% of these injuries were in children aged 5 to 14 years, and 10% were in children younger than 5 years [45]. Approximately 9400 injuries per year occur from lawn and garden equipment in children younger than 18 years; one-fourth of these injuries are in children younger than 5 years [46]. Pediatric lawnmower injuries, particularly due to riding mowers, are a highly preventable cause of morbidity and mortality [46,47]. Many of these sports are not prevalent in the non-Western nations and the injury patterns are likely to be different.

The epidemiology of animal bite injuries is available in many countries [48–50]. In the United States, an estimated 300,000 to 4.5 million dog bites each year result in 1% of all emergency department visits [48]. Children seen in emergency departments are more likely than older persons to be bitten on the face, neck, and head. It is estimated that, for each United States dog-bite fatality, there are about 670 hospitalizations and 16,000 emergency department visits [51–53]. Dog-bite injuries are an important source of injury among children. Similar observations were seen in a Hong Kong study [50]. Children are more likely to be bitten because of their smaller size, relative inability to defend themselves, interest in animals, and unintentional (or intentional) abuse of animals. The highest frequency of dog bites comes from dogs that are younger than 1 year old, male, and unneutered. German shepherds, pit bulls, and chow chows are the most common dogs that bite [48,50,51,54,55]. Deaths from dog bites are usually from pit bull–type dogs and rottweilers [51,54,55].

In the United States, approximately 1000 children aged 15 years and younger die in residential fires [3,56]. Children are still being injured by fireworks [57]. An estimated 85,800 pediatric fireworks-related injuries were treated in United States emergency departments during a 14-year study period [58]. Consumer fireworks cause serious preventable injuries among pediatric fireworks users and bystanders in the United States [58].

Racial Considerations

Interracial differences in morbidity and mortality have been observed [11]. Research studies have consistently shown that American Indian and Alaskan Native children are at a higher risk of unintentional injury than children of other races in the United States [59]. These ethnic groups also have a higher rate of injury-related death, which remains almost double the rate for all children in the United States.

African American children have the highest rates of death secondary to drowning, firearms, and other violence-related injuries [11,60]. Saluja and colleagues [61] studied the circumstances surrounding swimming pool drowning among United States residents aged 5 to 24 years. During the study period, 678 United States residents aged 5 to 24 years drowned in pools.

Drowning rates were highest among black males; most black victims (51%) drowned in public pools, most white victims (55%) drowned in residential pools, and most Hispanic victims (35%) drowned in neighborhood pools. Foreign-born males also had an increased risk for drowning compared with American-born males [61]. In a study of 7,778 children with moderate or severe traumatic brain injuries, Haider and colleagues [60] found that Hispanics (n = 1041) had outcomes comparable with whites (n = 4762). Black children (n = 1238) had significantly increased premorbidities, penetrating trauma, and violent intent. They also had higher unadjusted mortality and longer mean intensive care unit (ICU) and floor stays. Black patients were more likely to be discharged to an inpatient rehabilitation facility and had increased odds of possessing a functional deficit at discharge. Black children with TBI had worse clinical and functional outcomes at discharge compared with equivalently injured white children [60]. In a separate study, African American infants had 3.5 times the risk of death from preventable injuries compared with white infants [62]. This disparity persisted despite controlling for type of health insurance, a surrogate for socioeconomic status. The investigators concluded that understanding these disparities and developing injury-prevention programs targeting high-risk mechanisms of injury such as abuse and suffocation among African American is critical toward eventually eliminating these preventable deaths [62]. In the study by Bennett and colleagues [63], standard statistical tests were conducted to determine homicide rates among children aged 0 to 4 years across the United States. These data showed that the 2003 and the 2004 homicide rates for children aged 0 to 4 years were 3.0 and 2.5 per 100,000 population, respectively [63]. In homicide, African Americans were 4.2 times as likely as whites to be victims [63]. Suspects were commonly parents/caregivers. Most infant/child homicides occurred in houses or apartments, using weapons that included household objects. The epidemiologic findings have important educational and practical implications in terms of policy about prevention.

MAJOR CATEGORIES OF INJURIES
RTAs
Injury due to RTA refers to injuries sustained on the road secondarily to traffic accidents. The term may be synonymous with motor vehicle accidents, although it carries a broader sense to involve trams, trains, and vehicles without a motor, such as bicycles and horse carriage. The primary cause of death of children in the United States and many countries is RTA [1,5,9,64,65]. Despite legal regulations, many children involved in motor vehicle crashes are unrestrained. Car safety seats for children are required in many countries and their proper use could significantly reduce vehicle-associated fatalities and hospitalizations [66–69]. The correct type of safety seat to be used is important [67]. It must be weight and age appropriate. Children should use a combination lap/shoulder belt when they have grown enough to properly fit the vehicle seat belts. A rear-facing car seat should not be

used in a seat with a passenger air bag [67]. A car seat should never be used if the child has outgrown the seat. In childhood RTA, the case fatality rate is 1% when a child is a passenger in a car crash [65,70]. The risk of fatality increases threefold for children hit by cars. Hence, pedestrian safety skills should be taught to children early in childhood [64]. Nevertheless, teaching cannot replace parental supervision of children near roadways. Furthermore, studies have indicated that using a cellular telephone while driving is associated with a fourfold increase in motor vehicle crashes [71,72]. Parents and teenage drivers should be made aware of the law that prohibits the usage of hand-held cellular phones while driving.

Injury from a motor vehicle collision is the leading cause of death in individuals aged 1 to 19 years, and accounts for many deaths annually [1,5,9]. In the United States in the year 2002, 2542 children younger than 5 years died in motor vehicle collisions [15]. Almost half were unrestrained, and many more were inappropriately restrained [73,74].

In a motor vehicle collision, children are 3 times more likely to die in a pickup truck than in another type of automobile [64,75]. Compared with a properly restrained cabin passenger, a child in the cargo area of a pickup truck is 8 times more likely to die in a crash [75].

Bicycle Injuries

Bicycle injuries can be considered a form of RTA but deserve separate consideration [17,76,77]. Bicycling remains one of the most popular recreational sports among children in the United States and is the leading cause of recreational sports injuries treated in emergency departments [17]. Bicycle injuries involving children and adolescents are common. Head trauma accounts for most bicycle-related fatality; most such brain injuries can be prevented through the use of bicycle helmets [78]. Hence, bike riders should wear a helmet every time they ride. However, helmet-use rates remain low in many communities [17,79]. An estimated 44 million children and adolescents younger than 21 years in the United States ride bicycles [17]. Facial injuries to cyclists occur at a rate nearly identical to that of head injuries [80]. Sosin and colleagues [16] reported that an average of 247 TBI deaths and 140,000 head injuries among individuals younger than 20 years were related to bicycle crashes each year in the United States. As many as 184 deaths and 116,000 head injuries might have been prevented annually if these riders had worn helmets. An additional 19,000 mouth and chin injuries were treated each year. The youngest age groups had the highest proportions of head and mouth injuries. The use of a bicycle helmet can reduce the occurrence of serious brain injuries by 88% [16,17,81]. However, it is estimated that only 20% of children in the United States wear bicycle helmets. Theoretical frameworks for interventions aimed at increasing bicycle helmet use in children and adolescents have been considered [82]. An Australian study reaffirmed that social norms, perceptions of control, and past behavior significantly predicted intentions to use helmets, and perceptions of control and past behavior predicted actual helmet use [81].

The investigators concluded that strengthening the routine of helmet use and building young people's confidence can overcome any perceived barriers to helmet use and will increase helmet wearing. The frequency of helmet use in children rises if helmets are worn by parents, caregivers, friends, or other relatives. Community helmet campaigns with incentives and school-based interventions have been created to promote helmet use, but these have had mixed success. Laws mandating helmet use are being enforced in local communities. Helmets need to be replaced if they have been involved in a crash.

Falls

Falls are common [12]. In metropolitan cities with high-rise buildings, morbidity and mortality from window falls can result in high morbidity and mortality [22,83]. Although most minor falls do not require medical care, some victims suffer from major sequelae. The results of closed head injuries following falls may range in severity from minor asymptomatic trauma to death. Neuropsychiatric sequelae may occur even following apparently minor closed head injury. Any form of fall may result in injury to the spine. Children may sustain irreversible injury following a seemingly minor fall. A seemingly minor fall of 50 cm onto a mattress can result in permanent paraplegia [84].

Fire, Burn, and Scald Injuries

Thermal injury is a major cause of accidental death and disfigurement in children. Pain, morbidity, the association with child abuse, and the preventable nature of burns constitute an area of major concern in pediatrics. Common causes include hot water or food, appliances, flames, grills, vehicle-related burns, and curling irons. Burns occur commonly in toddlers, and in boys more frequently than in girls.

Fires and burns are the leading cause of injury-related deaths in the home. Categories of burn injury include smoke inhalation; flame contact; scalding; and electrical, chemical, and ultraviolet burns.

Scalding is the most common type of burn in children. Most scalds involve hot foods and beverages, but nearly one-fourth of scalds are with hot tap water. It is recommended that hot-water heaters should be set to less than 54°C (130°F) [29,85–87].

Sunburn is another form of common thermal injury. Symptoms of excessive sun exposure usually do not begin until after the skin has been damaged. Sunburn and excessive sun exposure are associated with skin cancers in Whites.

Even brief contact with a high-voltage source will result in a contact burn. When an infant or toddler bites an electric cord, burns to the commissure of the lips occur that appear gray and necrotic, with surrounding erythema. If an arc is created with passage of current through the body, the pattern of the thermal injury will depend on the path of the current; therefore, it is important to search for an exit wound and internal injuries. Excessive damage to deep tissue may occur. Current transversing the heart may cause nonperfusing arrhythmias. Neurologic effects of electrical burns can be immediate (eg, confusion, disorientation, peripheral nerve injury), delayed (nerve damage in the thrombosed limb after compartment syndrome), or late (impaired concentration or memory).

Firearm Injuries and Violence

Firearm injuries are uniquely prevalent in the United States and are often reported on national and international news. The American Academy of Pediatrics periodically issues statements and reviewed data, trends, prevention, and intervention strategies in firearm-related injuries affecting the pediatric population [32]. The United States has a higher rate of firearm-related death than any other industrialized country. Injuries from firearms are more frequent for young people age 15 to 24 years than for any other age group, and black males are especially vulnerable [32]. Some gun deaths may be accidental but most are the results of homicide or suicide. A gun in the home doubles the likelihood of a lethal attempt. Although handguns are often kept in homes for protection, a gun is more likely to kill a family member or a friend than an intruder. The most effective way to prevent firearm injuries is to remove guns from the home and community. Families who keep firearms at home should lock them in a cabinet or drawer and store ammunition in a separate locked location.

Physical Abuse and NAI

NAIs have profound effect on the well-being of children. Reported NAIs may represent only a small proportion of the children who suffer from maltreatment. Physicians are mandated by law to protect children by identifying and reporting all cases of suspected child abuse. It is then the responsibility of child protection services to investigate reports of suspected abuse to determine whether abuse has occurred and to ensure the ongoing safety of the child.

Drowning and Near-drowning

Drowning is also a leading cause of injury-related death in children in the United States and many Western nations [7,88–91]. Toddlers have the highest rate of drowning [90–92]. It has been shown that for every death by drowning, 6 children are hospitalized for near-drowning and up to 10% of survivors experience severe brain damage [90,91]. The sites of drowning are relevant in preventive education. Children younger than 1 year are most likely to drown in the bathtub. Buckets filled with water also present a risk of drowning to the older infant or toddler [92]. For children 1 to 4 years old, drowning or near-drowning occurs most often in home swimming pools, and for school-aged children and teens, drowning occurs most often in large bodies of water such as swimming pools or pen water. After the age of 5 years, the risk of drowning in a swimming pool is much greater for black males than white males [61,90,91]. Similar demographic data are also observed in an Asian study in Hong Kong [92]. Hon and colleagues [92] noted that the top-loading washing machine represented an unusual mechanism of drowning.

Poisoning

Poisoning is a category that needs to be discussed separately because it is a non-trauma form of injury [8,28,93–100]. Poisoning and ingestions account for numerous visits to emergency departments and pediatric hospitals each year. Most childhood poisoning cases are trivial and many do not require medical care. Ingestion or poisoning can be unintentional or intentional. In a review of children hospitalized for ingestion and poisoning at a tertiary center, Hon and colleagues [94] noted that most of these admissions involved unintentional poisoning. Compared with unintentional poisoning, patients who intentionally poisoned themselves were significantly older and were predominantly female. In most admissions, the patients ingested a single substance. Tablets and pills, especially in adolescents who attempted suicide, were more commonly ingested than syrups. The spectrum of substances ingested was vast, but paracetamol, cough or cold medicines, and common adult household medications and agents accounted for most of the medications ingested. The substances ingested were obtained at home in half of the cases and as over-the-counter medication in one-fifth of the cases. Most patients presented within 24 hours of ingestion. Paracetamol poisoning was common. Nearly 30% of patients who ingested paracetamol as a suicidal gesture had toxic levels and required antidote treatment with N-acetyl cysteine. A history of previous poisoning was more common and subsequent follow-up was offered to 74% of patients [94]. Accidental poisoning can be serious and might require intensive care support [101]. Life-threatening poisonings requiring ICU support can pose diagnostic difficulties and challenges to frontline medical officers at the emergency department. Children from all age groups can be affected. Prompt diagnosis is based on relevant history, careful clinical examination, and a high index of suspicion in patients known to be at risk. Young boys are at greater risk of unintentional ingestion, possibly due to curiosity, whereas adolescent girls are more likely to ingest medications as a gesture of suicide. Occasionally, poisoning may occur in a cluster [102]. A detailed description of individual types of poisoning is beyond the scope of this article and is available in most standard textbooks in pediatrics, emergency medicine, intensive care medicine, and toxicology. Nevertheless, knowledge of common toxidromes is advantageous in facilitating a prompt diagnosis.

Animal and Human Bites

Bites account for a large number of visits to the emergency department. Most fatalities are due to dog bites [50,103]. A small number of animal bites are due to cats and other mammals. However, most infected bite wounds are from human and cat bites. In dog bites, boys are bitten more frequently than girls, and the dog is known by the victim in most cases. Younger children have a higher incidence of head and neck wounds, whereas school-aged children are most often bitten on the upper extremities. In cat bites, girls are frequently involved, and the principal complication is infection. The infection risk is higher in cat bites than in dog bites because cat bites are more likely to produce a puncture wound. Scratches or bites from cats may also result in cat-scratch fever. Most cat-scratch disease (CSD) begins with a scratch from the claw or tooth of a kitten less than 1 year of age, although it can also be caught from an adult cat. In California, about 40% of cats carry *Bartonella* [104]. Most cases of CSD occur in children between the ages of 2 and 14 years, and in veterinarians (those most likely to be scratched by a cat). For reasons yet to be determined, most cases occur in the fall or winter months. CSD is a common, zoonotic, infectious disease transmitted by young cats that serve as passive vectors for the bacillus *Bartonella henselae*. Although CSD can affect persons of any age, the condition is most common in previously healthy children and adolescents. Clients with CSD generally present with a positive history of contact with young cats; an inoculation skin papule; and proximal, regional lymphadenitis that can persist for several months. Each year, an estimated 22,000 case of CSD occur in the United States, with 2000 of those cases requiring hospitalization for complications of the disease [105]. Reports indicate that CSD is seasonal, with peaks of the disease occurring in the fall and winter months in temperate climates and extending to July and August in warmer climates. CSD occurs worldwide and all ethnic groups are affected. Males seem to contract the disease more often than females, and the affected families often have at least 1 cat, and most often kittens. The bacillus *B henselae* is most frequently isolated in young, male cats that are not ill and require no treatment, but that serve as passive vectors in transmitting the disease to humans [105–107]. Fleas and ticks have also been associated with the transmission of CSD, although more evidence is required to establish ticks as vectors. Transmission of CSD occurs from a bite, scratch, or petting, as a result of direct contact with the cat's saliva. The saliva is deposited on an infected cat's fur and claws from self-grooming [107].

Most human bites occur during fights. Bites may occur during playing among young children [108–110]. Alternatively, victims may be bitten by mentally retarded children. Cultures most commonly grow streptococci, anaerobes, staphylococci, and *Eikenella corrodens*. Severe insect or reptile bites represent another major category of bite injuries, but the mechanism of injury is different from that of mammalian bites. Venoms are often involved and antivenoms may be needed in their management. Scorpion stings are common in arid areas of the south-western United States [111–113]. Scorpion venom is more toxic than most snake venoms, but only minute amounts are injected. Although neurologic manifestations may last a week, most clinical signs subside within 24 to 48 hours. Local symptoms include pain or paresthesias. Systemic manifestations include hypersalivation, restlessness, muscular fasciculations, abdominal cramps, opisthotonos, convulsions, urinary incontinence, and respiratory failure.

Another important group that inflict human injuries is spiders [113]. Spiders that are of medical importance include the black widow (*Latrodectus mactans*) and the North American brown recluse (violin) spider (*Loxosceles reclusa*). Positive identification of the spider is helpful, because many spider bites may mimic those of the brown recluse spider.

In snake bites, human morbidity and mortality are low [113–115]. The outcome depends on the size of the child, the site of the bite, the degree of envenomation, the type of snake, and the effectiveness of treatment.

Suffocation and Strangulation

Suffocation and strangulations are unusual childhood injuries [4,116–118]. Nevertheless, suffocation is the leading cause of mortality for infants [4]. Strangulation is the cause of death in more than 50% of all playground fatalities [118]. Neurologic damage and death are often caused by airway obstruction and venous congestion leading to hypoxia, acidosis, brain congestion, and brain cell death [116]. Spinal cord injury has not been found in survivors. The mortality in strangulation is high. These injuries have medicolegal implications. At the PICU, the principal author managed a case of fatal strangulation when a 10-year-old boy was unhappy during a festival season and hanged himself with a towel. Physicians caring for the family of these cases need to be aware of the emotional and medicolegal implications.

PREVENTION AND INTERVENTIONS

Severe injuries may result in instantaneous fatality or grave, irreversible sequelae if the victims survive the initial insults. It is sensible for a society to implement measures to prevent injuries. Injury control presents constant challenges and must be evidence based [119–124]. Three forms of injury-preventive interventions have been proposed [125,126]. Active intervention requires an action taken on the part of the host (child or parent) to prevent injury. One example is the storage of medications out of the child's reach. In passive intervention, no action is required for the intervention to be successful. An example is the packaging of medications in nonlethal amounts so that harm is not inflicted even if the medications are accidental taken by the child. Most often, mixed interventions, partly active and partly passive, are used. As an illustration, bike helmets inherently protect the cyclist's head, but they must be worn correctly. Generally, the more effort required on the part of the child or parent, the less successful is the intervention. The 3 fundamental aspects of injury-prevention science are epidemiology, biomechanics, and behavioral science [120,121,127]. Epidemiology provides an understanding of the nonrandom distribution of injury risk among populations of children so that areas of concern can be identified and targeted interventions can be designed and implemented [124]. Biomechanics provides an understanding of human vulnerability and resilience to limit energy transfer in a potentially injurious event. For example, biomechanics researchers and engineers have continually challenged and updated designs of infant car seats to provide protection in motor vehicle collisions. Behavioral science provides knowledge about effective and ineffective ways of altering the risk of injury by manipulating behaviors of children, adolescents, adults, and communities [119]. For example, laws that require the use of seat belts in automobiles can be analyzed for effectiveness in curtailing childhood injury and death.

A fundamental concept of the science of epidemiology is the phase-factor matrix, introduced in 1972 by William Haddon [128]. The matrix is a conceptual framework that combines the epidemiologic components (host, agent, and social environments) with 3 stages of event-related modifiable risk factors (before, during, or after the event). Taking RTA as an example, pre-event factors refer to separating bicyclists from traffic. Event factors refer to protection from head injuries with helmet use while bicycling. Postevent factors consider availability of emergency services and trauma centers after an injury. A framework for how intervention can be applied within each cell of the matrix can be derived when taking these elements into account.

Reducing the risk and severity of injuries are the simultaneous goals of biomechanics research and development. Energy is the primary enemy of injury-prevention efforts. Energy can be mechanical, thermal, chemical, or electrical, or in the form of ionizing radiation. Mechanical energy is responsible for most injury-related morbidity and mortality in children. Examples of strategies to minimize the effects of mechanical energy include seat belts and car seats in motor vehicles, properly worn bicycle helmets, and energy-absorbing surfaces under playground equipment [16,17,40,80]. Questions such as whether an infant would be safer in the event of a motor vehicle collision if he or she were seated facing the rear are being investigated and challenged through biomechanics research. It has been concluded that impact direction in a motor vehicle collision is an important determinant of infant morbidity and mortality. For example, lateral impacts to the head cause more axonal injury than impacts from other directions; therefore, side-impact airbags have been developed in cars. Because most severe car collisions are frontal, infant safety seats should face backward.

Persons at risk of injury may be persuaded to alter their behavior (eg, to wear seat belts, to install smoke detectors, not to smoke at home). However, this has proven to be an intractable problem. Many health behavioral change interventions do not succeed because they fail to take into account the habitual quality of most health and safety–related behavior. A more complete model of behavioral change based on a better understanding of the role of habit should be considered [129]. Requiring behavioral change by law (eg, seat belt and motorcycle helmet laws, building codes for fire exits and smoke detectors) is an attempt by government bodies to force healthy decisions to be made by society to improve public health. Advocacy groups use behavioral techniques in public service announcements and other outlets to provide education to parents and children in an attempt to encourage good decision-making. Behavioral science deals mostly with active injury-prevention strategies or strategies that require the parent or child to actively alter his or her activity or make a healthy decision such as purchasing, wearing, and replacing bicycle helmets.

Injury-prevention counseling is an important component and should be reinforced during health supervision visits [130]. Counseling should focus on problems that are frequent and age appropriate. Passive strategies of prevention should be emphasized, because these are more effective than active strategies.

Encouraging the use of childproof cupboard latches to prevent poisoning (passive strategy) will be more effective than instructing parents and caregivers (active strategy).

As mentioned earlier, the leading cause of injuries in children and adolescents is RTA and most victims are pedestrians [76,131]. Public education through local media should be in force in an attempt to modify the habits of pedestrians and drivers. As with many other types of injuries, modification of external factors, such as traffic engineering modification, seems to be the most practical solution [131]. The safest place in a motor vehicle for an infant or child is in the back seat. In all 50 of the United States, the law requires that infants be in a car seat while riding in a motor vehicle. An infant should never be placed in a rear-facing car seat in the front seat of a car equipped with a passenger-side air bag [74,132,133]. If a child must sit in the front seat, the seat should be moved back as far as possible, away from a passenger-side air bag, and the child should be properly belted in a booster seat [73]. Children are at a higher risk for air bag–related injuries because of their size and the positioning of their seat belts, which expose the child's face and neck to the full velocity of a deploying airbag [74,132,133]. The National Highway Traffic Safety Administration regularly publishes statistics regarding incidents in which deployment of an airbag resulted in a fatal injury, and many incidents in which children were not properly restrained in a rear-facing safety seat [133]. Front airbags seem to offer more harm than protection to children younger than 13 years who are seated in the front seat. Infants younger than 1 year and weighing less than 9 kg (20 lb) should be placed in the back seat in a rear-facing child-restraint car seat [69,133,134]. Forward-facing car seats can be used for children older than 1 year and weighing more than 9 kg until the child is aged 4 years and weighs at least 18 kg (40 lb). To ensure that the installed seat belt is properly used by children younger than 8 years who do not require a car seat, booster seats placed in the back seat are recommended [73]. In some communities, car seat safety checks are periodically available so that parents can have their car seat installation checked. A good car seat is the correct size for the infant or child, fits into the car appropriately, works with the car's seat belt system, is easy for the parent to install, meets all federal safety standards, and has not previously been in a car that was involved in a collision.

Societal changes have begun to improve safety in regards to child restraints. Ongoing improvements of new vehicle safety restraints have been developed, including side-impact air bags and Lower Anchors and Tethers for Children (LATCH) [135]. LATCH is a system that allows the installation of child safety seats without the use of the vehicle's seat belt. However, it is important to continue to educate parents, caretakers, and technicians about proper restraint use. Also, local and national resources are available to aid parents in proper restraint use. Nevertheless, reports have indicated that the use of booster seats is still inadequate [73].

Children should be brought up to observe safe pedestrian habits. Young children should hold hands with an adult at all times when near traffic. Deaths have occurred in the driveway of the home when a family member or guest unintentionally reversed a car over a child.

In bicycle-related injuries, the strict implementation of laws on use of helmets while cycling may prevent or reduce the incidence of severe head injuries [17,77–79,136,137].

Home safety is an important issue because most children are injured in indoor environments. In urban families, implementation of the safety practices recommended by the American Academy of Pediatrics is low [138]. The structural design of urban homes may be a significant barrier to home safety–product use [138]. Home childproofing should be encouraged for parents with a young child. Important strategies to encourage include covering outlets, padding table corners, placing stair gates to prevent falls, and eliminating hot exposures. In many metropolitan cities, most residents live in high-rise buildings. A fall from a window, roof, or balcony can injure or kill a child [22,83]. In Hong Kong, fatal falls of toddlers from windows are frequently reported in the media. Window guards that keep children in but allow for egress during a fire are recommended. To minimize falls from windows, the maximum spacing in railings has been set at 10 cm (4 in). Almost all children younger than 6 years can fit through a railing with 15-cm (6-in) spacing, and almost no child older than 1 year can fit through a railing with 10-cm spacing. Parents should not leave doors open or unlocked at night, especially in winter. Toddlers can get out of bed and leave the home unattended. In the case of head injury following a fall, children should be evaluated for neurologic symptoms. After a period of observation, patients with mild head injury may be discharged with detailed written instructions if physical examination remains normal and parental supervision and follow-up are adequate. Children with persistent neurologic deficits require admission or prolonged observation. Computed tomography (CT) scan and neurosurgical consultation are indicated if the child's mental state deteriorates. Patients with severe head injuries require prompt treatment and evaluation by a neurosurgeon in a hospital.

Most fire-related deaths result from smoke inhalation. Smoke detectors can prevent most injuries and deaths caused by fires at home [23,24]. Families should practice emergency evacuation of the home.

Excessive sun exposure during childhood has been associated with subsequent development of skin cancers. Prevention of sunburn is best achieved by sun avoidance, particularly during the hours of 10 AM to 3 PM [139,140]. Sunscreen with a sun protection factor of 15 or greater extends the period of time that a child can spend in the sun without sunburn. Hats, sunglasses, and special precautions for fair-skinned individuals and infants are also important aspects of safe sun exposure.

Like falls, scalding is a common mode of injury in the home environment. Although not as often fatal as head injuries in falls or motor vehicle accidents, scalding by hot liquids may cause misery, pain, and disfigurement. To prevent scalding injuries, toddlers must not be allowed in kitchen areas where scald injury can easily occur. Fires and burns combined are a common cause of unintentional severe childhood injuries [9]. Smoke detectors should be installed near each sleeping area, and regularly checked for proper functioning. In practice, smoker detectors are only installed in major corridors of high-rise residential apartments in many cities. Families should develop a home-escape plan for use in the event of a fire. Children should be taught to feel a door for warmth; to stay close to the ground if smoke is present; and to stop, drop, and roll if their clothing begins to burn. Burns should be treated as soon as possible by cooling with cool running water and by applying a clean dressing. Burn severity is described in terms of degrees. Medical attention should be sought. The risk of scalding burns can be lowered by instructing parents to set the hot-water heater in the home to 49°C (120°F) or cooler [29,85–87]. Before 1980, manufacturers routinely set water-heater temperatures at 60°C (140°F) or hotter. At this temperature, a full-thickness burn in an adult would occur in about 2 to 5 seconds; only about 0.5 to 2 seconds is required for a similar burn in a child. Health care providers should inform parents about the dangers of hot-water burns to children and advise setting maximum water temperatures to 49°C (120°F) as recommended by the American Academy of Pediatrics [29,85–87].

Fireworks are dangerous for individuals of any age, but particularly for young children [57,58]. Consumer fireworks cause serious preventable injuries among pediatric fireworks users and bystanders. Parents should be advised to take their children to safer public fireworks displays rather than allowing consumer fireworks to be used by or near their children. A national restriction of consumer fireworks, in accordance with the policy recommendations of the American Academy of Pediatrics, should be implemented to reduce the burden of fireworks-related injuries among children.

Poisoning and ingestion is a large category. A lot of epidemiologic information has been generated and preventive recommendations derived [8,12,94–97,101,141]. Severe poisoning usually involves careless disposition of poisons or medications [101]. Children should be protected from all dangerous chemicals and substances found in the home. These should be put out of the reach of children, and the use of child-protective devices to prevent opening of cabinets should be encouraged [142,143]. Medications and poisons should not be kept in refrigerators. In particular, chemicals must not be kept in bottles or containers normally used for common proprietary food or drinks. A variety of foodstuffs can cause fatal aspiration and choking when the food material obstructs the airway or the esophagus. Infants and toddlers should avoid small objects and foods because of the threat of choking [144]. Batteries, buttons, jewelry (especially necklaces and hoop earrings), coins, certain holiday decorations, and small toys should be eliminated from the small child's environment. The most dangerous foods include peanuts, popcorn, bread, whole grapes, raisins, bites of apple and meat, carrots, candy, and fish bones.

The phone number of a poison control center should be known to all parents, schools, or services caring for children and should be readily available in the case of poison ingestion. The American Academy of Pediatrics recommends that ipecac no longer be routinely used as a poison treatment intervention in the home, and pediatricians should advise parents who do have ipecac at home to dispose of it [145,146]. Inducing a child to vomit certain chemicals can make the condition worse. In some situations, giving a child ipecac delays presentation to the emergency department, and in some cases has delayed the use of more effective substances such as activated charcoal. Parents and caregivers should always call the poison control center before administering any therapy to a child with a toxic ingestion. Parents should take their child to the nearest medical care facility for evaluation. Unintentional acetaminophen toxicity in children can occur, and counseling for parents by pediatricians on the correct dosing procedures for all over-the-counter drugs, including acetaminophen, is recommended [94]. Medications used by family members are a particularly common source of ingestion by children. Parents should be cautioned to make sure that each home in which the child spends substantial time is safe.

Submersion injuries are an important but avoidable cause of mortality and morbidity in children [8,89,92,147,148]. Fencing laws have been instituted in many nations and the incidence of submersion injury has been decreasing [89]. Unlike many Western nations, domestic swimming pools are uncommon in many Asian cities, and near-drowning or drowning rarely occurs in these settings [92]. Although outdoor submersion injuries are more common, indoor submersion injuries seem to be associated with worse outcomes [92]. The amounts of water involved are often small. Nevertheless, severe sequelae may occur. Supervised environments such as public swimming pools rarely produce in tragic sequelae. Fencing domestic swimming pools has been an important preventive measure overseas, but this is not relevant in cities where domestic swimming pools are not popular [92,149]. The median age for patients with indoor submersion injury is significantly lower than that of outdoor submersion injury. It seems that young children are curious but unaware of potential dangers in their home environment. They may also be unable to extricate themselves from the small amount of water when they are submerged [92]. Therefore, buckets of water or any unused containers of water in the home should be drained if toddlers or young children are present. Infants and children need to be watched at all times when around water. Instances of toddlers drowning in containers of water as small as a bucket have been reported [91,92]. Because they are top heavy, children who put their heads into a bucket may be unable to right themselves and can easily drown in the water (or whatever liquid the bucket contains). Leaving a child unattended while he or she is bathing is a particularly common, yet dangerous, occurrence. Many childhood drowning episodes occur in bathtubs. To increase awareness of water safety, swimming lessons are generally encouraged for older children. Swimming programs with proper supervision are encouraged for infants and toddlers, but they have not been shown to decrease the risk of drowning. Parents should not feel secure that their child is safe in water or safe from drowning after participating in such programs. Young children should receive constant, close supervision by an adult while in and around water [150,151]. Of recreational activities, swimming carries the highest risk for children. School-aged children should be taught to swim, and recreational swimming should always be supervised. Public swimming pools should have a lifeguard in attendance. Private swimming pools should be fenced securely so that unsupervised and vulnerable toddlers cannot gain entrance [91,149,152,153]. Recommendations are that the fence should be 1.2 m (4 ft) tall or higher, the distance between the bottom of the fence and the ground should be less than 10 cm (4 in), and the gate of the pool fence should be self-latching and self-closing. Parents should also know how to perform cardiopulmonary resuscitation [89–91].

Regarding animal and insect bites, young children should not be left alone in the presence of a dog. Children should be taught about dog behavior, and the public should be educated about the selection of dogs and their training, care, and socialization. Dog bites are treated similarly to other wounds, with high-pressure, high-volume irrigation with normal saline, debridement of any devitalized tissue, removal of foreign matter, and tetanus prophylaxis. The risk of rabies from dog bite is low in developed countries. Nevertheless, rabies prophylaxis should be considered when appropriate [103]. Animal rabies can be controlled by proper induction of herd immunity (domestic dogs should be regularly taken to a veterinarian to minimize the chance of acquiring and spreading disease via a bite), humane removal of stray animals, promotion of responsible pet ownership through education, and enactment of leash laws. Pre-exposure vaccination with modern cell culture rabies vaccine is recommended for people at high risk of exposure to rabies and for travelers who spend longer than 1 month in countries where rabies is a threat, or for those who travel in a country where immediate access to appropriate care is limited. Postexposure prophylaxis consists of prompt and thorough wound cleansing and immunization with modern cell culture rabies vaccine, together with administration of rabies immune globulin to those individuals who have not previously received pre-exposure prophylaxis [103]. Wounds should be sutured only if necessary for cosmetic reasons, because wound closure increases the risk of infection. Prophylactic antibiotics have not been proven to decrease rates of infection in low-risk dog-bite wounds not involving the hands or feet. If a bite involves a joint, periosteum, or neurovascular bundle, prompt orthopedic surgery consultation should be obtained. The most common pathogens isolated from a dog-bite wound are *Pasteurella multocida, Capnocytophaga canimorsus,* streptococci, staphylococci, and anaerobes [154]. Infected dog bites can be treated with penicillin for *P multocida,* and broad-spectrum coverage can be provided by amoxicillin and clavulanic acid or cephalexin. Complications of dog bites include scarring, CNS infections, septic arthritis, osteomyelitis, endocarditis, and sepsis.

Cat wounds should not be sutured except when absolutely necessary for cosmetic reasons. *P multocida* is the most common pathogen. Cat bites create a puncture-wound inoculum, and prophylaxis antibiotics (penicillin plus cephaxin, or amoxycillin and clavulanic acid) are recommended. High dosage to ensure adequate tissue penetration is recommended. The typical course of CSD is usually self-limiting and requires only supportive therapy.

A major complication of human bite wounds is infection of the metacarpophalangeal joints [109]. A hand surgeon should evaluate clenched-fist injuries from human bites. If necessary, operative debridement is followed in many cases by intravenous antibiotics. Although antibiotics are often used, studies have shown that most human bites in children are superficial and do not become infected [109,110]. Antibiotics do not seem to be useful in prophylaxis for minor bite wounds seen shortly after injury. Nevertheless, follow-up is necessary for all bite wounds, because serious infection may develop, or an established, seemingly minor infection may worsen. Hand wounds and deep wounds should be treated with antibiotic coverage against *E corrodens* and gram-positive pathogens by a penicillinase-resistant antibiotic. Only severe lacerations involving the face should be sutured. Other wounds can be managed by delayed primary closure or healing by second intention.

Children should be discouraged from exposing themselves to potentially dangerous environments. Snake bites commonly involve curious males who go out in the evening without wearing proper shoes [114,115]. Children in snake-infested areas should wear boots and long trousers, should not walk barefooted, and should be cautioned not to explore under ledges or in holes [114,115]. Snake venoms may be coagulopathic or neurotoxic. Antivenoms may be required for severe local symptoms such as compartment syndrome or for systemic symptoms [113–115]. For scorpion bites, sedation is the primary therapy [111]. Antivenom is reserved for severe poisoning [112]. In severe cases, patients may require endotracheal intubation, and treatment of seizures, hypertension, or tachycardia. The prognosis is good if the patient's airway is managed appropriately. In black widow spider bites, death of the victims is extremely rare. If available, antivenom should be reserved for severe cases in which the therapies discussed earlier have failed. Local treatment of the bite is not helpful. In brown recluse spider bites, fatalities are rare but fatal disseminated intravascular coagulopathy has been reported.

A nonviolent environment should be provided to all children [32]. Secure parent-infant attachments, social and conflict-resolution skills, and the avoidance of violence (on television or actual) all have a role in promoting nonviolence. Most unintentional firearm-related deaths are caused by children who are unsupervised in a home with a handgun (70%) [9]. Risk factors associated with childhood firearm death include exposure to family violence, history of antisocial behavior, depression, suicidal ideation, drug and alcohol use, poor school performance, bullying, withdrawal, and isolation from peer groups. Guns are strictly forbidden in many nations or cities and there have been no pediatric deaths related to gunshot in these cities. At the time of writing, there is a report in the news that a mother accidentally discharged a toy gun when she was waving it playfully on the face her own 7-month-old daughter. The lead bullet went through the eye into the daughter's brain and the infant was left in a critical condition (http://appledaily.atnext.com/template/apple/art_main.cfm?iss_id=20090110&sec_id=15335&subsec_id=15336&art_id=12073196). This case illustrates that even a toy gun may do harm to children. Other than the United States and some western nations, most countries have strict laws prohibiting the possession of a gun by civilians. The laws are welcome by most parents and they should be reinforced.

Product manufacturers are charged with making products safe for children and are held to safety standards and regulations. For consumer product and toy safety, many items available for purchase or use must meet safety standards before marketing. For example, items such as bunk beds, gas grills, garage-door openers, hair dryers, infant carriers, shopping carts, and self-locking toy chests all carry specific hazards for children. Mobile infant walkers are not recommended by the American Academy of Pediatrics [44]. These walkers do not help an infant learn to walk, and they pose a serious danger of falls down stairs. Stationary infant activity centers are recommended as an alternative to mobile infant walkers. Trampolines are so strongly associated with childhood injury that the American Academy of Pediatrics has advised that no parent consider purchasing one [45]. Most of the serious injuries involve bone fractures. Trampoline injuries that are fatal usually involve spinal cord and head trauma. Lawn and garden equipment should be used with caution. Lawnmowers pose a threat to toddlers who do not realize their danger. Home safety education in a clinical setting or at home, especially with the provision of safety equipment, is effective in increasing a range of safety practices [29]. However, there is a lack of evidence regarding its effect on child injury rates. There is no consistent evidence that home safety education, with or without the provision of safety equipment, is less effective in safeguarding those at greater risk of injury [29].

Communities and government bodies are responsible for reinforcing child protection laws. The current roles of injury-prevention laws and manufacturing practices in enhancing child safety are often inadequate. Health professionals should continue to raise the issue by campaigning for legislative and engineering changes to reduce childhood injuries [155]. Citizens who witness violations of child safety laws should alert the appropriate authorities. In certain situations, citizens can be held responsible for not reporting a neglectful or abusive action. Researchers constantly examine the state of child safety and the prevailing statistics to identify areas of concern and apply methods to improve injury prevention.

Studies of sports injuries show that the most dangerous sports for children are football, gymnastics, wrestling, and ice hockey. Proper coaching and instruction, as well as proper use of protective gear, including helmets, face masks, and mouth guards, are essential to help prevent injury. Concussions during football games are common, and the proper treatment of a player with a concussion is the responsibility of the coaches and trainers for the team. Concussion-scoring systems exist to help a coach or trainer properly assess the severity and to decide on a plan for return to play, if appropriate. Baseball is a popular sport in the United States. Soft baseballs lessen the impact and potentially decrease the injury from being hit by one. The American Academy of Pediatrics Committee on Sports Medicine outlines the risk of injury from baseball and softball in children 5 to 14 years of age [35,36,39]. Soft baseballs can potentially decrease the risk of commotio cordis. This is the syndrome associated with a youth baseball player being hit in the chest and experiencing the often-fatal ventricular fibrillation [36,39]. Researchers believe that children are more prone to this phenomenon because their thoraces are more elastic and more easily compressed by an impact than those of an adult. Soft baseballs should be considered for use by children aged 14 years and younger. Padded chest protectors are also undergoing testing, but not enough is known about them for them to be universally recommended. Catchers must wear protective gear to protect themselves from the pitched ball and swinging bat. All youth baseball players should also wear batting helmets. Baseball is the leading cause of sports-related eye injuries. Polycarbonate plastic lenses and frames that are sturdy and impact resistant provide optimal protection. They are recommended for batting helmets and should be required for any player with a history of eye surgery or single-eye blindness [156,157]. Breakaway bases are encouraged, and headfirst slides are discouraged. Benches and dugouts should be protected, and the use of an on-deck circle should be discouraged, unless it is enclosed by a fence. Little-league elbow is an injury that is mainly seen in pitchers who are not yet skeletally mature. Medial elbow pain develops in these athletes. Many guidelines are available to determine the appropriate age to start throwing certain pitches, how many pitches to throw, and how much rest is needed between pitching outings. Gymnastics injuries can be minimized with good coaching and floor padding around equipment. Most injuries involve upper and lower extremities and include fractures, dislocations, avulsions, and lacerations. Because cheerleading styles have changed to include more gymnastic moves, there is also a risk of concussion, neck injuries, and closed head injuries. It is recommended that coaches complete a safety training and certification program. Youth ice hockey players are advised to avoid checking until they are at least 16 years old. Soccer is a fairly safe sport; almost all deaths reported occurred because of an impact with a goal post [158–160]. From 1979 to 1993, 18 fatalities due to a blow caused by a falling soccer goalpost resulting from improper installation were reported in the United States [161]. Soccer is second only to basketball in the number of orofacial and dental injuries. Whether heading the ball in soccer causes cognitive deficits remains controversial. Skateboarding, scootering, inline skating, snowboarding, and skiing are increasingly popular recreational sports that require proper equipment and protective gear to adequately protect children from injury. For skateboard and scooter safety, avoiding traffic, wearing proper protective gear, and having adequate supervision are advised. No child younger than 10 years should be allowed to skateboard unsupervised, and no child younger than 8 years should be allowed to ride a scooter without supervision [37]. Inline skating has become popular. Snowmobiling is a particularly dangerous sport for teenagers and younger children. It is not recommended for anyone younger than 16 years because of the coordination and upper body strength required to manipulate the machine. Most snowmobile injuries are head injuries, and most deaths associated with snowmobiles are from head injuries. Personal watercraft, such as jet skis, should be operated only by individuals aged 16 years or older. Individual states have laws outlining specific regulations regarding the operation of watercraft. Some require completion of a water safety course before operating a motorized watercraft, depending on the individual's age. Children participating in horseback riding should be encouraged to wear a proper helmet to protect against head injury. Another example of injury prevention in sports is fencing, which is an open-skilled combat sport that has also become popular [162]. The physical demands of fencing competitions are high, involving the aerobic and anaerobic alactic and lactic metabolisms, and are also affected by age, sex, level of training, and technical and tactical models used in relation to the adversary. The anthropometric characteristics of fencers show a typical asymmetry of the limbs as a result of the practice of an asymmetric sport activity. Fencing produces typical functional asymmetries that emphasize the high level of specific function, strength, and control required in this sport. Although fencing is not particularly dangerous, there is a fine line between a fatal lesion and a simple wound from a broken blade. The suggestions for injury prevention are in 3 primary areas: (1) actions that can be taken by participants, (2) improvements in equipment and facilities, and (3) administration of fencing competitions. As in every other sport, the prevention of accidents must be accomplished at various levels and must involve the institutions that are responsible for safety in sports [162]. Schools and daycare facilities are held to state safety regulations. Protecting children on playgrounds is a particular challenge. Supervision is crucial. Padded or soft surfaces under playground equipment are helpful [163–166].

Injuries that occur in abusive or neglectful environments are difficult to prevent. Parents can be counseled on the harm of shaking a baby, and they can be taught strategies for diffusing a stressful situation without resorting to harming the child.

More aggressive education to make parents aware about the risk of injury should be implemented so that more families will invest their time in injury prevention [130,167]. Successful injury-prevention strategies often include multifaceted approaches such as education, incentives for safe human behavior, legislation/enforcement, and environmental changes [9]. Careful evaluation for effectiveness of injury-prevention programs, with weighing of societal and economic values, continues to be a challenge. Generally, passive measures such as improved engineering are more effective than measures that require modification of human behaviors. Critical care providers can actively engage in preventive efforts and improved acute care of the severely injured child. Data suggest that preventive efforts should especially target educating parents with young children about home safety. The primary care provider is also in an ideal position to identify high-risk situations and to intervene before injury occurs.

Pediatric injury prevention is one of the most important and challenging aspects of child health care. Young children inherently lack mature decision-making skills to protect themselves from injury, whereas some older children and adolescents engage in risky behaviors in attempts to rebel against adult advice. No child is immune from all dangers that pose a threat to his or her health and safety. Prevention of childhood injury–related deaths is the responsibility of society, caregivers, and physicians. Pediatricians, during a patient's health maintenance visit, should address injury prevention with parents and caregivers, as well as with the children themselves, when appropriate. Parents need to take an active role in preventing childhood injury in all settings. Schools and daycare providers are responsible for minimizing hazards and providing a safe environment.

In medical office–based education and counseling, the pediatrician plays a pivotal role in influencing parental behavior to reduce the risk of injury [124,130]. Effective counseling should be developmentally focused and understandable, prioritizing injuries for the particular age group receiving counseling. It engages the parent, patient, or both in a dialog so that a sense of responsibility and importance can be developed. Other than office-based counseling, home visiting programs have the potential to reduce significantly the rates of childhood injury [167]. Parents with younger children must be convinced that the active injury-prevention intervention is worthwhile. Home safety education, provided most commonly as one-to-one, face-to-face education, in a clinical setting or at home, especially with the provision of safety equipment, is effective in increasing a range of safety practices. At present, there is a lack of evidence regarding its effect on child injury rates.

SUMMARY

The causes of severe childhood injuries are heterogeneous. These injuries occur most commonly indoors. Cardiopulmonary or neurologic/neurosurgical supports are often required, and outcomes may be fatal or disastrous. Epidemiology findings have important implications and serve to heighten public awareness, especially of home safety in the prevention of childhood accidents. Each city should study its own epidemiologic data and individualize preventive policy. The most devastating injuries to children come from the environment in which the child lives. Although children cannot be protected totally, the risk can be lessened with common sense. This begins with knowing what the risks are and then minimizing and removing them [3].

References

[1] Roberts I, DiGuiseppi C, Ward H. Childhood injuries: extent of the problem, epidemiological trends, and costs. Inj Prev 1998;4(Suppl 4):S10–6.

[2] Agran PF, Winn D, Anderson C, et al. Rates of pediatric and adolescent injuries by year of age. Pediatrics 2001;108:E45.

[3] McLone DG. The risk. Pediatr Neurosurg 2001;34:169–71.

[4] Pan SY, Ugnat AM, Semenciw R, et al. Trends in childhood injury mortality in Canada, 1979–2002. Inj Prev 2006;12:155–60.

[5] Sonkin B. Walking, cycling and transport safety: an analysis of child road deaths. J R Soc Med 2006;99:402–5.

[6] Kibel SM, Bradshaw D, Joubert G. Trends in childhood injury mortality in three South African population groups, 1968–1985 Suid-Afrikaanse Tydskrif Vir Geneeskunde. S Afr Med J 1990;78:392–7.

[7] Quan L, Kinder D. Pediatric submersions: prehospital predictors of outcome. Pediatrics 1992;90:909–13.

[8] Shannon M. Ingestion of toxic substances by children. N Engl J Med 2000;342:186–91.

[9] Dowd MD, Keenan HT, Bratton SL. Epidemiology and prevention of childhood injuries. Crit Care Med 2002;30(Suppl 11):S385–92.

[10] Ong ME, Ooi SB, Manning PG. A review of 2,517 childhood injuries seen in a Singapore emergency department in 1999–mechanisms and injury prevention suggestions. Singapore Med J 2003;44:12–9.

[11] Tomashek KM, Hsia J, Iyasu S. Trends in postneonatal mortality attributable to injury, United States, 1988–1998. Pediatrics 2003;111(5 Part 2):1219–25.

[12] Chan CC, Cheng JC, Wong TW, et al. An international comparison of childhood injuries in Hong Kong. Inj Prev 2000;6:20–3.

[13] Rates of homicide, suicide, and firearm-related death among children-26 industrialized countries. JAMA 1997;277:704–5.

[14] Vaca FE. National Highway Traffic Safety Administration (NHTSA) notes. Ann Emerg Med 2004;43:274–5.

[15] Kay MP. National highway traffic safety administration notes. Rehabilitation costs and long-term consequences of motor vehicle injuries. Ann Emerg Med 2007;49:817–8.

[16] Sosin DM, Sacks JJ, Webb KW. Pediatric head injuries and deaths from bicycling in the United States. Pediatrics 1996;98:868–70.

[17] American Academy of Pediatrics, Committee on Injury and Poison Prevention. Bicycle helmets. Pediatrics 2001;108:1030–2.

[18] Thompson RS, Rivara FP, Thompson DC. A case-control study of the effectiveness of bicycle safety helmets. N Engl J Med 1989;320:1361–7.

[19] Thompson DC, Thompson RS, Rivara FP, et al. A case-control study of the effectiveness of bicycle safety helmets in preventing facial injury. Am J Public Health 1990;80:1471–4.

[20] Sacks JJ, Holmgreen P, Smith SM, et al. Bicycle-associated head injuries and deaths in the United States from 1984 through 1988. How many are preventable? [see comment]. JAMA 1991;266:3016–8.

[21] Sacks JJ, Kresnow M, Houston B, et al. Bicycle helmet use among American children, 1994. Inj Prev 1996;2:258–62.

[22] Committee on Injury and Poison Prevention. American Academy of Pediatrics: falls from heights: windows, roofs, and balconies. Pediatrics 2001;107:1188–91.

[23] Runyan CW, Bangdiwala SI, Linzer MA, et al. Risk factors for fatal residential fires. N Engl J Med 1992;327:859–63.

[24] Onwuachi-Saunders C, Forjuoh SN, West P, et al. Child death reviews: a gold mine for injury prevention and control. Inj Prev 1999;5:276–9.

[25] Nagaraja J, Menkedick J, Phelan KJ, et al. Deaths from residential injuries in US children and adolescents, 1985–1997. Pediatrics 2005;116:454–61.

[26] Istre GR, McCoy M, Carlin DK, et al. Residential fire related deaths and injuries among children: fireplay, smoke alarms, and prevention. Inj Prev 2002;8:128–32.

[27] Marshall SW, Runyan CW, Bangdiwala SI, et al. Fatal residential fires: who dies and who survives? JAMA 1998;279:1633–7.

[28] Hon KL, Nelson EA. Gender disparity in paediatric hospital admissions. Ann Acad Med Singap 2006;35:882–8.

[29] Kendrick D, Coupland C, Mulvaney C, et al. Home safety education and provision of safety equipment for injury prevention. Cochrane Database Syst Rev 2007;1:CD005014.

[30] Adekoya N, Thurman DJ, White DD, et al. Surveillance for traumatic brain injury deaths–United States, 1989–1998 Surveillance Summaries. MMWR Morb Mortal Wkly Rep 2002;51:1–14.

[31] Guerrero JL, Thurman DJ, Sniezek JE. Emergency department visits associated with traumatic brain injury: United States, 1995–1996. Brain Inj 2000;14:181–6.

[32] Firearm-related injuries affecting the pediatric population. Committee on Injury and Poison Prevention. American Academy of Pediatrics. Pediatrics 2000;105(4 Pt 1):888–95.

[33] Ikeda RM, Gorwitz R, James SP, et al. Trends in fatal firearm-related injuries, United States, 1962–1993. Am J Prev Med 1997;13:396–400.

[34] Eber GB, Annest JL, Mercy JA, et al. Nonfatal and fatal firearm-related injuries among children aged 14 years and younger: United States, 1993–2000. Pediatrics 2004;113:1686–92.

[35] Risk of injury from baseball and softball in children 5 to 14 years of age. American Academy of Pediatrics Committee on Sports Medicine. Pediatrics 1994;93:690–2.

[36] Committee on Sports Medicine and Fitness. American Academy of Pediatrics: Risk of injury from baseball and softball in children. Pediatrics 2001;107:782–4.

[37] Committee on Injury and Poison Prevention, American Academy of Pediatrics. Skateboard and scooter injuries. Pediatrics 2002;109:542–3.

[38] Shields BJ, Smith GA. Cheerleading-related injuries to children 5 to 18 years of age: United States, 1990–2002. Pediatrics 2006;117:122–9.

[39] Flyger N, Button C, Rishiraj N. The science of softball: implications for performance and injury prevention. Sports Med 2006;36:797–816.

[40] Centers for Disease Control and Prevention. Playground safety–United States, 1998–1999. MMWR Morb Mortal Wkly Rep 1999;48:329–32.

[41] Phelan KJ, Khoury J, Kalkwarf HJ, et al. Trends and patterns of playground injuries in United States children and adolescents. Ambul Pediatr 2001;1:227–33.

[42] In-line skating injuries in children and adolescents. American Academy of Pediatrics. Committee on Injury and Poison Prevention and Committee on Sports Medicine and Fitness. Pediatrics 1998;101(4 Pt 1):720–2.

[43] Injuries associated with infant walkers. American Academy of Pediatrics Committee on Injury and Poison Prevention. Pediatrics 1995;95:778–80.

[44] American Academy of Pediatrics, Committee on Injury and Poison Prevention. Injuries associated with infant walkers. Pediatrics 2001;108:790–2.

[45] Trampolines at home, school, and recreational centers. American Academy of Pediatrics. Committee on Injury and Poison Prevention and Committee on Sports Medicine and Fitness. Pediatrics 1999;103(5 Pt 1):1053–6.

[46] Lau ST, Lee YH, Hess DJ, et al. Lawnmower injuries in children: a 10-year experience. Pediatr Surg Int 2006;22:209–14.

[47] Loder RT, Dikos GD, Taylor DA. Long-term lower extremity prosthetic costs in children with traumatic lawnmower amputations. Arch Pediatr Adolesc Med 2004;158:1177–81.

[48] Weiss HB, Friedman DI, Coben JH. Incidence of dog bite injuries treated in emergency departments. JAMA 1998;279:51–3.

[49] Bernardo LM, Gardner MJ, O'Connor J, et al. Dog bites in children treated in a pediatric emergency department. J Soc Pediatr Nurs 2000;5:87–95.

[50] Hon KL, Fu CC, Chor CM, et al. Issues associated with dog bite injuries in children and adolescents assessed at the emergency department. Pediatr Emerg Care 2007;23:445–9.

[51] Sacks JJ, Lockwood R, Hornreich J, et al. Fatal dog attacks, 1989–1994. Pediatrics 1996;97(6 Pt 1):891–5.

[52] From the Centers for Disease Control and Prevention. Dog-bite-related fatalities–United States, 1995–1996. JAMA 1997;278:278–9.

[53] Centers for Disease Control and Prevention. Dog-bite-related fatalities–United States, 1995–1996. MMWR Morb Mortal Wkly Rep 1997;46:463–7.

[54] Tsokos M, Byard RW, Puschel K. Extensive and mutilating craniofacial trauma involving de-fleshing and decapitation: unusual features of fatal dog attacks in the young. Am J Forensic Med Pathol 2007;28:131–6.

[55] Raghavan M. Fatal dog attacks in Canada, 1990–2007. Can Vet J 2008;49:577–81.

[56] Reducing the number of deaths and injuries from residential fires. Pediatrics 2000;105: 1355–7.

[57] Edwin AF, Cubison TC, Pape SA. The impact of recent legislation on paediatric fireworks injuries in the Newcastle upon Tyne region. Burns 2008;34:953–64.

[58] Witsaman RJ, Comstock RD, Smith GA. Pediatric fireworks-related injuries in the United States: 1990–2003. Pediatrics 2006;118:296–303.

[59] The prevention of unintentional injury among American Indian and Alaska Native children: a subject review. Committee on Native American Child Health and Committee on Injury and Poison Prevention. American Academy of Pediatrics [review]. Pediatrics 1999;104:1397–9.

[60] Haider AH, Efron DT, Haut ER, et al. Black children experience worse clinical and functional outcomes after traumatic brain injury: an analysis of the National Pediatric Trauma Registry. J Trauma 2007;62:1259–62.

[61] Saluja G, Brenner RA, Trumble AC, et al. Swimming pool drownings among US residents aged 5–24 years: understanding racial/ethnic disparities. Am J Public Health 2006;96: 728–33.

[62] Falcone RA Jr, Brown RL, Garcia VF. The epidemiology of infant injuries and alarming health disparities. J Pediatr Surg 2007;42:172–6.

[63] Bennett MD Jr, Hall J, Frazier L Jr, et al. Homicide of children aged 0–4 years, 2003–04: results from the National Violent Death Reporting System. Inj Prev 2006;12(Suppl 2): ii39–43.

[64] Wilson MH, Shock S. Preventing motor vehicle-occupant and pedestrian injuries in children and adolescents. Curr Opin Pediatr 1993;5:284–8.

[65] Durkin MS, Laraque D, Lubman I, et al. Epidemiology and prevention of traffic injuries to urban children and adolescents. Pediatrics 1999;103:e74.

[66] Selecting and using the most appropriate car safety seats for growing children: guidelines for counseling parents. American Academy of Pediatrics. Committee on Injury and Poison Prevention. Pediatrics 1996;97:761–3.

[67] Braver ER, Whitfield R, Ferguson SA. Seating positions and children's risk of dying in motor vehicle crashes. Inj Prev 1998;4:181–7.

[68] Segui-Gomez M, Glass R, Graham JD. Where children sit in motor vehicles: a comparison of selected European and American cities. Inj Prev 1998;4:98–102.

[69] Elliott MR, Kallan MJ, Durbin DR, et al. Effectiveness of child safety seats vs seat belts in reducing risk for death in children in passenger vehicle crashes [erratum appears in Arch Pediatr Adolesc Med 2006;160(9):952]. Arch Pediatr Adolesc Med 2006;160:617–21.

[70] de Sousa RM, Regis FC, Koizumi MS. [Traumatic brain injury: differences among pedestrians and motor vehicle occupants]. Revista de Saude Publica 1999;33:85–94 [in Portuguese].

[71] Yan X, Harb R, Radwan E. Analyses of factors of crash avoidance maneuvers using the general estimates system. Traffic Inj Prev 2008;9:173–80.

[72] Lam LT. Distractions and the risk of car crash injury: the effect of drivers' age. J Safety Res 2002;33:411–9.

[73] National Highway Traffic Safety Administration (NHTSA) Notes. Not enough children ages four through eight using booster seats. Ann Emerg Med 2005;45:157–9.

[74] McKay MP. National Highway Traffic Safety Administration (NHTSA) notes. Seat belt use in 2005: demographic results. Ann Emerg Med 2006;47:370–1.

[75] American Academy of Pediatrics Committee on Injury and Poison Prevention. Children in pickup trucks. American Academy of Pediatrics. Committee on Injury and Poison Prevention. Pediatrics 2000;106:857–9.

[76] Illingworth CM. 227 road accidents to children. Acta Paediatr Scand 1979;68:869–73.

[77] Spinks A, Turner C, McClure R, et al. Community-based programmes to promote use of bicycle helmets in children aged 0–14 years: a systematic review. Int J Inj Contr Saf Promot 2005;12:131–42.

[78] Leblanc JC, Beattie TL, Culligan C. Effect of legislation on the use of bicycle helmets. CMAJ 2002;166(5):592–5.

[79] Nykolyshyn K, Petruk JA, Wiebe N, et al. The use of bicycle helmets in a western Canadian province without legislation Revue Canadienne de Sante Publique. Can J Public Health 2003;94:144–8.

[80] Thompson DC, Rivara FP, Thompson R. Helmets for preventing head and facial injuries in bicyclists. Cochrane Database Syst Rev 2000;2:CD001855.

[81] O'Callaghan FV, Nausbaum S. Predicting bicycle helmet wearing intentions and behavior among adolescents. J Safety Res 2006;37:425–31.

[82] Weiss J, Okun M, Quay N. Predicting bicycle helmet stage-of-change among middle school, high school, and college cyclists from demographic, cognitive, and motivational variables. J Pediatr 2004;145:360–4.

[83] Spiegel CN, Lindaman FC. Children can't fly: a program to prevent childhood morbidity and mortality from window falls. Am J Public Health 1977;67:1143–7.

[84] Hon KL, Chan SY, Ng BK, et al. Spinal cord injury without radiographic abnormality (SCIWORA): a mere 50-cm fall that matters. Injury Extra 2006;37:364–70.

[85] Katcher ML, Landry GL, Shapiro MM. Liquid-crystal thermometer use in pediatric office counseling about tap water burn prevention. Pediatrics 1989;83:766–71.

[86] Erdmann TC, Feldman KW, Rivara FP, et al. Tap water burn prevention: the effect of legislation. Pediatrics 1991;88:572–7.

[87] Pichoff BE, Schydlower M, Stephenson SR. Children at risk for accidental burns from hot tap water. Tex Med 1994;90:54–8.

[88] Quan L. Drowning issues in resuscitation. Ann Emerg Med 1993;22(2 Pt 2):366–9.

[89] Brenner RA, Trumble AC, Smith BS, et al. Where children drown, United States, 1995. Pediatrics 2001;108:85–9.

[90] Brenner RA. Prevention of drowning in infants, children, and adolescents. Pediatrics 2003;112:440–5.

[91] American Academy of Pediatrics Committee on Injury, Violence, and Poison Prevention. Prevention of drowning in infants, children, and adolescents. Pediatrics 2003;112:437–9.

[92] Hon KL, Leung TF, Chan SY, et al. Indoor versus outdoor childhood submersion injury in a densely populated city. Acta Paediatr 2008;97:1261–4.

[93] American Academy of Pediatrics Committee on Injury, Violence, and Poison Prevention. Poison treatment in the home. American Academy of Pediatrics Committee on Injury, Violence, and Poison Prevention. Pediatrics 2003;112:1182–5.

[94] Hon KL, Ho JK, Leung TF, et al. Review of children hospitalised for ingestion and poisoning at a tertiary centre. Ann Acad Med Singap 2005;34:356–61.

[95] Litovitz T, Manoguerra A. Comparison of pediatric poisoning hazards: an analysis of 3.8 million exposure incidents. A report from the American Association of Poison Control Centers. Pediatrics 1992;89(6 Pt 1):999–1006.

[96] Litovitz TL, Klein-Schwartz W, Dyer KS, et al. 1997 annual report of the American Association of Poison Control Centers Toxic Exposure Surveillance System. Am J Emerg Med 1998;16:443–97.

[97] Litovitz TL, Klein-Schwartz W, Caravati EM, et al. 1998 Annual report of the American Association of Poison Control Centers Toxic Exposure Surveillance System. Am J Emerg Med 1999;17:435–87.

[98] Litovitz TL, Klein-Schwartz W, White SM, et al. 1999 Annual Report of the American Association of Poison Control Centers Toxic Exposure Surveillance System [special toxicology issue]. Am J Emerg Med 2000;18:517–74.

[99] Litovitz TL, Klein-Schwartz W, White SM, et al. 2000 Annual Report of the American Association of Poison Control Centers Toxic Exposure Surveillance System. Am J Emerg Med 2001;19:337–95.

[100] Litovitz TL, Klein-Schwartz W, Rodgers GC, et al. 2001 annual report of the American Association of Poison Control Centers Toxic Exposure Surveillance System. Am J Emerg Med 2002;20:391–452.

[101] Hon KL, Ho JK, Hung EC, et al. Poisoning necessitating pediatric ICU admissions: size of pupils does matter. J Natl Med Assoc 2008;100:952–6.

[102] Hon KL, Yeung WL, Ho CH, et al. Neurologic and radiologic manifestations of three girls surviving acute carbon monoxide poisoning. J Child Neurol 2006;21:737–41.

[103] Leung AK, Davies HD, Hon KL. Rabies: epidemiology, pathogenesis, and prophylaxis. Adv Ther 2007;24:1340–7.

[104] Jameson P, Greene C, Regnery R, et al. Prevalence of Bartonella henselae antibodies in pet cats throughout regions of North America. J Infect Dis 1995;172:1145–9.

[105] Jackson LA, Perkins BA, Wenger JD. Cat scratch disease in the United States: an analysis of three national databases. Am J Public Health 1993;83:1707–11.

[106] Carithers HA. Cat-scratch disease. An overview based on a study of 1,200 patients. Am J Dis Child 1985;139:1124–33.

[107] August JR. Cat scratch disease. J Am Vet Med Assoc 1988;193:312–5.

[108] Baker MD, Moore SE. Human bites in children. A six-year experience. Am J Dis Child 1987;141:1285–90.

[109] Leung AK, Robson WL. Human bites in children. Pediatr Emerg Care 1992;8:255–7.

[110] Schweich P, Fleisher G. Human bites in children. Pediatr Emerg Care 1985;1:51–3.

[111] Gibly RM. Continuous intravenous midazolam infusion for Centruroides exilicauda scorpion envenomation. Ann Emerg Med 1999;34:620–5.

[112] LoVecchio FD. Incidence of immediate and delayed hypersensitivity to Centruroides antivenom. Ann Emerg Med 1999;34:615–9.

[113] Bond GR. Snake, spider, and scorpion envenomation in North America. Pediatr Rev 1999;20:147–50.

[114] Hon KL. Snakebites in children in the densely populated city of Hong Kong: a 10-year survey. Acta Paediatr 2004;93:270–2.

[115] Hon KL, Chow CM, Cheung KL, et al. Snakebite in a child: could we avoid the anaphylaxis or the fasciotomies? Ann Acad Med Singap 2005;34:454–6.

[116] Hanigan WC, Aldag J, Sabo RA, et al. Strangulation injuries in children. Part 2. Cerebrovascular hemodynamics. J Trauma 1996;40:73–7.

[117] Sabo RA, Hanigan WC, Flessner K, et al. Strangulation injuries in children. Part 1. Clinical analysis. J Trauma 1996;40:68–72.

[118] Sep D, Thies KC. Strangulation injuries in children. Resuscitation 2007;74:386–91.

[119] Bass JL, Christoffel KK, Widome M, et al. Childhood injury prevention counseling in primary care settings: a critical review of the literature. Pediatrics 1993;92:544–50.

[120] Towner E, Dowswell T, Jarvis S. Updating the evidence. A systemic review of what works in preventing childhood unintentional injuries: part 2. Inj Prev 2001;7:249–53.

[121] Towner E, Dowswell T, Jarvis S. Updating the evidence. A systematic review of what works in preventing childhood unintentional injuries: part 1. Inj Prev 2001;7:161–4.

[122] Johnston BD, Rivara FP. Injury control: new challenges. Pediatr Rev 2003;24:111–8.

[123] Blackhall K, Ker K. Searching for studies for inclusion in Cochrane Systematic Reviews on injury prevention. Inj Prev 2008;14:137–8.

[124] Betz M, Li G. Injury prevention and control. Emerg Med Clin North Am 2000;25:901–14.

[125] Widome MD. Vehicle occupant safety: the pediatrician's responsibility. Pediatrics 1979;64:966–8.

[126] Widome MD. Pediatric injury prevention for the practitioner. Curr Probl Pediatr 1991;21:428–68.

[127] Dowswell T, Towner EM, Simpson G, et al. Preventing childhood unintentional injuries–what works? A literature review. Inj Prev 1996;2:140–9.
[128] Haddon W Jr. A logical framework for categorizing highway safety phenomena and activity. J Trauma 1972;12:193–207.
[129] Nilsen P, Bourne M, Verplanken B. Accounting for the role of habit in behavioural strategies for injury prevention. Int J Inj Contr Saf Promot 2008;15:33–40.
[130] Office-based counseling for injury prevention. American Academy of Pediatrics Committee on Injury and Poison Prevention. Pediatrics 1994;94(4 Pt 1):566–7.
[131] Rivara FP, Barber M. Demographic analysis of childhood pedestrian injuries. Pediatrics 1985;76:375–81.
[132] Centers for Disease Control and Prevention. Update: fatal air bag-related injuries to children–United States, 1993–1996 [erratum appears in MMWR Morb Mortal Wkly Rep 1997;46(2):40]. MMWR Morb Mortal Wkly Rep 1996;45:1073–6.
[133] Martinez R. Air bag-related injuries. Ann Emerg Med 2003;42:285–6.
[134] Sherwood CP, Abdelilah Y, Crandall JR, et al. The performance of various rear facing child restraint systems in a frontal crash. Annu Proc Assoc Adv Automot Med 2004;48:303–21.
[135] Decina LE, Lococo KH. Observed LATCH use and misuse characteristics of child restraint systems in seven states. J Safety Res 2007;38:273–81.
[136] Curnow WJ. The Cochrane collaboration and bicycle helmets. Accid Anal Prev 2005;37:569–73.
[137] Curnow WJ. Bicycle helmets and public health in Australia. Health Promot J Austr 2008;19:10–5.
[138] Stone KE, Eastman EM, Gielen AC, et al. Home safety in inner cities: prevalence and feasibility of home safety-product use in inner-city housing. Pediatrics 2007;120:e346–53.
[139] Leung AK. Sunburn from the treatment of neonatal jaundice. Burns Incl Therm Inj 1986;12:291–2.
[140] Olson AL, Dietrich AJ, Sox CH, et al. Solar protection of children at the beach. Pediatrics 1997;99:E1.
[141] Scherz RG. Prevention of childhood poisoning. A community project. Pediatr Clin North Am 1970;17:713–27.
[142] Sibert JR, Craft AW, Jackson RH. Child-resistant packaging and accidental child poisoning. Lancet 1977;2(8032):289–90.
[143] Sibert JR, Clarke AJ, Mitchell MP. Improvements in child resistant containers. Arch Dis Child 1985;60:1155–7.
[144] Hon KL, Leung TF, Hung CW, et al. Food associated adverse events necessitating pediatric ICU admissions. Indian J Pediatr 2009;76:283–6.
[145] Krenzelok EP, McGuigan M, Lheur P. Position statement: ipecac syrup. American Academy of Clinical Toxicology; European Association of Poisons Centres and Clinical Toxicologists. J Toxicol Clin Toxicol 1997;35:699–709.
[146] Shannon M. The demise of ipecac. Pediatrics 2003;112:1180–1.
[147] Ibsen LM, Koch TM. Submersion and asphyxial injury Critical care considerations in pediatric trauma. Crit Care Med 2002;30:S402–8.
[148] Papa L, Hoelle R, Idris A. Systematic review of definitions for drowning incidents. Resuscitation 2005;65:255–64.
[149] Thompson DC, Rivara FP. Pool fencing for preventing drowning in children. Cochrane Database Syst Rev 2000;2:CD001047.
[150] Part 8: advanced challenges in resuscitation: section 3: special challenges in ECC: submersion or near-drowning. Circulation 2000;102:I233–6.
[151] Gladish K, Washington RL, Bull MJ. Swimming programs for infants and toddlers. Pediatrics 2002;109:168–9.
[152] Horwood LJ, Fergusson DM, Shannon FT. The safety standards of domestic swimming pools. N Z Med J 1981;94:417–9.

[153] Fergusson DM, Horwood LJ, Shannon FT. The safety standards of domestic swimming pools 1980–1982. N Z Med J 1983;96:93–5.

[154] Leung AK, Robson WL. Penile dog bite in an adolescent. Adv Ther 2005;22:363–7.

[155] Woods AJ. The role of health professionals in childhood injury prevention: a systematic review of the literature. Patient Educ Couns 2006;64(1–3):35–42.

[156] Stock JG, Cornell FM. Prevention of sports-related eye injury. Am Fam Physician 1991;44: 515–20.

[157] Napier SM, Baker RS, Sanford DG, et al. Eye injuries in athletics and recreation. Surv Ophthalmol 1996;41:229–44.

[158] Keller CS, Noyes FR, Buncher CR. The medical aspects of soccer injury epidemiology. Am J Sports Med 1987;15:230–7.

[159] Raschka VC, Roth J, Sitte T, et al. [Fatal soccer injury as an unfortunate sequela of collision]. Sportverletz Sportschaden 1995;9:24–6 [in German].

[160] Blond L, Hansen LB. Injuries caused by falling soccer goalposts in Denmark. Br J Sports Med 1999;33:110–2.

[161] Centers for Disease Control and Prevention. Injuries associated with soccer goalposts–United States, 1979–1993. MMWR Morb Mortal Wkly Rep 1994;43:153–5.

[162] Roi GS, Bianchedi D. The science of fencing: implications for performance and injury prevention. Sports Med 2008;38:465–81.

[163] Leung AK, Robson WL, Lim SH, et al. Playground safety. J R Soc Health 1993;113:320–3.

[164] Cradock AL, Kawachi I, Colditz GA, et al. Playground safety and access in Boston neighborhoods. Am J Prev Med 2005;28:357–63.

[165] Mitchell R, Sherker S, Cavanagh M, et al. Falls from playground equipment: will the new Australian playground safety standard make a difference and how will we tell? Health Promot J Austr 2007;18:98–104.

[166] Hudson SD, Olsen HM, Thompson D. An investigation of school playground safety practices as reported by school nurses. J Sch Nurs 2008;24:138–44.

[167] Roberts I, Kramer MS, Suissa S. Does home visiting prevent childhood injury? A systematic review of randomised controlled trials. BMJ 1996;312:29–33.

Advances in Pediatrics 57 (2010) 63–83

ELSEVIER
MOSBY

ADVANCES IN PEDIATRICS

Controversies in the Evaluation of Young Children with Fractures

Melissa K. Egge, MD[a],*, Carol D. Berkowitz, MD[b,c]

[a]Department of Pediatrics, Harbor-UCLA Medical Center, 1000 West Carson Street, Box 437, Torrance, CA 90509, USA
[b]Department of Pediatrics, Harbor-UCLA Medical Center, Torrance, CA, USA
[c]David Geffen School of Medicine at UCLA, Los Angeles, CA, USA

The differential diagnosis for a young child with 1 or more fractures is extensive and should be given careful consideration. Because inflicted trauma is a frequent cause, the question is best rephrased as "What is a reasonable differential diagnosis for the young child with fracture(s) and the cost-effective approach to the evaluation of such a child?" This article focuses on diagnoses introduced into the forensic assessment of the young child with multiple fractures. Is it appropriate to order tests simply to address possible differential diagnoses introduced by the defense? Are physicians who do not test making conclusions about child abuse prematurely? How does the analysis of injury biomechanics and fracture type help us? Does a delay in obtaining medical care affect the assessment of child abuse or neglect?

Defense attorneys may want to create reasonable doubt during a criminal prosecution when child abuse is being alleged and would prefer that testing not be done, so that the possibility of a medical explanation for the findings lingers. Prosecuting attorneys would prefer to eliminate that possibility of doubt, by having definitive tests that have excluded various medical/pathologic causes for the child's fracture(s). Physicians must be judicial in ordering tests and order them when it is medically reasonable to do so, rather than when they are legally indicated. Which medical conditions may predispose a child to fracture or be mistaken for trauma on imaging studies? At what point and at what cost is testing for these conditions appropriate?

Suspected child abuse and neglect require evaluation by a multidisciplinary team. It is the medical provider's job to report suspected child abuse while further diagnoses are being considered. There is immunity from civil and criminal liability on the presumption that the reporting party is acting in good faith. However, the inverse is not true; if the responsible party suspects child abuse and does not immediately report it, he or she is civilly and criminally liable for failure to report, which is punishable with a fine and/or imprisonment. Unless

*Corresponding author. E-mail address: melissa.egge@gmail.com

0065-3101/10/$ – see front matter
doi:10.1016/j.yapd.2010.08.002

suspected child abuse is reported, the physician may be unaware that there have been previous allegations. Also, if the report to child protective services (CPS) has not also been cross-reported to law enforcement, the team may be unaware of the criminal history of the caregivers.

CASE 1

A 3 month old is brought in by ambulance, called by the mother who perceived that the infant had left knee pain and swelling. The mother relates a vague history of trauma, after hearing the results of the leg radiograph. The parents are separated and each has a history of prior arrests. The infant's examination is remarkable only for crying and perceived pain with movement of the left leg and when the child is lifted or carried. A skeletal survey (SS) reveals an acute proximal tibia fracture and a corner metaphyseal lesion of the distal femur. The radiographs do not reveal any evidence of osteopenia or structural abnormalities of the bones. Laboratory testing shows normal electrolytes, calcium, phosphorus, and alkaline phosphatase levels. A radionucleotide bone scan additionally reveals findings suspicious for 3 right-sided rib fractures, 2 of which are anterolateral and 1 is posterior-medial (Fig. 1). A follow-up chest radiograph 10 days later confirms the 3 rib fractures (Fig. 2). The investigating detective asks whether we have ruled out the possibility of the infant having brittle bone disease. The detective reports that the criminal prosecutor wants to know.

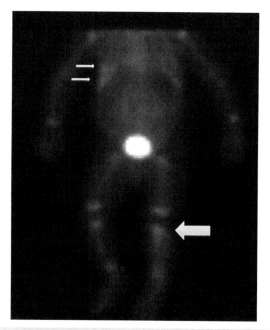

Fig. 1. Bone radionucleotide study shows increased uptake in the right ribs (*thin arrows*) and proximal left tibia (*thick arrow*).

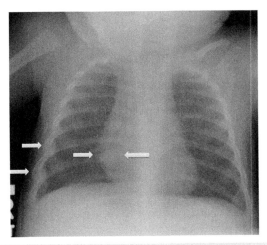

Fig. 2. Chest radiograph performed 10 days after admission reveals callus formation over 3 rib fractures (*arrows*). Initial chest radiograph was considered to be negative.

CASE 2

A 3 year old is referred to the clinic for suspicion of child abuse after sustaining a proximal ulna fracture at age 2 years (Fig. 3). The case was brought to the attention of CPS when a neighbor called the hotline after observing the child crying while guarding his arm all day. The child is brought in by a new foster parent who has no history on the child or his family. The child also has a history of a tibia/fibula fracture sustained at age 18 months, at which time an obese 12-year-old cousin fell on him (Fig. 4). The child is speech delayed and can offer no explanation for either injury. There have been 5 previous reports for child neglect, emotional abuse, caretaker absence, and physical abuse (3 unfounded and 2 substantiated). The mother is known to abuse crystal methamphetamine, and his youngest sibling was methamphetamine exposed at birth and died at 1 month in an overlay incident.

CASE 3

A baby who was a 25-week preemie was brought to the emergency department at age 8 months by her mother who reported decreased use of her right leg. During the evaluation, a frontal skull fracture was discovered in addition to healing fractures of the distal right tibia and proximal left radius. There were no explanations for any of the fractures. The infant had spent 4 months in the neonatal intensive care unit (NICU) where she was diagnosed with rickets based on increased alkaline phosphatase (1104 IU/L), craniotabes, rachitic rosary, and pathologic radius and rib fractures. Radiographs revealed diffuse osteopenia; periosteal changes; and cupped, frayed metaphyses.

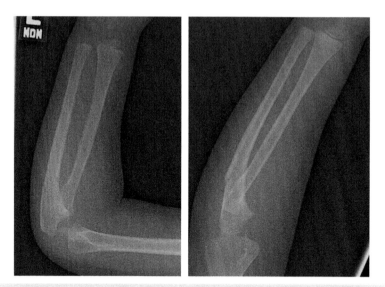

Fig. 3. Transverse fracture of ulna at 2 years old (case 2) after a minor trauma.

FRACTURES AND ABUSE

National Child Abuse and Neglect Data System data revealed that, in the United States in 2007, an estimated 794,000 children (1% of minors) were reported to CPS and substantiated as victims of maltreatment. More than one-half (59.0%) of victims suffered neglect, 13.1% of victims suffered from more than 1 type of maltreatment, and 10.8% suffered physical abuse [1]. There were many more victims who were not recognized or not reported.

Fractures are one of the leading presentations of child physical abuse, second to soft tissue injuries. Of children less than 12 months of age hospitalized with fractures, approximately 25% were attributed to abuse. Of children less than 36 months with fractures, the overall proportion leading to hospitalization because of abuse was 12% [2]. However, there are children initially believed to have been abused who have fractures that are common from accidents [3]. Kirschner and Stein [4], a forensic pathologist, described 10 cases reported as child abuse by inexperienced physicians that led to false allegations and failure to recognize serious medical conditions. Small but significant numbers of children who are deemed nonabuse have factors predisposing to bone fragility after assessment [5]. Wardinsky and colleagues [6], as part of a child abuse team, analyzed 504 consults and found 7% to have medical conditions, such as osteogenesis imperfecta (OI) or Ehlers-Danlos syndrome initially not considered . Dr Carole Jenny [7], in a clinical report on behalf of the American Academy of Pediatrics, discussed the differential diagnosis and medical evaluation of young children with fractures. She comments that parents of children later diagnosed with medical conditions leading to bone disease were at times mistakenly accused of child abuse [7].

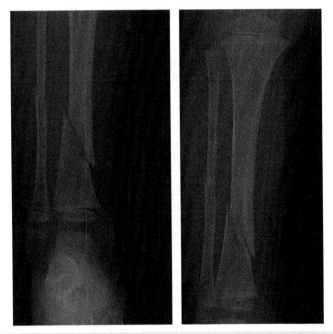

Fig. 4. Oblique fractures of the distal tibia and fibula at age 18 months (case 2) after a minor trauma.

SUSPICION AND REPORTING

Primary care pediatricians underreport and underdiagnose child abuse, especially compared with doctors with access to consultation with child abuse specialists [8–11]. Child abuse specialists in Toronto found that 20.5% of inflicted fracture cases were initially unrecognized as abuse related. The cases more likely to be missed were boys with extremity fractures who presented in the emergency department or to their pediatrician [12]. For many pediatricians, it is unfathomable that a parent could harm a child to such a degree. Some pediatricians deny that abuse is a possibility despite overwhelming signs that a child has been seriously injured, because they are so devoted to the families [13]. It is challenging for a general pediatrician who has an ongoing relationship with a family to suspect or accuse an outwardly loving caregiver of abusing a child. The opinion may be deferred to an unbiased expert in the field who does not have personal loyalties to the family.

WORK-UP AND EVALUATION

How can a price be placed on laboratory testing when the caregiver's and child's lives may be affected in such a drastic way? Who should pay for testing? Consequences may involve criminal, personal, and emotional costs that are priceless to the accused. Children are placed in protective custody, criminal charges are pressed, and major financial strains are imposed on the family.

CONSIDERING THE HISTORY OF TRAUMA WITH THE BIOMECHANICS

Recent studies of engineering principles have changed the way fractures are analyzed. When considering the history, the clinician must carefully consider the external forces imposed on the bone with characteristics of the fracture (type, location, number, and age) [14]. To consider the mechanism, a detailed history must be obtained, to translate which loading forces were involved to see whether the history and anticipated forces correlate (Table 1). Factors to consider are the movement of the child at the time of injury, the height of the fall, and the surface onto which the child fell. On occasion, a perpetrator may partially disclose the mechanism of injury. The fewer the details, or the more inconsistencies, the higher the suspicion of inflicted injury or neglect.

There are pure external forces, simply push (compression), pull (tension), and shear. However, most real-life injuries involve a combination of forces. All forces can be seen in accidental or inflicted trauma. A spiral fracture may occur by a twisting mechanism. An accidental spiral femur fracture is seen in toddlers who plant 1 foot as they are running and fall as they change their direction of motion. A torus fracture is a mild fracture caused during a sudden axial compression as with a fall on an outstretched arm from playground equipment. A transverse fracture may occur as a result of a direct blow perpendicular to the bone. One example is a 2-year-old child who was playing in the backyard in the middle of a construction site. The child pulled a large 10 cm × 10 cm panel of wood down causing a transverse fracture of the femur. In the same month, a 2 year old was punched in the leg by his father for running in the house. A nearly identical femur fracture resulted.

In case 1, the infant presented with acute rib fractures. The explanation the mother gave for the rib fractures was an incident 3 weeks earlier when the father allegedly closed a door on the mother while she was holding the infant against her chest. The infant being squeezed between the door and the mother's chest produced anterior-posterior compression and bending forces against the infant's rib cage. However, although the biomechanics may seem plausible, the timing does not.

Table 1 Fracture types and causative loading forces	
Loading force	Fracture type
Torsional	Spiral
Compressive/axial	Buckle/torus
Bending	Transverse
Compressive+bending	Oblique
Shear/tensile	Classic metaphyseal lesion

Data from Carlson KP. Child abuse or parent abuse? Pediatrics 2004;113:181–2; and Pierce MC, Bertocci GE, Vogeley E, et al. Evaluating long bone fractures in children: a biomechanical approach with illustrative cases. Child Abuse Negl 2004;28:505–24.

Intrinsic bone factors are equally important. Certain locations within the bone carry higher specificity for abuse because of the bone's intrinsic properties (ie, metaphysis vs diaphysis). The metaphysis has a cortex that is thinner and more porous, overlying trabecular bone that is spongy, making it weak compared with the diaphyseal portion of bone. The diaphysis has a much stronger cortex, with dense underlying bone. The transition zone between diaphysis and metaphysis is an inherently weak region, making it also susceptible to fracture [2,14].

DATING FRACTURES

Occasionally, dating the fracture assists with determining the plausibility of the history provided. Child abuse experts are frequently asked to narrow the timing of the injury to evaluate allegations of physical abuse or neglect. Prosser and colleagues [15] reviewed the literature in an attempt to create uniformity in a timetable of radiologic findings in children's fractures. However, because of the number of studies that included infants and young children, in conjunction with the lack of a uniform language, dating of fractures in children remains a difficult task. Those with a prosecutorial focus often need a much narrower time window than can be offered. Time frames for dating fractures are usually on the order of weeks, not days. For example, soft callus formation is seen between 10 to 21 days after injury, and hard callus may exist as early as 14 days and may persist until 90 days after injury. The studies that have documented radiographic healing processes have dealt with immobilized bones and may not be applicable [16] to fractures caused by abuse that are often left unattended for long periods of time [17]. Repeated injury to an existing abusive fracture extends the time frames and alters the appearance of some radiographic findings. If the abused child expires, histologic examination of the fracture may elucidate the timing of the injury or show a chronic fracture or one that has been repeatedly injured [18].

CORRELATION OF ABUSE BY FRACTURE LOCATION

Some bones carry a higher specificity for abuse (eg, ribs, scapula, sternum, acromion), but no fracture is pathognomonic. A meta-analysis reviewed 32 studies that sought to determine whether some bones are more often associated with abuse than with other mechanisms of accidental injury. Kemp used strict criteria for confirmed abuse that required perpetrator admission, witnessed event, or abuse confirmed through court proceedings or by a multidisciplinary team. Abused children commonly had more than 1 broken bone. Rib fractures (71%) carried the highest probability for abuse. Probability of abuse was lower in femur fractures and skull fractures (28% and 30% respectively), although the probabilities increase in nonambulatory children. The probability of confirmed abuse was higher in the humerus (48%), especially for midshaft fractures [19].

Preambulatory children rarely sustain extremity fractures. Long bone fractures are strongly associated with abuse in infants less than 12 months of age

[20]. However, children who are capable of rolling and crawling do sustain fractures of the skull with a short fall. A simple, linear parietal skull fracture is a familiar sequela after a fall from a bed or couch onto a hardwood or tile floor. Skull fractures can be difficult to judge. In cases of both inflicted and accidental trauma, the parietal bone is the most frequently fractured part of the skull. Characteristics of abusive fractures include those that are multiple, bilateral, and that cross suture lines [21].

Studies have shown the high specificity of rib fractures for abuse in a young child. One study found that the positive predictive value of rib fractures being inflicted in children less than 3 years old was 95%. Another group retrospectively studied 39 infants with rib fractures: 32 were caused by abuse, 3 were caused by major accidental trauma, 1 was the result of birth trauma, and 3 were attributed to bone fragility. The causes of bone fragility were OI and rickets (1 nutritional and 1 ex-preemie) [22]. Although rib fractures may strengthen an argument for abuse, alternative causes must be contemplated. Rib fractures are not obvious on plain chest films, even on follow-up after the standard 2 weeks. In a postmortem study of 11 infants with 84 rib fractures, only 30 healing fractures were discernible on the SS. Twenty-three rib fractures were acute and incognito; a reminder that a repeat SS at 2 weeks follow-up may increase the yield in identifying occult injuries [23].

DISORDERS OF COLLAGEN FORMATION
OI

OI is a well-recognized inherited clinical entity characterized by bone fragility and predisposition to fractures [24]. The milder forms of OI, types I and IV, may be considered in the differential diagnosis of children with multiple fractures or fractures after seemingly minor trauma. Both OI and abuse may present with multiple fractures in various stages of healing and children with OI may also be abused. Some of the physical findings of OI are not apparent in the young infant, so genetic testing should be performed when it cannot be ruled out [25]. The incidence of OI has been estimated as 1:10,000 to 1:20,000 live births. In children less than 3 years old, abuse is 24 times more likely to be the cause of a fracture than OI [16]. A careful history of the injury should be sought. Ideally, a family member will have witnessed an apparently minor trauma and would be able to explain the details of the timing, location, and other circumstances. The family history may reveal other family members who have sustained fractures after minor trauma, are short or deaf, and who have blue sclera. However, the genetic mutation in collagen is more often de novo and the family history is negative. Physical examination may reveal classic signs of OI in infancy (Table 2). However, many of the examination findings in mild forms of OI are not evident in infancy. The hearing impairment, short stature, bone deformities, and dentinogenesis imperfecta associated with OI may not be evident until well after infancy but should be inquired about in the family. Alternatively, blue sclerae are a common finding in many infants because their sclerae are thinner and reveal the underlying uveal

Table 2
Characteristics of OI in infancy, in which child abuse may be in the differential diagnosis

OI type	Possible clinical features in infants	Incidence
I	Blue sclera	4:100,000
	Wide fontanelle+delayed closure	
	Wormian bones	
	Normal or near-normal stature	
	Thin, easily bruised skin	
	Fractures are rare in neonatal period	
	Normal teeth	
	Mild osteopenia with femoral bowing	
II	Lethal in utero	1:100,000
III	Born with multiple fractures	1:100,000
	Diagnosed on prenatal ultrasound	
IV	White sclera	4:100,000
	Short stature	
	Triangular facies	
	Fractures are seen in neonatal period	
	DI	
V	Fractures in the first year of life	7 reported cases
	White sclera; normal teeth	
VI	First fractures documented after age 4 months	8 reported cases
	No wormian bones or DI	
	White sclera or faintly blue	
VII	Multiple fractures at birth; rhizomelia	8 reported cases
VIII	Multiple fractures at birth	5 reported cases

OMIM #166200, #166210, #166220, #259420, #610682, #610915, #610967, #610968.
Abbreviation: DI, dentinogenesis imperfecta.

tissue. Review of radiographs may raise suspicion of OI if osteopenia is appreciated in the long bones or more than 10 wormian bones on the skull radiograph are noted [26]. With normal bone density, OI is excluded, but bone density can be difficult to ascertain. In the absence of abuse, classic metaphyseal lesions and symmetric rib fractures are rarely seen with OI [27]. In the absence of clinical or radiologic signs of OI or family history in an infant, it has been estimated to have a likelihood of 1 in a million of being the cause of a fracture.

Ninety percent of OI cases are the result of a mutation in 1 of 2 genes: COL1A1 or COL1A2. These genes are the blueprints for the production of type IA1 and IA2 procollagens. A trimer of the 2 types of procollagen forms collagen, the basic structural protein of bone. If there is an error (mutation) in the blueprint or processing of collagen, the structure of bone is not sound. There may be mutations that result in shortened or disfigured proteins; either may lead to bone fragility. The disfigured proteins cause more instability to bone than do the shortened proteins [28,29].

There are 2 types of laboratory tests that are used to diagnose OI: fibroblast tissue culture ($1350) or serum DNA sequencing ($2300), and each identifies about 90% of patients with OI [30,31]. The fibroblast culture may have a greater usefulness in mild cases with low suspicion; however, it requires a skin biopsy. If there are enough clinical signs, including a family history, a geneticist may make the diagnosis clinically or order the serum DNA sequencing. Both tests give results in approximately 6 to 8 weeks. In practice, DNA sequencing is the test of choice because it is technically much easier to obtain and is less traumatic to the child than a skin biopsy.

Testing is often requested by non–medically trained professionals. Testing may result in few positives, but even a single positive result is significant for the family affected. In a study by Steiner and colleagues [32], 6/48 children had abnormal collagen synthesized by dermal fibroblasts. In 88% of the cases, testing was requested by child protection service workers, attorneys, or courts.

One might expect a greater probability of a positive OI test in children referred for DNA analysis through a geneticist. Byers and colleagues [25] reviewed 262 children who underwent genetic testing during investigations for abuse. Of those, only 11 (4.2%) tested positive for OI. Three of the 11 children had no indication of OI apart from their fractures. The study found that, despite the children being referred by doctors with training in clinical genetics, the predicted incidence of OI was no higher than expected if there had been no clinical screening. One reason for the low percentage of positive OI tests is that a significant number of children were referred by CPS or by the court, and the geneticist's role was to facilitate testing. In addition, OI is a difficult diagnosis to exclude clinically in infancy. The study did validate the exclusion of children with other findings of abuse (eg, burns, bruises, bites) from genetic testing.

Ten percent of OI cases are not detected by current genetic testing. A geneticist, after reviewing a case, can render a clinical diagnosis if there is enough supporting evidence.

Not considering the diagnosis of OI can have devastating emotional effects on families. There are reports from patients initially diagnosed with nonaccidental trauma who were subsequently diagnosed with OI [4,33]. Kocher, an orthopedic surgeon, reported on his ongoing review of misdiagnosed child abuse at the annual meeting of the American Academy of Orthopaedic Surgeons in 2007 [34]. Kocher and colleagues gathered retrospective data from self-reported questionnaires of families of children formally diagnosed with OI [34]. The 33 families (who were affiliated with Protect our Families, an organization that represents parents who have been accused of child abuse) answered a questionnaire about their children's presenting symptoms. The children presented with clinical symptoms of fractures at ages 1 to 23 months (average 7.1 months). There was no known accident in 14 of the 33 children. Multiple fractures (average 7) were found in 28/33 children, often in multiple stages of healing. Twenty-three of the children were removed from their families during the investigation of the fractures. Nearly one-third of the families sued the doctors, hospitals, or CPS. It was not stated whether their lawsuits were successful [34]. Although the removal of the child from the home can be difficult, it is the goal of CPS to prevent another serious injury or the death of the child.

There are descriptions of new types of OI, named types V, VI, VII and VIII, which are subtypes of IV based on the Sillence classification system. These newly described types of OI are rare and have unique clinical, histologic, and radiographic features (see Table 2) [35]. Types V to VIII exhibit severe bone deformities. Patients with type VI all had vertebral compression fractures [36]. Type VII is an autosomal recessive form of OI localized to an isolated group of 8 affected family members in Quebec [37]. There are 5 reported cases of type VIII, another form of OI that is autosomal recessive, who exhibit severely affected bones [38]. It is believed that types V, VI, and VII may comprise approximately 8% of patients with OI [24].

Copper Deficiency

Acquired

Acquired copper deficiency has been proposed as predisposing an infant to multiple fractures; however, documented cases are rare. Standard formulas now have adequate copper and there are no reports of a breastfed infant who has suffered from nutritional copper deficiency. Ex-premies are at increased risk, manifesting symptoms at ages 6 to 12 months with a history of prolonged parenteral nutrition. Neutropenia ($<1.5 \times 10^9/L$) is the first and most common sign of copper deficiency, but a sideroblastic anemia resistant to iron treatment is also prevalent [39]. Less often (11/51 in 1 study), infants with acquired copper deficiency present with fractures [40]. There have only been a few reported cases in full-term babies. Radiographs show changes similar to rickets, with symmetric cupping and fraying of the metaphyses and osteopenia [41]. Low serum copper (<0.45 mg/L) and ceruloplasmin concentrations (<200 mg/L) may not always be evident, but of the 2 values, ceruloplasmin is the first to be reduced [39,42].

Infants who present before the age of 1 year were being fed a nonstandard formula or had a history of prolonged parenteral nutrition. The ex-premature infants present earlier with a copper concentration less than 0.33 mg/L. The full-term infant presents later at approximately 8 months old. Common presenting signs, in addition to the abnormal laboratory values mentioned earlier, are psychomotor retardation hypotonia, pallor, hypopigmented skin and hair, and prominent scalp veins [41].

Menkes disease

Menkes disease (MD) is an X-linked recessive disorder of copper metabolism that is usually lethal by 3 years of age, although there are milder forms. The classic form of MD, with an incidence of 1:300,000, should not be confused with abuse because the fractures are the result of diffuse osteoporosis and there are concomitant clinical features [43]. The radiologic findings overlap with copper deficiency. Seizures develop by 3 months of age and, at about the same time, the diagnostic steel-wool hair is noticed. The mildest form is occipital horn syndrome (OHS), named for characteristic bony protuberances from the occipital bone that appear after age 1 year. Patients with OHS have chronic diarrhea and urinary tract infections [44].

DISORDERS OF MINERALIZATION
Rickets and Vitamin D Deficiency

The clinical and radiographic signs of classic rickets are apparent to an experienced clinician and pediatric radiologist actively considering it in the differential diagnosis. Radiographic findings of rickets should be symmetric and are first evident with cupping and fraying of the costochondral junctions and long bone metaphyses. Subperiosteal new bone forms in both rickets and from trauma. Other findings used to help differentiate the 2 entities are generalized osteopenia and insufficiency fractures, found in rickets but not in child abuse [45]. Dr Paul Kleinman [46] recently acknowledged that a small metaphyseal bony fragment in rickets can look like a classic metaphyseal lesion caused by abuse. The diagnosis may be unclear if the infant has been partially treated with vitamin D. Clinical and laboratory evaluation should clarify this rare scenario. Strouse [47] implores us to create prospective studies to further investigate the question of congenital rickets: "There is no concrete evidence in the literature that vitamin D deficiency in infants younger than 6 months of age renders them susceptible to the same types of fractures as have been accepted to bear high specificity for child abuse" [47].

As was pointed out in a recent commentary, the medical definition of rickets involves radiologic findings. Therefore, deficiency of vitamin D without radiographic signs of rickets is not rickets. There are 3 radiologic findings in rickets: osteopenia, physeal and metaphyseal changes, and osteomalacia [48]. However, in a recent study of healthy infants and toddlers, 7.5% of children who were deficient in vitamin D (25-hydroxyvitamin D [25OHD] <20 ng/mL) had rachitic changes on radiographs, and 32.5% showed demineralization [49].

As with OI, there are anecdotal and case reports of infants supposedly misdiagnosed with abuse-related fractures when vitamin D deficiency rickets was apparent [50–52]. Most of these reports by individuals who frequently testify provide selectively sparse and inaccurate details of history, tests, and images [53]. However, many of the children in these cases had unexplained bruising, a finding not commonly attributable to vitamin D deficiency. In 1 case, a 6-week-old infant presented with a seizure and widened sutures without mention of evaluation for intracranial hemorrhage or retinal hemorrhages [54]. The clinical record should be evaluated in its entirety with an attempt to explain all findings, some of which may be highly associated with inflicted trauma. Carole Jenny [55], in an extensive report on her experience, found no children (out of several thousand) who were thoroughly evaluated for maltreatment to have rickets or vitamin D deficiency when they presented exclusively with fractures [55].

Vitamin D deficiency and associated rickets is a significant issue in infants who are solely breastfed, especially by mothers with inadequate ultraviolet B radiation and diet. The American Academy of Pediatrics recommends vitamin D supplementation of 400 IU for all infants and children, beginning soon after birth [56]. Testing for rickets must be considered if dietary history, clinical examination, or radiographs raise suspicion. The serum phosphorus level is usually less than 4 mg/dL, but the alkaline phosphatase level is often increased for age in both rickets and fractures. A serum 25OHD less than 20 ng/mL is suggestive, and parathyroid hormone levels reactively increase only in older infants and children in the presence of rickets.

Osteopenia of Prematurity

Osteopenia of prematurity is a well-described clinical entity with a peak incidence of 6 to 12 weeks postnatal age known to predispose infants to fracture. Laboratory studies of calcium, inorganic phosphate, and alkaline phosphatase are routinely performed beginning at 6 weeks postnatal age to screen for early rickets while the infant is in the NICU. Rickets tests should be repeated on a weekly or bimonthly basis. Birth records and laboratory studies should be obtained when considering whether an infant's fractures may be the result of prematurity. Premature infants in the very low birth weight (VLBW; birth weight <1500 g) and extremely low birth weight (ELBW; birth weight <1000 g) groups have increased susceptibility to fractures for a variety of reasons, all stemming from poor bone mineralization. For various periods of time, these infants are sustained on parenteral nutrition [57], are deprived of physical stimulation [58], and are given diuretics to treat lung disease associated with prematurity. In addition, 80% of an infant's calcium and phosphorus deposition occurs in the third trimester, leaving preterm infants seriously deficient in total body store [57]. It has been estimated that up to 24% of VLBW infants sustain a fracture in the first year of life because of osteopenia of prematurity [59,60].

Nutritional deficits

When evaluating a preemie with suspected osteopenia, information about calcium, phosphate, alkaline phosphatase, or vitamin D levels ordered in the newborn period should be compared with known normal values for term and preterm babies. Backstrom and colleagues [61] showed that using a minimum alkaline phosphatase level of 900 IU/L and a maximum inorganic phosphate level of 1.8 mmol/L detects all premature infants with osteopenia. However, nutritional supplementation does not overcome all of the influences leading to weaker bones of the premature infant. Chronic lung disease and related use of diuretics further depletes the infant of calcium stores. An orthopedic group assessed 247 VLBW infants for rickets and discovered that 10.5% sustained fractures at around 2.5 months of age. Infants averaged about 4 fractures each, most commonly in the ribs. As mentioned earlier, risk factors for sustaining a fracture included parenteral nutrition, diuretic use, cholestatic disease, chest physical therapy, and passive range-of-motion exercises. However, nutritional supplementation does not overcome all of the external influences leading to weaker bones of the premature infant [60,62].

Mechanical deprivation

Mechanical stimulation occurs in the third trimester as the infant kicks and pushes against the uterus. The stress and strain on the bones induced by movement stimulates bone growth and development [63]. The immobility and lack of external (uterine) stress causes increased bone resorption and demineralization. Premature infants do exhibit some adaptive catch-up mineralization when bone density increases more rapidly than in full-term infants from 40 to 60 weeks after menstruation, so that, between 65 and 100 week after menstruation, all infants have comparable bone mineral content [64]. Therefore, up to 65 weeks after menstruation must be considered as a time for increased susceptibility for fractures in preterm infants. However, each case should be considered for its unique risk factors [60].

Chronic lung disease
Another consideration in ex-preemies may be prolonged mechanical ventilation and use of diuretics. In the past, steroid use further exacerbated bone demineralization, but steroids are no longer commonly used in premature infants as part of standard therapy for chronic lung disease [60].

BIRTH-RELATED FRACTURES
The forceful process of delivery is a common cause for fractures in the newborn period. It is important to understand the characteristics of such birth trauma. Commonly fractured bones include clavicle, humerus, and femur. Skull fractures and rib fractures have been documented after traumatic vaginal deliveries [65]. Cumming studied the radiologic characteristics of 23 neonates with clavicle, humerus, and femur fractures that resulted from delivery and found that the earliest calcification occurred at 7 days after birth, but all had radiologic evidence of periosteal reaction by 11 days [66]. Some parents may have videorecorded the infant during the first examination in the newborn nursery. At times it is helpful for the consultant to view the video because it may provide insight as to whether a fracture may have been present at birth (ie, asymmetric moro reflex may imply a clavicle or humerus fracture).

NONFRACTURE MIMICS
Scurvy
Scurvy is a nutritional vitamin deficiency rarely seen in children from the United States or other developed countries. There are few case reports in infants from developed countries in recent decades [67–69]. The usual age at presentation is 6 to 24 months, and the affected infant seems ill, with significant pain leading to pseudoparalysis. Surface examination may reveal petechiae, ecchymoses, and mucosal hemorrhage. It is a clinical and radiologic diagnosis in which a diet deficient in vitamin C should be documented [70]. Getting a detailed diet history at presentation eliminates confusion later. Practitioners should be alert for future cases of congenital scurvy in solely breastfed babies whose mothers have a restricted diet. The recent case reports have exhibited unique diets: 1 ketogenic diet to control a severe seizure disorder and 1 prescribed by the Church of Scientology, both devoid of fruits and vegetables. Vitamin C levels are not routinely sent because of the protein's lability. Vitamin C is heat labile and has been deficient in infants whose milk was boiled. Radiologic findings in scurvy are subtle but distinct from abusive injuries. Cortices are notably thin and the

epiphyses appear osteopenic with denser outlines. During the repair phase of scurvy, as vitamin C is replenished, subperiosteal and soft tissue hemorrhage appear similar to healing trauma. In addition, the metaphyseal irregularities are similar to those seen in abused children.

Congenital Syphilitic Periostitis

Prenatal clinical testing does not rule out congenital syphilis. Untreated primary syphilis infection is almost always transmitted to the fetus. About two-thirds of infants are asymptomatic at birth, but untreated infants develop symptoms within weeks to months. The common early signs include jaundice, hepatosplenogmegaly, transaminitis, anemia, and thrombocytopenia, but radiologic findings may precede clinical manifestations in up to 20% of those asymptomatic infants [49]. Radiologic findings are diffuse but irregular and commonly involve the proximal tibia, distal femur, and humerus [31]. Bony lesions show metaphyseal erosions or rat bite lesions, which may be confused with classic metaphyseal lesions.

Vitamin A Toxicity and Other Causes of Periosteal Reactions

A careful history of diet, medications, and supplements may alert the treating physician to the possibility of hypervitaminosis A in the face of pathologic periosteal bone formation. Additional radiologic findings with excess vitamin A intake include premature closure of the epiphyses and cortical hyperostis, which occurs after 6 months of age [71]. Other causes of periosteal reactions include Caffey disease, prostaglandin administration, physiologic, leukemia, and osteomyelitis. The children with excess vitamin A and Caffey disease should have normal metaphyses and no fractures [42]. Osteomyelitis can appear as metaphyseal lesions, but not corner fractures, and young infants may not have systemic signs of infection. Osteomyelitis has been shown in the setting of fatal child abuse [72].

TEMPORARY BRITTLE BONE DISEASE

Although there has been controversy around a condition called temporary brittle bone disease (TBBD), there is no accepted medical evidence that such an entity exists. The impetus for such a condition seems to be the legal motivation to explain multiple fractures in a young infant that spontaneously resolve when a child is removed from the home environment. Paterson [73] first described this hypothetical entity of transient copper deficiency. The fractures sustained by the 39 infants in the article had fractures highly specific for abuse, such as ribs and metaphyseal lesions. There was little mention of the results of evaluations for nonaccidental trauma in the infants. The retrospective review did not adhere to any scientific method. A second group has supported a similar idea of TBBD in which the bones are briefly demineralized ,and reported 26 cases attributed to decreased and restricted fetal movement, as reported by the mothers. Again, there was no mention of the evaluations for inflicted injury. Their methods for measuring bone density have not been validated. Many experts from a wide background of subspecialties have dissected TBBD and exposed it as a sham [74–76].

IMAGING OF FRACTURES

The complete medical assessment of suspected child physical abuse cases was delivered in a clinical report by Nancy Kellogg in 2007 [77]. Studies have shown that use of the SS in conjunction with bone scinitigraphy (BS) is the best method of detecting occult fractures in a young child [78].

SS

When considering radiation, the SS is a low quantity. It is recommended that a SS be done on all children less than 2 years old with a suspicious injury or with any fracture. The current recommended views are skull, chest (including oblique views), humeri, forearms, femurs, lower legs, hands, feet, cervical and lumbar spine, and pelvis. A babygram (single view of the entire skeleton) is suboptimal and should never suffice as a method for detecting occult fractures. The yield on SSs revealing other healing fractures is significant. A follow-up SS 2 weeks after the initial study increases the yield of additional findings [79]. Kleinman and colleagues [80] detected new findings in 61% of cases in which a repeat SS was performed. When head trauma is suspected, a computed tomography (CT) scan of the head is the preferred method of detecting skull fractures and underlying acute injury. The three-dimensional reconstruction of the head CT may help delineate the skull fracture.

> Pros: detects epiphyseal, metaphyseal, and skull fractures
> Cons: misses acute and healing rib fractures.

Bone Scan

Acute rib fractures may be missed on a chest radiographs. A repeat chest radiograph in 10 to 14 days may reveal some, but not all, occult fractures. Bone scintigraphy should be performed when the suspicion of abuse is great and a complete assessment is needed [81].

> Pros: detects acute and healing occult rib fractures
> Cons: requires intravenous line placement, sedation, radiation exposure; findings are nonspecific for trauma (may be positive in areas of increased metabolic demand (ie, infection).

VARIABILITY IN DIAGNOSING CHILD ABUSE

Knowledgeable opinions are variable, even among child abuse experts [82]. What constitutes medical certainty, the standard set in court for an expert opinion? Child abuse specialists use varying degrees of vague language to impart their wisdom. The terms possible, probable, consistent with, indicative of, and more likely than not are frequently used in medical assessments. Less frequently used are terms like not concerning for, definite, or diagnostic of inflicted injury. It is important to consider the choice of language and how it may relate to the burden of proof in each type of hearing. In a civil hearing, in which dependency court decides who will care for the children, the burden of proof is a preponderance of evidence, whereas in criminal court the accused may be on trial for consequences that may include a death sentence or life in prison. There, the burden of proof is much greater; it must be beyond a reasonable doubt.

CASE RESOLUTIONS

Case 1: the calcium, alkaline phosphatase, and phosphorus were within normal limits for age. The opinion of the pediatric radiologist was that the bones appear to be of normal density and did not appear suspicious for any metabolic disease or vitamin deficiency. The infant was otherwise thriving on an appropriate standard formula, which provides approximately 400 IU of vitamin D daily. Multiple altercations between the parents were witnessed by nurses and staff during the infant's hospitalization. The father was arrested for assaulting the mother outside the hospital. No further testing was done. The infant was placed in protective custody and has sustained no further fractures.

Case 2: on examining the child, blue sclerae were noted. Further history revealed an autosomal dominant pattern of fractures with minor trauma on the father's side. The child was referred to genetics clinic where the clinical diagnosis of OI was made and DNA sequencing confirmed a null mutation in the COL1A1 gene. OI type I was confirmed. Allegations of neglect were substantiated because of the delay in seeking medical care.

Case 3: because of the infant's well-documented history of severe rickets, the team reasoned that much less force would be required to cause fractures in this susceptible infant. As an outpatient, the infant was being treated with 12,000 IU of vitamin D daily. It would have been interesting to check a 25OHD level on the infant as a measure of compliance with therapy. The skull fracture was caused by an impact trauma to the head that was unexplained, but believed to have required less force given the history of craniotabes. It is often difficult to know whether neglect or abuse has played a role. However, the head CT and ophthalmologic examinations did not reveal other signs of inflicted trauma.

SUMMARY

It is important for the general pediatrician to consider abuse in the differential diagnosis each time a child presents with a fracture. When appropriate, the primary care doctor should order ancillary tests to rule out conditions that may predispose the young child to fracture, interpret the results of the tests, and refer the case to a child abuse specialist if expert opinion is sought. Child abuse specialists may be used to objectively evaluate cases of suspected abuse and neglect [83]. General pediatricians should not be asked to perform forensic examinations on children they have known and parents they have befriended. Knowingly or not, their opinions are biased. Suspected cases should be referred to forensic centers by law enforcement, CPS, and generalists.

Fractures and many other forms of abuse must be evaluated in the consideration of broad differentials, but ordering of tests should be judicious. The specialist must take a careful history, perform the forensic examination, and consider prudent testing. When evaluating the history and injury, consideration must be given to the biomechanics of both the potential forces involved and the tissues injured. Home investigations are done on families after a fractured bone cannot be explained in a way that is biomechanically rational. The need to protect children must be balanced with the emotional turmoil of disrupting families or making false allegations. The child abuse expert must impart medical wisdom to law enforcement, attorneys, and CPS, keeping in mind the burden of proof in each court. Child abuse and pathologic disease are not mutually exclusive causes of fractures in young children. Children with known disability may be at greater risk for victimization by their caregivers [84].

Future efforts in prevention of child physical abuse are needed. Parents need education regarding age-appropriate discipline and guidance for anger management. High-risk parents should receive training to prepare them for various scenarios that may lead to frustration, anger, and physical harm of their child. In addition, general pediatricians should continue education in detecting the warning signs and symptoms of an abused child.

TAKE-HOME POINTS

- A thorough multidisciplinary team approach is essential to every case of suspected child abuse
- Every case of suspected physical abuse should be reported to CPS and cross-reported to law enforcement
- Obtain a detailed diet history on presentation, from birth, including maternal sun exposure
- Ex-premature infants have several comorbidities that may predispose them to fractures; examine the NICU records
- Judicious testing to rule out diagnoses should be used when the pediatrician (in collaboration with the pediatric radiologist) deems it reasonable to do so
- OI can present in infancy with few signs
- Consider whether neglect played a role in the injury
- No differential diagnosis is mutually exclusive of maltreatment.

References

[1] National Child Abuse and Neglect Data System, 2007. Available at: http://www.acf.hhs.gov/programs/cb/pubs/cm07/cm07.pdf. Accessed August 13, 2010.

[2] Leventhal JM, Martin KD, Asnes AG. Incidence of fractures attributable to abuse in young hospitalized children: results from analysis of a United States database. Pediatrics 2008;122(3):599–604.

[3] Wheeler DM, Hobbs CJ. Mistakes in diagnosing non-accidental injury: 10 years' experience. BMJ 1988;296:1233–6.

[4] Kirschner RH, Stein RJ. The mistaken diagnosis of child abuse: a form of medical abuse? Am J Dis Child 1985;139(9):873–5.

[5] McClelland CQ, Heiple KG. Fractures in the first year of life. A diagnostic dilemma. Am J Dis Child 1982;136(1):26–9.

[6] Wardinsky TD, Vizcarrondo FE, Cruz BK. The mistaken diagnosis of child abuse: a three-year USAF Medical Center analysis and literature review. Mil Med 1995;160(1):15–20.

[7] Jenny C, American Academy of Pediatrics, Committee on Child Abuse and Neglect. Evaluating infants and young children with multiple fractures. Pediatrics 2006;188:1299–303.

[8] Trokel M, Waddimba A, Griffith J, et al. Variation in the diagnosis of child abuse in severely injured infants. Pediatrics 2006;117:722–8.

[9] O'Keefe L. Uncovering child abuse. AAP news 2007;28(6):9.

[10] Flaherty EG, Sege RD, Griffith J, et al. From suspicion of physical child abuse to reporting: primary care clinician decision-making. Pediatrics 2008;122:611–9.

[11] Dalton HJ, Slovis T, Helfer RE, et al. Undiagnosed abuse in children younger than 3 years with femoral fracture. Am J Dis Child 1990;144(8):875–8.

[12] Ravichandiran N, Schuh S, Bejuk M, et al. Delayed identification of pediatric abuse-related fractures. Pediatrics 2010;125(1):57–63.

[13] Carlson KP. Child abuse or parent abuse? Pediatrics 2004;113:181–2.

[14] Pierce MC, Bertocci G. Fractures resulting from inflicted trauma: assessing injury and history compatibility. Clin Pediatr Emerg Med 2006;7:143–8.

[15] Prosser I, Maguire S, Harrison SK, et al. How old is this fracture? Radiologic dating of fractures in children: a systematic review. AJR Am J Roentgenol 2005;184(4):1282–6.

[16] Islam O, Soboleski D, Symons S, et al. Development and duration of radiographic signs of bone healing in children. AJR Am J Roentgenol 2000;175:75–8.

[17] Chapman S. The radiological dating of injuries. Arch Dis Child 1992;67:1063–5.

[18] O'Connor JF, Cohen J. Dating fractures. In: Kleinman PK, editor. Diagnostic imaging of child abuse. 2nd edition. St. Louis (MO): Mosby; 1998. p. 168–77.

[19] Kemp AM, Dunstan F, Harrison S, et al. Patterns of skeletal fractures in child abuse: systematic review. BMJ 2008;337:a1518.

[20] Thomas SA, Rosenfield NS, Leventhal JM, et al. Long-bone fractures in young children: distinguishing accidental injuries from child abuse. Pediatrics 1991;88:471–6.

[21] Meservy CJ, Towbin R, McLaurin RL, et al. Radiographic characteristics of skull fractures resulting from child abuse. AJR Am J Roentgenol 1987;149:173–5.

[22] Bulloch B, Schubert CJ, Brophy PD, et al. Cause and clinical characteristics of rib fractures in infants. Pediatrics 2000;105:e48.

[23] Kleinman PK, Marks SC Jr, Nimkin K, et al. Rib fractures in 31 abused infants: postmortem radiologic-histopathologic study. Radiology 1996;200:807–10.

[24] Sillence DO, Senn A, Danks DM. Genetic heterogeneity in osteogenesis imperfecta. J Med Genet 1979;16:101–16.

[25] Marlowe A, Pepin MG, Byers PH. Testing for osteogenesis imperfecta in cases of suspected non-accidental injury. J Med Gent 2002;39:382–6.

[26] Cremin B, Goodman H, Spranger J, et al. Wormian bones in osteogenesis imperfecta and other disorders. Skeletal Radiol 1982;8(1):35–8.

[27] Lachman RS, Krakow D, Kleinman PK. Differential diagnosis II: osteogenesis imperfecta. In: Kleinman PK, editor. Diagnostic imaging of child abuse. 2nd edition. St. Louis (MO): Mosby; 1998. p. 197–212.

[28] Byers PH, Krakow D, Nunes ME, et al. Genetic evaluation of suspected osteogenesis imperfecta (OI). Genet Med 2006;8:383–8.

[29] Basel D, Steiner RD. Osteogenesis imperfecta: recent findings shed new light on this once well-understood condition. Genet Med 2009;11(6):375–85.

[30] Wenstrup RJ, Willing MC, Starman BJ, et al. Distinct biochemical phenotypes predict clinical severity in nonlethal variants of osteogenesis imperfecta. Am J Hum Genet 1990;46:975–82.

[31] Korkko J, Ala-Kokko L, De Paepe A, et al. Analysis of the COL1A1 and COL1A2 genes by PCR amplification and scanning by conformation-sensitive gel electrophoresis identifies only COL1A1 mutations in 15 patients with osteogenesis imperfecta type I: identification of common sequences of null-allele mutations. Am J Hum Genet 1998;62:98–110.

[32] Steiner R, Pepin M, Byers P. Studies of collagen synthesis and structure in the differentiation of child abuse from osteogenesis imperfecta. J Pediatr 1996;128:542–7.

[33] Ojima K, Matsumoto H, Hayase T, et al. An autopsy case of osteogenesis imperfecta initially suspected as child abuse. Forensic Sci Int 1994;65:97–104.

[34] McKee J. Is it osteogenesis imperfecta or child abuse? AAOS Now July 2007. Available at: http://www.aaos.org/news/bulletin/jul07/clinical6.asp. Accessed August 13, 2010.

[35] Glorieux FH, Rauch F, Plotkin H, et al. Type V osteogenesis imperfecta: a new form of brittle bone disease. J Bone Miner Res 2000;15(9):1650–8.

[36] Glorieux FH, Ward LM, Rauch F, et al. Osteogenesis imperfecta type VI: a form of brittle bone disease with a mineralization defect. J Bone Miner Res 2002;17(1):30–8.

[37] Ward LM, Rauch F, Travers R, et al. Osteogenesis type VII: an autosomal recessive form of brittle bone disease. Bone 2002;31(1):12–8.

[38] Cabral WA, Chang W, Barnes AM, et al. Prolyl 3-hydroxylase 1 deficiency causes a recessive metabolic bone disorder resembling lethal/severe osteogenesis imperfecta. Nat Genet 2007;29(3):359–65.

[39] Cordano A. Clinical manifestations of nutritional copper deficiency in infants and children. Am J Clin Nutr 1998;67(Suppl):1012S–6S.

[40] Shaw JCL. Copper deficiency and non-accidental injury. Arch Dis Child 1988;63:448–55.

[41] Carty H. Brittle or battered. Arch Dis Child 1988;63:350–2.

[42] Manser JL, Crawford CS, Tyrala EE, et al. Serum Cu concentrations in sick and well preterm infants. J Pediatr 1980;97:795–9.

[43] Bacopoulou F, Henderson L, Philip SH. Menkes disease mimicking non-accidental injury. Arch Dis Child 2006;91:919.

[44] Turner Z, Moller LB. Menkes disease. Eur J Hum Genet 2010;18:511–8.

[45] Brill PW, Winchester P, Kleinman PK, et al. Differential diagnosis I: diseases simulating abuse. In: Kleinman PK, editor. Diagnostic imaging of child abuse. 2nd edition. St. Louis (MO): Mosby; 1998. p. 178–96.

[46] Kleinman PK. Problems in the diagnosis of metaphyseal fractures. Pediatr Radiol 2008;38 (Suppl 3):S388–94.

[47] Strouse PJ. Vitamin D deficiency vs. child abuse: what do we know now and where do we go? Pediatr Radiol 2009;39:1033.

[48] Slovis TH, Chapman S. Evaluating the data concerning vitamin D insufficiency/deficiency and child abuse. Pediatr Radiol 2008;38:1221–4.

[49] Gordon CM, Feldman HA, Sinclair L, et al. Prevalence of vitamin D deficiency among healthy infants and toddlers. Arch Pediatr Adolesc Med 2008;162(6):505–12.

[50] Senniappan S, Elazabi A, Doughty I, et al. Fractures in under-6-month-old exclusively breast-fed infants born to immigrant parents: non-accidental injury? Acta Paediatr 2008;97: 836–7, 992–3.

[51] Keller KA, Barnes PD. Rickets vs. abuse: a national and international epidemic. Pediatr Radiol 2008;388:1210–6.

[52] Paterson CR. Rickets or child abuse? Acta Paediatr 2009;98:2008–12.

[53] Feldman K. Commentary on "Congenital Rickets" article. Pediatr Radiol 2009;39:1127–9.

[54] Paterson CR. Vitamin D deficiency rickets and allegations of non-accidental injury. Acta Paediatr 2009;98:2008–12.

[55] Jenny C. Rickets or abuse? Pediatr Radiol 2008;38:1219–20.

[56] Wagner CL, Greer FR, American Academy of Pediatrics Section on Breastfeeding, et al. Prevention of rickets and vitamin D deficiency in infants, children, and adolescents. Pediatrics 2008;122:1142–52.

[57] Shah MD, Shah SR. Nutrient deficiencies in the premature infant. Pediatr Clin North Am 2009;56:1069–83.

[58] Moyer-Mileur LJ, Brunstetter V, McNaught TP, et al. Daily physical activity program increases bone mineralization and growth in preterm very low birth weight infants. Pediatrics 2000;106:1088–92.

[59] Koo WW, Sherman R, Succop P, et al. Fractures and rickets in very low birth weight infants: conservative management and outcome. J Pediatr Orthop 1989;9:326–30.

[60] Carroll DM, Doria AS, Paul BS. Clinical-radiological features of fractures in premature infants–a review. J Perinat Med 2007;35(5):366–75.
[61] Backstrom MC, Kourt I, Kuusela AL, et al. Bone isoenzyme of serum alkaline phosphatase and serum inorganic phosphate in metabolic bone disease of prematurity. Acta Paediatr 2000;89:867–73.
[62] Dabezies EJ, Warren PD. Fractures in very low birth weight infants with rickets. Clin Orthop Relat Res 1997;335:233–9.
[63] Frost HM. Bone's mechanostat: a 2003 update. Anat Rec A Discov Mol Cell Evol Biol 2003;275:1081.
[64] Horsman A, Ryan SW, Congdon PJ, et al. Bone mineral content and body size 65–100 weeks' postconception in preterm and full term infants. Arch Dis Child 1989;64:1579–86.
[65] Van Rijn RR, Bilo RA, Robben SG. Birth-related mid-posterior rib fractures in neonates: a report of three cases (and a possible fourth case) and a review of the literature. Pediatr Radiol 2009;39:30–4.
[66] Cumming W. Neonatal skeletal fractures: birth trauma or child abuse? J Can Assoc Radiol 1979;30:30–3.
[67] Hirsch M, Mogle P, Barkli Y. Neonatal scurvy: report of a case. Pediatr Radiol 1976;4: 251–3.
[68] Riepe FG, Eichmann D, Oppermann HC, et al. Picture of the month. Arch Pediatr Adolesc Med 2001;155:607–8.
[69] Boeve WJ, Martijn A. Case Report 406. Skeletal Radiol 1987;16:67–9.
[70] Heird WC. Vitamin deficiencies and excesses. In: Behrman RE, Kliegman RM, Jenson HB, editors. Nelson textbook of pediatrics. 17th edition. Philadelphia: WB Saunders; 2004. p. 177–90.
[71] Ved N, Haller JO. Periosteal reaction with normal-appearing underlying bone: a child abuse mimicker. Emerg Radiol 2002;9:278–82.
[72] Ribe JK, Changsri C. A case of traumatic osteomyelitis in a victim of child abuse. Am J Forensic Med Pathol 2008;29(2):164–6.
[73] Paterson CR. Osteogenesis imperfecta and other bone disorders in the differential diagnosis of unexplained fractures. Journal of the Royal Society of Medicine 1990;83:72–4.
[74] Chapman S, Hall CM. Non-accidental injury or brittle bones. Pediatr Radiol 1997;27: 106–10.
[75] Mendelson KL. Critical review of 'temporary brittle bone disease'. Pediatr Radiol 2005;35: 1036–40.
[76] Hicks R. Relating to methodological shortcomings and the concept of temporary brittle bone disease. Calcif Tissue Int 2001;68(5):316–9.
[77] Kellogg ND, Committee on Child Abuse and Neglect. Evaluation of suspected child physical abuse. Pediatrics 2007;119:1232–41.
[78] Kemp AM, Butler A, Morris S, et al. Which radiological investigations should be performed to identify fractures in suspected child abuse? Clin Radiol 2006;61(9):723–36.
[79] Zimmerman S, Makoroff K, Care M, et al. Utility of follow-up skeletal surveys in suspected child physical abuse evaluations. Child Abuse Negl 2005;29:1075–83.
[80] Kleinman PD, Nimkin K, Spevak MR, et al. Follow-up skeletal surveys in suspected child abuse. Am J Roentgenol 1996;167(4):893–6.
[81] Slovis TL, Smith W, Kushner DC, et al. Imaging the child with suspected physical abuse. American College of Radiology. ACR appropriateness criteria. Radiology 2000;215 (Suppl):805–9.
[82] Lindberg DM, Lindsell CJ, Shapiro FA. Variability in expert assessments of child physical abuse likelihood. Pediatrics 2008;121:e945–53.
[83] Block RW, Palusci VJ. Child abuse pediatrics: a new pediatrics subspecialty. J Pediatr 2006;148:711–2.
[84] Sullivan PM, Knutson JF. Maltreatment and disabilities: a population-based epidemiological study. Child Abuse Negl 2000;24(10):1257–73.

Advances in Pediatrics 57 (2010) 85–140

ADVANCES IN PEDIATRICS

ELSEVIER
MOSBY

Pediatric Nonalcoholic Fatty Liver Disease: A Comprehensive Review

Sarah M. Lindbäck, MD, MPH[a], Charles Gabbert, MD[a,b],
Benjamin L. Johnson, MEd[c], Emmanuil Smorodinsky, MD[b,c],
Claude B. Sirlin, MD[c], Natalie Garcia, MD[b],
Perrie E. Pardee, BS[a], Kristin D. Kistler, PhD[a],
Jeffrey B. Schwimmer, MD[a,c,d],*

[a]Division of Gastroenterology, Hepatology, and Nutrition, Department of Pediatrics, University of California, San Diego School of Medicine, 200 West Arbor Drive, San Diego, CA 92103-8450, USA
[b]Department of Medicine, University of California, San Diego School of Medicine, 9500 Gilman Drive La Jolla, CA 92093-0671, USA
[c]Liver Imaging Group, Department of Radiology, University of California, San Diego School of Medicine, 200 West Arbor Drive San Diego, CA 92103, USA
[d]Department of Gastroenterology, Rady Children's Hospital San Diego, 3020 Children's Way - MC 5030 San Diego, CA 92123, USA

N onalcoholic fatty liver disease (NAFLD) rapidly emerged from a relatively unknown condition to become the most common form of chronic liver disease in the pediatric population. This change was due in large part to the rapid, widespread increase in child and adolescent overweight and obesity. Not only is obesity a major risk factor for NAFLD, but the intensive investigation of obesity advanced the knowledge base for many comorbidities of obesity including NAFLD. The phenotype of NAFLD has both overlapping and nonoverlapping elements with obesity, and these are described in this article. In its progressive form, nonalcoholic steatohepatitis (NASH), some children will develop cirrhosis and end-stage liver disease.

    Funding: This work was funded in part by grants from the National Institutes of Health including R21 DK71486 from the National Institute of Diabetes and Digestive and Kidney Diseases, P60 MD00220 for the San Diego EXPORT Center from the National Center of Minority Health and Health Disparities, M01 RR000827 from the National Center for Research Resources for the General Clinical Research Center at UCSD, and DK080506 for the UCSD Digestive Diseases Research Development Center. The funders did not participate in the writing, review, or approval of the manuscript. The contents of this work are solely the responsibility of the authors and do not necessarily represent the official views of the National Institutes of Health.

*Corresponding author. Division of Gastroenterology, Hepatology, and Nutrition, Department of Pediatrics, University of California, San Diego, 200 West Arbor Drive, San Diego, CA 92103-8450. E-mail address: jschwimmer@ucsd.edu

0065-3101/10/$ – see front matter
doi:10.1016/j.yapd.2010.08.006

NAFLD also is a risk factor for adverse cardiovascular, endocrine, and psychological outcomes. The aim of this review is to provide a comprehensive understanding of the current knowledge on NAFLD in children and adolescents. Increased attention is given to those with the most recent advances in key aspects including diagnosis (histopathology, biomarkers, imaging), epidemiology, pathogenesis, clinical presentation, and treatment. A concise, practical guide to pediatric NAFLD may be found in Box 1.

LITERATURE SEARCH

In November 2009, PubMed was searched using the terms "nonalcoholic fatty liver disease," "nonalcoholic steatohepatitis," "quality of life," "health related quality of life," "physical activity," "treatment," and combinations of these search terms. Results were limited to studies in humans, English language, and the age groups infant, preschool child, child, and adolescent. A summary of articles referenced multiple times in this review is provided in Table 1.

DIAGNOSIS

Clinical suspicion for liver disease provides the initial impetus for the diagnosis of NAFLD. Such may be suggested by hepatomegaly, an elevated ALT, and/or abnormal imaging consistent with excess fat in the liver. None are sufficient for diagnosis, however, and at the current time, liver histology is required to confirm the diagnosis of NAFLD, or suggest other possible causes for the clinical findings. Furthermore, liver biopsy remains the only means to evaluate the severity of necroinflammation and fibrosis, as well as possible architectural remodeling of the parenchyma. Thus the diagnosis of steatohepatitis, which has prognostic significance, can only be made by liver biopsy. The following sections discuss histologic evaluation of NAFLD as well as other modalities that are being developed to aid in the detection of NAFLD, such as serum markers and imaging modalities.

Histology

NAFLD encompasses a broad spectrum of liver disease ranging from steatosis to steatohepatitis, fibrosis, and cirrhosis with or without residual NAFLD [1,2]. At a minimum, diagnosis requires that 5% or more hepatocytes have macrovesicular steatosis, and that other liver diseases such as viral hepatitis, autoimmune hepatitis, Wilson disease, and α1-antitypsin disease are excluded [3]. Wilson disease may not necessarily be excluded by biopsy evaluation, thus in the proper setting further testing of the liver biopsy tissue for quantitative copper can be requested. Histologic patterns of advanced disease in pediatric NAFLD continue to be defined. Several iterative studies have produced a set of criteria for the diagnosis of steatohepatitis [4–7]. The diagnosis rests on a constellation of histologic findings in which global assessment remains essential, as there are meaningful implications for patient outcomes that can only be derived from liver histopathologic evaluation. A summary of key articles describing pediatric NAFLD histopathology is given in Table 2.

Box 1: Summary of key points as a guide for the general pediatrician

- Nonalcoholic fatty liver disease (NAFLD) represents a spectrum of liver pathology ranging from isolated steatosis to steatohepatitis to cirrhosis in the absence of other infectious or autoimmune etiology
- Signs and Symptoms

  May be asymptomatic but often will have some level of abdominal pain, irritability, and/or fatigue

  Quality of life often lower than healthy children

  Notable physical examination features can include obesity, hepatomegaly, acanthosis nigricans, and hypertension
- Laboratory Evaluation

  Initial screening includes alanine aminotransferase (ALT) and aspartate aminotransferase (AST)
- Differential Diagnosis

  Viral hepatitis, Wilson disease, α1-antitrypsin deficiency, autoimmune hepatitis, medication toxicity
- Diagnosis

  Histology is critically important in making an accurate diagnosis and monitoring disease progression

  Diagnosis requires at least $\geq 5\%$ hepatocytes with macrovesicular steatosis and exclusion of other liver diseases

  Noninvasive tests (biochemistry, imaging) are not sufficient alone or in combination for the diagnosis of NAFLD
- Screening

  Expert Committee Guidelines recommend screening AST and ALT for obese children as well as for overweight children with additional risk factors

  Children diagnosed with NAFLD should be screened for other comorbid disorders including dyslipidemia, diabetes mellitus, hypertension, and obstructive sleep apnea
- Risk Factors & Outcomes

  Children with NAFLD may progress to end-stage liver disease and/or hepatocellular carcinoma (HCC)

  When cirrhosis is present, screening for HCC is recommended and is best done by magnetic resonance imaging (MRI)

  Children with NAFLD are at increased risk for cardiovascular disease and type 2 diabetes
- Treatment

  Lifestyle optimization including healthy diet and adequate physical activity are universally recommended

  Pharmacologic approaches to treatment are under active investigation

  Weight loss surgery can be an important element of therapy for some adolescents; however, optimal timing of surgical intervention (age and disease severity) remains to be determined

Table 1
Recent studies in pediatric nonalcoholic fatty liver disease foundational to the current review

Study	Year	N	Age range (years)	Location	Study design	Study evaluated
Schwimmer et al [23]	2003	43	2–17	San Diego, USA	Retrospective review of children with biopsy-proven NAFLD evaluated between 1999 and 2002	Biomarkers Histopathology Epidemiology
Schwimmer et al [12]	2005	100	2–18	San Diego, USA	Retrospective chart review of children who had undergone liver biopsy between 1997 and 2003	Biomarkers Histopathology Epidemiology
Schwimmer et al [145]	2005	127	17–18	USA, multicenter	Cohort of obese 12-graders from larger school-based randomized trial (Child and Adolescent Trial for Cardiovascular Health)	Biomarkers Epidemiology
Nobili et al [13]	2006	84	3–18	Rome, Italy	Prospective study of consecutive children evaluated in Liver Unit for elevated aminotransferase levels	Biomarkers Histopathology Treatment
Nobili et al [24]	2006	72	9–18	Rome, Italy	Retrospective chart review of children who had undergone liver biopsy between 2002 and 2004	Biomarkers Pathogenesis Risk factors
Schwimmer et al [133]	2006	742	2–19	San Diego, USA	Retrospective, population-based study of pediatric autopsies in San Diego County	Histopathology Epidemiology

Study	Year	Number	Age (y)	Location	Description	Topics
Manco et al [155]	2008	197	3–19	Rome, Italy	Cross-sectional study of consecutive children seen in gastroenterology clinic for biopsy-proven NAFLD	Biomarkers, Histopathology, Risk factors
Patton et al [25]	2008	176	6–17	USA, multicenter	Observational study of subjects enrolled in NASH CRN	Biomarkers, Histopathology, Epidemiology
Schwimmer et al [159]	2008	300	5–17	San Diego, USA	Prospective, case-controlled study with subjects obtained from clinical research database of children 5–17 years old referred to a pediatric gastroenterology clinic	Biomarkers
Carter-Kent et al [14]	2009	130	4–18	USA, multicenter	Multicenter, retrospective study of children with biopsy proven NAFLD	Biomarkers, Histopathology, Epidemiology
Nobili et al [34]	2009	112	3–17	Rome, Italy	Observational study of consecutive children evaluated in Liver Unit for elevated aminotransferase levels	Biomarkers
Kistler et al [149]	2009	239	5–17	USA, multicenter	Subjects enrolled in cohort study (NASH CRN)	Clinical presentation

Abbreviation: CRN, Clinical Research Network.

Table 2
Histopathologic features of pediatric NAFLD

Study	Year	Location	N	Age in years (mean)	Mean BMI (kg/m²)	Portal inflammation or injury (%)	Bridging fibrosis & cirrhosis (%)	Histopathologic findings by type (%)		
								Type 1	Type 2	Mixed
Schwimmer et al [12]	2005	USA	100	2–18 (12)	31.6	70	8	17	51	16
Nobili et al [13]	2006	Italy	84	3–18 (11.7)	26.3	69	5	2	29	52
Carter-Kent et al [14]	2009	USA	130	4–18 (12)	31	85	20	6	7	82
Ko et al [15]	2009	South Korea	80	6–15 (12)	27.6	43	9	34	44	–

The lesions most frequently observed in the spectrum of NAFLD include steatosis, inflammation, hepatocellular ballooning, and fibrosis [8]. Steatosis is predominantly macrovesicular, although it may consist of large and small droplets of fat. Steatosis severity and zonal location may vary in children; different patterns of steatosis may correlate with increased risk for NASH [9]. Inflammation is also variable, ranging from mild to severe in both lobular and/or portal distributions. Discordance in the interpretation of histologic patterns has been reported [5]; this is greatest in pediatric biopsies, but has only been studied in small series. There remains a need for a systematic approach by an experienced pathologist to observe and integrate the histologic features of NAFLD.

One feature of particular discordance is hepatocellular ballooning [5]. Currently without a precise definition, "ballooning" indicates cellular injury in the form of hepatocyte enlargement and cytoplasmic alterations [8,10]. There is no specific size "cut-off" and most pathologists rely on the flocculent appearance of the cytoplasm as well as presence of cytoskeletal aggregates known as Mallory's hyaline, or more recently, as Mallory-Denk bodies. In pediatric biopsies, Mallory-Denk bodies are uncommon [11]. Loss of the 2 cytoskeletal filaments of hepatocytes, keratins 8 and 18, has been reported as useful in adult biopsies, but has yet to be tested in pediatric cases [11].

Histologic interpretation of fibrosis is less controversial, and is usually defined by its location as well as distribution as perisinusoidal or portal in early stages, and bridging (central-central, central-portal, portal-portal) in later stages. The evaluation of fibrosis severity is based on the degree of involvement as well as the disruption of hepatic architecture [4]. Fibrosis severity, particularly once there is bridging fibrosis or greater, portends a worse patient outcome.

While the pathologist's approach to liver histology is not age-specific, histologic features observed in the pediatric population are often different than those observed in adults. NAFLD in adults is frequently characterized by zone 3 macrovesicular steatosis and ballooning. Additional features observed in adults are Mallory-Denk bodies, megamitochondria, and parenchymal inflammation with or without zone 3 fibrosis. A study performed by the authors' research group, in which 2 pathologists analyzed 100 liver biopsies in children with NAFLD [12], was the first systematic attempt at categorizing histologic features observed in pediatric NAFLD (see Table 1). Hierarchical cluster analysis revealed 2 subtypes. A pattern characterized by steatosis with ballooning and/or perisinusoidal fibrosis was observed in 17% of children. Because of the similarity with NASH in adults, this constellation of features was termed Type 1 NASH. In these patients, portal inflammation was notably absent. A second histologic subtype, found in 51% of children studied, was characterized by predominant zone 1 macrovesicular steatosis and portal inflammation, with or without portal fibrosis. This pattern of histopathology was termed type 2 NASH. Of those children with advanced fibrosis, the majority displayed this pattern. In this initial classification scheme, the diagnosis of type 2 NASH required the absence of ballooning. Type 2 NASH was associated with nonwhite race. While type 2 NASH was predominant in this study, subsequent studies on children with different demographics found a higher prevalence of an overlapping pattern. A study of 84 children in Rome, Italy, found an overlap of type 1 and type 2 NASH to be the predominant histology [13] (see Table 1). Of those children who did not demonstrate a mixed pattern, type 2 NASH was most frequently observed. Ballooning was notably present in 49% of the children studied. A recent multicenter study of children in the midwestern United States and Canada also found overlap of type 1 and type 2 NASH in 82% of patients [14] (see Table 1). Children with significant fibrosis were found to have increased portal and lobular inflammation. Ballooning was present in 73% of the population, albeit "low-grade" in the majority of cases. It is possible that racial and ethnic differences contribute to the variability in observed NASH patterns among pediatric populations. In addition, differences in histologic interpretation may account for some of the observed discrepancies, particularly with respect to ballooning. A recent Korean study that categorized biopsies as types 1 or 2 found type 2 NASH (44%) to be more common than type 1 (34%) in a pediatric population that was predominantly male and obese [15]. In this study, type 2 NASH was similarly associated with a greater severity of fibrosis.

Despite the histologic variability of NASH observed in such populations, the findings of zone 1 steatosis and portal inflammation have been repeatedly observed in pediatric fatty liver. Subsequent to the initial findings of the authors' group [12], a study from Rome demonstrated that portal features were found in the vast majority of subjects [13]. Kleiner and colleagues [5] confirmed a histologic pattern distinct to children and reported that portal fibrosis is 4 times more likely to be seen in children than adults. In a study of 41 obese adolescents undergoing bariatric surgery, intraoperative liver biopsy demonstrated portal inflammation to be common [16]. Taken collectively, these studies demonstrate that portal-based injury is a frequent finding in pediatric NASH. Recent research has attempted to further elucidate a correlation between levels of portal inflammation and features of advanced disease. From the NASH Clinical Research Network (CRN) dataset, Brunt and colleagues [17] found "more than mild" amounts of portal inflammation to be associated with steatosis location and increased stage of fibrosis. Further data are warranted to determine whether the degree of inflammation can serve as a predictor of disease progression.

In an attempt to quantify histologic disease severity, the NAFLD activity score (NAS) was developed. This ordinal scoring system was designed and validated by the NASH CRN Pathology Committee for use of comparative features in clinical trials. This system has become, at present, the most widely accepted scoring system to describe the histologic severity of NAFLD [5]. The NAS is defined as an unweighted sum of scores for steatosis (0–3), lobular inflammation (0–3), and ballooning (0–2), where a higher score reflects more active disease. Other features such as foci of pure microvesicular steatosis, portal and lobular lipogranulomas, and Mallory hyaline (Mallory-Denk bodies) are qualitatively assessed as present or absent. Portal chronic inflammation is either none, mild, or "more than mild." Perhaps because this system was developed specifically for comparisons of biopsies in clinical trials, clinical application of this system remains challenging. There are some concerns regarding the use of this system for daily practice, such as subjectivity in grading and that reporting averages may not signify true disease activity. More outcomes data are warranted to better define the scoring of histologic features, so as to accurately predict risk for improvement and progression.

Biomarkers

Although liver biopsy remains the standard for clinical evaluation and diagnosis of NAFLD in both children and adults [18–21], there are times when this diagnostic standard is not practical [22]. Research efforts have focused on developing accurate, precise, and practical noninvasive methods for evaluating NAFLD that are complementary to histologic analysis. Both serologic tests and radiologic techniques have potential for such a role. An ideal noninvasive test would be strongly correlated with the presence of NAFLD and would allow for the distinction between clinically relevant entities, such as isolated steatosis versus steatohepatitis. To develop noninvasive biomarkers, potential candidates must be tested in the context of liver histology. For this reason, the following sections are limited to those studies that compare biomarkers directly to liver histology. Table 3 summarizes recent studies that aimed to identify serum biomarkers for pediatric NAFLD.

Table 3
Serum biomarkers of pediatric NAFLD

		Biomarker associated with			
Study	Year	Steatosis	Inflammation	Fibrosis	
Schwimmer et al [23]	2003	QUICKI ↑ Age Ethnicity	↑ ALT ↑ Fasting Insulin	Perisinusoidal: AST Fasting insulin BMI Z score	Portal: RUQ pain HOMA-IR
Schwimmer et al [12]	2005			↑ GGT ↓ Age ↑ Insulin resistance	
Nobili et al [24]	2006	↑ Leptin	↑ Leptin	↑ Leptin	
Patton et al [25]	2008		↑ AST ↑ GGT	↑ AST ↑ WBC ↓ Hct	
Nobili et al [34]	2009			ELF score	

Abbreviations: ALT, alanine aminotransferase; AST, aspartate aminotransferase; BMI, body mass index; ELF, Enhanced Liver Fibrosis; GGT, γ-glutamyl transferase; Hct, hematocrit; HOMA-IR, homeostatic model assessment of insulin resistance; RUQ, right upper quadrant; QUICKI, Quantitative insulin-sensitivity check index; WBC, white blood cells.

Biomarkers of hepatic steatosis

Steatosis, or accumulation of fat within hepatocytes, is widely believed to be the inciting event in NAFLD. For this reason, detection of steatosis could potentially lead to earlier diagnosis of NAFLD. Unfortunately, few studies in the pediatric population have identified biomarkers for isolated steatosis. In a predominately obese, male, and Hispanic group of children with NAFLD, the authors' research group found that a combination of insulin sensitivity (assessed by Quantitative insulin-sensitivity check index [QUICKI]), age, and ethnicity predicted the grade of steatosis [23] (see Table 1). In Italy, a study of 72 children with NAFLD found that serum leptin concentration, controlled for age, sex, and body mass index (BMI; calculated as [weight (kg)]/[height (m)]^2), was directly correlated with the ordinal steatosis score [24] (see Table 1). Data from histologic studies should be pooled with data from MR studies to further develop biomarkers for steatosis.

Biomarkers of NASH

Given the clinical relevance of identifying children with steatohepatitis, several studies have described biomarkers associated with pediatric NASH. In 2003, the authors took the approach of finding correlates of the individual features that are components of NASH. The presence of portal inflammation was predicted by the combination of serum ALT and fasting insulin [23]. In a NASH CRN study, Patton and colleagues [25] demonstrated that the mean values of aspartate aminotransferase (AST) and γ-glutamyl transferase (GGT) were significantly different between children grouped as having NAFLD but not NASH, versus those with borderline steatohepatitis, versus definite steatohepatitis (see Table 1). In addition, a study by Nobili and colleagues [26] evaluated children with NAFLD for variations in retinol binding protein 4 (RBP4), an adipocytokine thought to be involved in the pathogenesis of insulin resistance, and found RBP4 levels to be inversely correlated with NAS score. Collectively, such studies suggest a role for serologic biomarkers in predicting steatohepatitis; however, more research is necessary to elucidate the markers with greatest sensitivity and specificity.

In adults, 2 studies have employed a combination of biomarkers to predict the presence of NASH. In 2006, Poynard and colleagues [27] developed a proprietary algorithm to predict the presence of NASH using 13 parameters including age, sex, height, and weight, along with serum levels of triglycerides, total cholesterol, α2-macroglobulin, apolipoprotein A1, haptoglobin, GGT, ALT, AST, and total bilirubin. This test resulted in a high specificity for detection of NASH (94%) but had a poor sensitivity (33%). A small pilot discovery study by Miele and colleagues [28] suggested that the combination of hyaluronic acid (HA), tissue inhibitor of metalloproteinase-1 (TIMP-1), and age may be useful for identifying the subpopulation of patients who have NASH out of a population of people undergoing liver biopsy for suspected NAFLD.

Studies in adults have also implicated hepatocyte apoptosis in the pathogenesis of NASH [29]. For this reason, many research groups have examined apoptosis biomarkers for their ability to predict NASH. One such biomarker is cytokeratin-18 (CK-18), an intermediate filament protein found in the liver that is cleaved by caspases activated during apoptosis [30]. In a study of adults undergoing liver biopsy for suspected NAFLD, Weickowska and colleagues [31] found CK-18 to be significantly higher in those subjects with a NAS of 5 or greater compared with subjects with a NAS of 3 or less. In a large, multi-center confirmatory study, CK-18 was shown to be associated with the presence of NASH independent of age and aminotransferase levels [32]. Furthermore, preliminary data from 21 children with NAFLD suggested that CK-18 levels are associated with NAS score [33].

Biomarkers of hepatic fibrosis
Biomarkers have also been used to predict liver fibrosis type and severity among children with NAFLD. In a study by the authors' research group, perisinusoidal fibrosis was found to be predicted by a combination of AST, fasting insulin, and BMI Z-score in a population of 43 children with biopsy-proven NAFLD [23]. In the same population, portal fibrosis was predicted by a combination of right upper quadrant abdominal pain and insulin resistance [23]. In a second study by the authors' group, children with advanced fibrosis were found to be younger and more insulin resistant, and to have significantly higher serum GGT levels than children without advanced fibrosis [12]. Similarly, Patton and colleagues [25] found that higher levels of ALT, AST, and GGT were associated with more severe fibrosis. Lastly, Nobili and colleagues [34] tested the "Enhanced Liver Fibrosis" (ELF) score, originally devised using data from the adult population, to predict fibrosis in a population of children with NAFLD (see Table 1). The ELF score is an algorithm that combines serum levels of HA, amino-terminal propeptide of type III collagen, and TIMP-1 levels to predict the presence and severity of fibrosis in NAFLD. Their study, which examined children aged 3 to 17 with NAFLD, determined ELF score cut-off values for the prediction of fibrosis stages 1b, 1c, 2, and 3. None of these studies have predicted fibrosis location or extent with a high degree of accuracy. As shown here, the ability to predict hepatic fibrosis by serologic biomarkers is inadequate and the current literature lacks consistency between studies.

Biomarkers: future directions
At present, no single biomarker or combination of biomarkers has demonstrated sufficient utility and practicality to be incorporated into standard clinical care. To develop such biomarkers, it will be necessary create representative test populations and to employ well-designed validation studies to demonstrate the utility and accuracy of a given biomarker in the clinical context in which they would be used. In addition to cross-sectional validation, those biomarkers intended for monitoring will need to demonstrate longitudinal validation.

Radiologic Evaluation
For more than 2 decades, imaging modalities have been studied and used to noninvasively assess NAFLD across its clinical spectrum. Techniques in

ultrasonography, computed tomography (CT), and MRI have demonstrated varying abilities in evaluating NAFLD. Whereas some techniques are either investigational or only of research utility, others have been used regularly for clinical purposes. A summary of the imaging modalities used to evaluate NAFLD is shown in Table 4. Other more novel techniques show promise as accurate, precise measures of NAFLD features, specifically steatosis and fibrosis.

Radiologic evaluation of steatosis
All major radiologic modalities have been used in an attempt to detect and quantify steatosis, although with variable success. At present, the most widely employed modality to evaluate steatosis is ultrasonography, though new MR techniques are proving to be more accurate across a wider range of liver fat. Unfortunately, there is limited research on steatosis in the pediatric population. Although it is clear that NAFLD differs in the pediatric and adult populations, the principles underlying the imaging techniques are nonetheless applicable in children.

Sonography
Ultrasonography is the most widely used imaging tool for the evaluation of hepatic steatosis, due mainly to its low cost, excellent safety profile, and wide availability. Ultrasound (US) technology uses the characteristics of wave prop-agation to differentiate fatty tissue from normal hepatic tissue; fatty tissue scat-ters the US beam, causing more echoes to return to the US transducer and resulting in a brighter more echogenic liver. Qualitatively, the brightness of the liver can be compared with the brightness of the kidney, because the kidney is known to have an echogenicity similar to normal hepatic tissue [35,36]. In addition to changing echogenicity, hepatic steatosis attenuates the US beam. In mild steatosis, the attenuation is relatively small and may be unnoticeable. As the amount of steatosis increases, the degree of attenuation increases, causing vessels and other intrahepatic structures to become blurry and, eventu-ally, difficult to visualize. As the attenuation becomes more pronounced, there is loss of echogenicity in the far field and diminished visibility of the liver-dia-phragm interface. This depth-dependent reduction of hepatic echogenicity is referred to as posterior shadowing [35,37,38]. Investigators have attempted to use a combination of the degree of liver brightness, vascular blurring, and posterior shadowing to assess hepatic steatosis qualitatively [38]. Pediatric vali-dation studies are yet to be done, though a recent study compared the ability of ultrasonography and MRI to correlate with clinical and metabolic characteris-tics of 50 obese children [39]. In this study, ultrasonography proved unreliable for grading steatosis severity. Computer-based analysis of US images to quan-tify hepatic steatosis by objectively measuring beam backscatter and attenua-tion are under development and are currently available for use exclusively in research settings [39,40].

Despite its wide use, several limitations make ultrasonography inappropriate for diagnosis and monitoring of pediatric NAFLD. Hepatic pathology, such as fibrosis and inflammation frequently present in NAFLD, can increase liver echogenicity [41–43]. Obesity affects the ability of ultrasonography to evaluate steatosis, because extrahepatic fat attenuates the US beam before it reaches the liver. In morbidly obese adults, the sensitivity and specificity of ultrasonography decreased to 49% and 75% respectively, for detection on hepatic steatosis [38,44]. The ability of ultrasonography to detect steatosis also decreases significantly with lower levels of fat accumulation [38,45–47]. Another limitation of ultrasonography is interoperator and interinterpreter variability, resulting in compromised repeatability and reliability [38,48]. Given these limitations, the authors recommend ultrasonographic evaluation of hepatic steatosis be interpreted with caution, and do not recommend the routine use of ultrasonography as a diagnostic or monitoring tool for NAFLD in children.

Computed tomography

Whereas studies in adults have shown CT techniques to be more sensitive and specific than ultrasonography in the detection of fatty liver [49,50], the amount of ionizing radiation associated with an abdominal CT scan makes it an inappropriate modality for evaluating NAFLD in children. Furthermore, safer imaging modalities, such as MRI, have proven to be more accurate than CT at estimating liver fat. CT is subject to several confounders such as iron, copper, glycogen, fibrosis, and edema [51]. Though not useful as a primary study in children, qualitative [52,53] and quantitative [52,54] information regarding hepatic steatosis can be obtained from abdominal CT scans incidentally performed on children for other purposes.

MR spectroscopy

At present, magnetic resonance spectroscopy (MRS) is accepted as the most accurate radiologic tool for estimating hepatic steatosis. MRS measures the frequencies at which hydrogen protons resonate, which vary depending on the intrinsic electrochemical environment of the molecules in which they reside [55]. Hydrogen protons in water molecules have a dominant frequency in the MR spectrum at 4.7 ppm whereas hydrogen protons in triglyceride molecules have a dominant frequency peak at 1.2 ppm [56]. Furthermore, the hydrogen protons within triglyceride molecules are subject to different electrochemical environments depending on their position in the fat molecule itself, each electrochemical environment being associated with its own frequency peak. Consequently, triglyceride produces a spectrum of multiple frequency peaks, versus the single large peak created by water. In the absence of steatosis, the dominant water peak is clear, without evidence of additional peaks corresponding to triglyceride. When liver fat is present, the area under the water peak versus the area under that fat peaks allows for estimation of a hepatic fat fraction [20,57–59]. This technique has been validated in animal models, and studies in adults have demonstrated a diagnostic accuracy of 80% to 85% [60,61]. A unique strength of MRS is its ability to accurately quantify fat fractions in livers with less than 10% steatosis [20,62,63]. A recent study of adult liver samples compared MRS estimates of steatosis to biochemical and histologic

Table 4
Summary of imaging modalities to evaluate pediatric NAFLD

Feature	Ultrasound	Fibroscan	CT	MRI					MRS
	US for steatosis			Dixon IP/OP MRI	Advanced MRI addressing confounders	Double-contrast MRI	MR elastography	Diffusion-weighted imaging	
Steatosis									
Qualitative assessment	Only for moderate to severe	No	Only for moderate to severe	Yes	Yes	No	No	No	No
Quantitative assessment	No effective methods	No	Yes but with confounders	Yes but with confounders	More accurate than Dixon, overall accuracy still being validated	No	No	No	Yes, currently most accurate
Spatial distribution	Low fidelity and distal shadowing in obese patients	Steatosis not measured with fibroscan	Yes, can compare whole liver to other organs	High-fidelity whole liver scans in single breath hold	High-fidelity whole liver scans captured in single breath hold	No	No	No	Single voxel only, usually 2 × 2 × 2 cm, 2-dimensional MRS imaging in early development

Fibrosis

Qualitative assessment	Poor	No	Poor	Poor	Yes	No	Yes	No
Quantitative assessment	No	Yes (Young's Elastic Modulus), confounded by steatosis and inflammation	No	No	Yes	Yes (Shear Elastic Modulus), confounded by steatosis and inflammation	Some via ADC indirect measurement of fibrosis	No
Spatial distribution	Low fidelity and distal shadowing in obese patients	No, TE is a 1-dimensional technique	Yes but not easy to quantify	High-fidelity whole liver scans in single breath hold	High-fidelity whole liver scans in single breath hold	Possibly; produces a whole liver elastogram, but fidelity of spatial distribution not yet validated	Unclear	Single voxel, not currently used for fibrosis measurement

Abbreviations: ADC, apparent diffusion coefficient; IP, in-phase; OP, out-of-phase; TE, transient elastography.

assessments, which demonstrated a significant correlation between MRS-derived fat fractions and both histologic steatosis grading (r = 0.61) and triglyceride content (r = 0.63) across a wide clinical range of liver fat from less than 5% to more than 33% [64]. MRS-derived fat fractions have been used in studies of both adults and children as a clinical end-point measure of steatosis [62,63,65–67].

MRS is able to accurately estimate fat fractions across the entire steatosis spectrum [20,58,59]. If performed properly, MRS can accurately quantify liver fat across a range of steatosis and is sensitive even to trace liver fat accumulation. In addition, it has less operator dependence and interobserver variability than ultrasonography. Despite these strengths, MRS does have important limitations. As emphasized by Hamilton and colleagues [68], many commonly used spectroscopy techniques do not address confounding variables and lead to inaccurate estimates. Further, current MRS techniques analyze a single voxel covering 0.5% of the liver, about 8 cm^3, and no anatomic images are simultaneously obtained, causing MRS to be susceptible to sampling variability. Two-dimensional MRS imaging techniques that would allow whole liver analysis are still in early phases of development [69]. A final limitation of MRS is the complicated and time-consuming analysis of the spectra.

MR imaging to evaluate steatosis

Whereas MRS allows estimation of fat fraction in a single voxel through analysis of that voxel's frequency spectrum, MRI provides information in the form of a structural image, which allows fat heterogeneity to be assessed within the entire liver. MRI techniques for estimating hepatic fat have been in use for 25 years [70]. The Dixon technique, also known as chemical shift imaging, uses "echo times" at which signals from fat protons and water protons are nominally out-of-phase or in-phase [71]; by comparing the signal intensities on the out-of-phase and in-phase images, it is possible to generate a fat fraction map across the entire organ [72]. The ability to decompose the overall hepatic signal to its water and fat components gives MRI a key advantage over other approaches in that it generates a quantitative map of hepatic fat content [73–75]. Over the years, chemical shift imaging has been refined to improve accuracy and decrease scan times, demonstrating excellent correlation between MRI fat fraction and fat measured by biopsy histology or MRS [73,75–78].

Because MRI techniques estimate fat fraction from the MRI signal, any variable that affects either the water or fat signal will lead to inaccurate estimates of hepatic fat fractions. In recent years, confounders in conventional chemical shift imaging have been identified, including T1 weighting, T2* relaxation, and signal interference from the multiple spectral components of fat molecules, particularly at low fat fractions in the presence of iron [75,78]. Failure to address these confounders leads to errors in fat fraction estimation [69]. Recently, researchers at the authors' center [79], the University of Wisconsin [80], the University of Michigan [78], and others have developed techniques that use small flip angles to avoid T1 weighting that overestimates hepatic fat content [79–81] and measure T2* relaxation with additional acquisitions so that it can be corrected in the fat fraction maps [78,79,81]. In addition, shorter echo times are used to lessen T2* corruption, and spectral modeling takes the spectral complexity of fat into consideration, leading to fat fractions that agree closely with MRS derived fat fractions [69,79,81–84]. When compared with more conventional chemical-shift imaging and MRS, advanced MRI techniques can accurately and precisely estimate known fat fractions in phantom experiments [85]. These techniques, though advanced, are easily implemented with software that is currently available at research centers. Such techniques are likely to be available on commercial systems soon, although further validation studies are needed prior to their widespread implementation.

Radiologic evaluation of hepatic fibrosis
Conventional cross-sectional imaging techniques have limited capability to detect and assess hepatic fibrosis. The characteristic morphologic changes in the cirrhotic liver include surface nodularity, segmental atrophy or enlargement, and extrahepatic complications such as portal hypertension. Unfortunately, these morphologic and physiologic abnormalities are features of very advanced disease and their evaluation does not contribute to early detection of hepatic fibrosis. An ideal imaging technique to evaluate hepatic fibrosis would not only provide qualitative diagnostic information but also quantitative fibrosis staging to be used in longitudinal monitoring of hepatic disease.

To address this need, new techniques have been developed to noninvasively detect and grade hepatic fibrosis across its entire spectrum of severity. The majority of these techniques rely on indirect markers of fibrosis. Ultrasonography and MR elastography (MRE) are 2 techniques that noninvasively assess liver stiffness, which has been shown to correlate with the degree of fibrosis [12]. Functional imaging modalities have allowed for improved fibrosis imaging, such as diffusion-weighted MRI that quantifies water proton diffusivity and perfusion MRI that allows for evaluation of tissue perfusion. Double-contrast MRI aims to evaluate hepatic fibrosis by looking directly at textural abnormalities of the liver.

Ultrasound elastography to evaluate hepatic fibrosis
US elastography, also known as transient elastography, uses a small probe with a US transducer to produce elastic mechanical waves that propagate throughout the liver. The probe also emits a pulse-echo US wave, which is used to determine the velocity of the wave. This velocity is directly related to the liver stiffness, which has been shown to have a nonlinear relationship to degree of fibrosis [86–89]. Transient elastography does not produce an image. It is a 1-dimensional technique that provides average elasticity estimates (measured in kPa) of a cylinder of liver tissue 25 to 45 mm below the skin surface, which may not reach the liver in obese children [87].

Although transient elastography has been extensively studied in patients with chronic liver disease, including NAFLD, only one study evaluated its use in a pediatric setting [90]. In a study of 52 children with biopsy-proven

NAFLD, transient elastography was shown to be promising. These results were similar to a study of 97 adults with NAFLD in Japan [89]. Neither study was able to accurately discriminate between stages of fibrosis.

Obesity, narrow intercostal spaces, and the presence of ascites have been reported to affect the sensitivity and specificity of transient elastography [87,91]. In patients with NAFLD, cited failure rates of obtaining transient elastography measurements in pediatric and adult patients were 4% and 5%, respectively. These failure rates are considerably higher in larger studies that did not specifically focus on NAFLD [89,90]. Factors that alter liver stiffness, such as inflammation or congestive heart failure, have been shown to affect the diagnostic accuracy of transient elastography in grading fibrosis [92,93]. Mild steatosis has a minimal effect on diagnostic accuracy, but the presence of moderate to severe steatosis decreases interobserver agreement [86,89,91,94].

Conventional MRI to evaluate hepatic fibrosis

Morphologic abnormalities that occur in the context of severe fibrosis can easily be visualized by MRI. In advanced cirrhosis, MRI is able to depict the large fibrotic bridges and septa [95,96]. However, MRI lacks the sensitivity to detect early fibrosis. The liver parenchyma in precirrhosis and early cirrhosis has a normal appearance on conventional MRI or may exhibit only subtle abnormalities on unenhanced or single-agent enhanced images [96,97]. For this reason, advanced MRI techniques are being studied for their ability to more effectively evaluate hepatic fibrosis.

Double-contrast enhanced MRI to evaluate hepatic fibrosis

Although individual contrast agents have limited efficacy in improving the visibility of fibrosis on MRI, recent research has shown that combining contrast agents produces synergistic effects [98,99]. Two agents that depict fibrosis through different but complementary mechanisms are gadolinium chelates and superparamagnetic iron oxide (SPIO) [100]. Gadolinium-based contrast agents freely diffuse into the extracellular space, and as a result preferentially accumulate and cause signal enhancement in tissues with large extracellular compartments, such as fibrotic liver tissue [101]. In contrast, SPIO particles accumulate in Kupffer cells, which are found in normal liver cells but are diminished or dysfunctional in fibrotic tissues [102–104]. Tissues with reduced Kupffer cell density such as fibrotic scars do not accumulate iron oxides, do not lose signal intensity, and appear relatively bright on MR images. With this technique, Aguirre and colleagues [98] were able to detect advanced hepatic fibrosis and differentiate it from absent or mild fibrosis accuracy. Whereas the other techniques discussed here mainly rely on indirect markers of fibrosis, double-contrast enhanced MRI allows direct visualization of textural abnormalities without the requirement of extra equipment. Furthermore, by imaging the entire liver, sampling variability is avoided and concurrent detection of other pathology is possible [105]. While promising, further validation of this technique is required.

MR elastography to evaluate hepatic fibrosis
In recent years, MRE has been studied as a tool to detect and stage fibrosis across a wide spectrum of chronic liver diseases; however, few studies have evaluated its use in NAFLD, and no studies have evaluated MRE in the context of pediatric NAFLD. Despite this, MRE is discussed here, given its possible advantages over transient elastography and its superior ability to discriminate between stages of fibrosis, particularly in mild liver disease [86,106].

MRE can be implemented on a standard MR system by placing a mechanical driver against a person's abdominal wall to generate shear waves that propagate with a velocity and wavelength directly related to the tissue stiffness. The tiny physical displacements caused by the mechanical waves are imaged using a specialized phase-contrast MRI sequence and subsequently processed to generate an "elastogram," which is a quantitative map of liver stiffness. Each pixel in an elastogram has an associated stiffness value (in kPa) and may be displayed using a color scale throughout the entire liver. It is important be aware that elasticity values measured by MR elastography and transient elastography are not interchangeable. By generating images that display the spatial distribution of stiffness throughout the liver, MR elastography is superior to US transient elastography, which produces a single average stiffness value for each measurement.

In a head-to-head comparison of MRE and transient elastography in a mixed population (N = 146) of chronic liver disease, MRE had a greater area under the receiver operator characteristic curve for detection of all stages of fibrosis [86]. With respect to diagnostic accuracy, the advantage of MRE is most profound in the earlier stages of fibrosis where the difference in stiffness between stages is smaller [86,107,108].

Because MRE performance is not influenced by presence of ascites or obesity, it has a higher success rate than transient elastography [86,109]. Furthermore, MRE does not require an acoustic window or administration of contrast, and it analyzes large liver volumes, thus reducing potential for sampling variability [86,107]. Finally, MRE can be included in a comprehensive MR examination that allows detection of morphologic abnormalities, hepatocellular carcinoma, and extrahepatic complications of liver disease. As with transient elastography, MRE measures an indirect marker of fibrosis and is therefore confounded by any process that affects liver stiffness [92,93]. MRE cannot be performed on livers with iron overload because of signal-to-noise limitations [108].

PATHOGENESIS

Most studies on the pathogenesis of NAFLD have been in the adult population. While pediatric and adult NAFLD share many characteristics, known differences between the two, including histologic differences, indicate variation in the development of pediatric versus adult NAFLD [17,110]. Although our understanding of the pathogenesis is in its infancy, obesity, central adiposity, and insulin resistance are strongly associated with pediatric NAFLD and inflammation with progression to NASH.

Insulin Resistance

Insulin resistance may be defined as the state in which a given concentration of insulin is associated with a lower than normal response in glucose level. Insulin resistance is also associated with multiple metabolic abnormalities including metabolic syndrome, abnormal glucose metabolism, reproductive abnormalities in women, and cutaneous abnormalities including acanthosis nigricans and skin tags [111–113]. Systemic insulin resistance is thought to be critical to the pathogenesis of pediatric NAFLD, and has been demonstrated to be present in 95% of children with biopsy-proven NAFLD at the authors' center [23]. Studies in animals provide insight to the physiologic link between insulin resistance and fatty liver; hyperinsulinemia and insulin resistance result in increased adipose tissue lipogenesis and very low density lipoprotein uptake, resulting in increased adipocyte fat sequestration and obesity [114].

Insulin resistance in both adipose and liver tissue may be integral to the development of NAFLD. Insulin suppresses glucose output by the normal liver through inhibition of glycogen phosphorylase, decreasing glycogenolysis, and indirect inhibition of gluconeogenesis. The latter effect is in part mediated by decreasing the flux of free fatty acids (FFAs) to the liver. Elevated circulating FFAs derived from adipose tissue are the primary source of intrahepatic triglycerides [115,116]. In a small study (N = 18) of obese children with evidence of steatosis measured by MRS, children with higher intrahepatic triglyceride levels and insulin resistance demonstrated increased adipose lipolytic activity and elevated serum FFA levels consistent with impaired insulin-mediated suppression of adipose lipolysis [117]. In rat models of NAFLD, circulating FFAs inhibit insulin signaling, leading to intrahepatic insulin resistance through activation of the nuclear factor κB (NF-κB) pathway with subsequently increased intrahepatic triacylglyceride levels [118]. In addition, insulin-resistant organs, including the liver, demonstrate increased de novo lipogenesis [23]. The combination of elevated circulating FFA and increased hepatic de novo lipogenesis promotes the development of steatosis.

Inflammatory Cytokines

Elevated systemic and intrahepatic inflammatory cytokines have been demonstrated in patients with NAFLD. Adipocyte-derived cytokines including tumor necrosis factor-α (TNF-α) and resistin promote both systemic and hepatic insulin resistance and inflammation through activation of c-Jun NH$_2$-terminal kinase (JNK-1) and NF-κB pathway [119,120]. The activation of JNK-1 results in increased synthesis of cytokines including TNF-α, interleukin (IL)-1β, IL-6, and monocyte chemoattractant protein-1. The NF-κB pathway leads to inactivation of systemic and intrahepatic insulin receptor signaling. Furthermore, in mouse models, neutralization of IL-6 with IL-6 antibodies improved insulin resistance and led to decreased NF-κB target gene mRNA levels [119]. Taken together, there is a complex systemic and intrahepatic feedback loop involving adipokines, intrahepatic cytokines, and systemic and hepatic insulin resistance.

FFAs also contribute to the elevated levels of intrahepatic inflammatory cytokines observed in NAFLD. In mouse models, intrahepatic, saturated FFAs overwhelmed the oxidative capabilities of mitochondria, leading to nonoxidative metabolism with the development of toxic metabolites, the generation of reactive oxygen species, and activation of inflammatory pathways including the release of cathepsin B, a lysosomal cysteine protease [121]. In the same study, cathepsin B knock-out mice fed a high-carbohydrate diet developed significant steatosis compared with wild-type mice on the same diet. As such, elevated circulating FFAs are integral to the development of intrahepatic inflammation observed in NAFLD.

Inflammatory cytokines including IL-6, TNF-α, and leptin have been implicated in the progression of steatosis to steatohepatitis and the promotion of hepatic fibrinogenesis through activation of hepatic stellate cells and dendritic cells [122–124]. In a study examining the complex interplay between Kupffer cells and hepatic stellate cells, the latter were incubated in the presence of recombinant rat IL-6, resulting in elevated extracellular collagen-I when compared with controls [123]. This study also demonstrated that reactive oxygen species may be crucial to the development of fibrosis, as increased catalase levels resulted in near basal levels of intracellular and extracellular collagen-I. In another in vitro study, increased expression of genes encoding collagen-I, TIMP-1, transforming growth factor-β1, and connective tissue growth factor was found when hepatic stellate cells were cultured with medium from Kupffer cells incubated with leptin [124]. In addition, researchers noted exaggerated proliferation of hepatic stellate cells when cultured with leptin.

Whereas leptin, IL-6, and TNF-α appear to contribute to inflammation, adiponectin may be protective. In a study of 30 children subdivided into groups of nonobese, obese with normal ALT, and obese with elevated ALT, children who were obese with elevated ALT had significantly lower adiponectin levels than the control groups [125]. In one study of 72 obese adolescents with hepatic fat fraction estimated by MRI, a higher hepatic fat fraction was associated with lower adiponectin levels [126]. Adiponectin may be involved at several steps in the pathogenesis of NAFLD and NASH, as was demonstrated in a comparison of adiponectin-knock-out with wild-type mice. The adiponectin-knockout mice had increased hepatic TNF-α and procollagen-α expression, increased intrahepatic triglyceride content, and marked hepatocyte ballooning, necrosis, and fibrosis [127]. In addition, administration of adiponectin via adenovirus-mediated expression prevented the development of steatohepatitis in adiponectin knock-out mice [128].

Studies have revealed potentially adaptive mechanisms in NAFLD and may help explain the variation in disease progression in patients. A recent study compared 50 lean adult controls with normal ultrasonography and serum aminotransferases to 25 patients with steatosis and 50 patients with NASH [128]. Patients with NASH were noted to have lower serum stearic acid and higher palmitoleic acid levels. This finding was interpreted as reflecting alterations in lipogenesis and FFA metabolism and is a possible adaptive mechanism in patients.

Although important advances have been made in understanding the pathogenesis of pediatric NAFLD, much remains unclear. For instance, in a study using mouse models of the disease, inhibition of hepatic triglyceride synthesis decreased steatosis but aggravated necroinflammation [129]. Similarly, while elevated circulating FFAs have been consistently demonstrated in both adult and pediatric NAFLD patients, hepatic FFA uptake inhibition with acipimox in adult patients acutely improved hepatic injury and insulin sensitivity without affecting liver triglyceride stores [130].

In Utero Environment

The in utero environment may be important to the development of NAFLD in children and has been investigated in animal models. In mice, measurement of hepatic gene expression in the offspring of mothers fed a prenatal, high-fat diet revealed higher levels of lipogenesis and genes involved in oxidative stress and inflammation than the offspring of mice fed a control chow diet [131]. In addition, genes involved in fatty acid, triacylglycerol, and cardiolipin synthesis were also upregulated in the high-fat/control offspring and even more so in the high-fat/high-fat offspring. This latter observation was subsequently confirmed in the offspring of high-fat dams fed a high-fat diet after weaning, using reverse transcription/polymerase chain reaction to measure the rate-limiting enzymes in de novo lipogenesis and triglyceride synthesis. Levels of these enzymes were higher in the high-fat/high-fat offspring than the control/high-fat mice. In addition, steatosis and progression to steatohepatitis, evaluated at 15 and 30 weeks of age, were more pronounced in this group. Taken together, these findings suggest that the prenatal environment affects subsequent lipid homeostasis.

A study of the offspring of both lean and obese nonhuman primates fed a high-fat diet found similar results [132]. Offspring demonstrated higher intrahepatic triglyceride levels and markers of oxidative stress such a p-JNK1. In addition, 4 enzymes in the gluconeogenesis pathway demonstrated increased expression in offspring of mothers fed a high-fat diet, which correlated with higher intrahepatic triglyceride levels. Of note, in both the mice and primate models, fatty liver disease in offspring of mothers on a high-fat diet persisted beyond the immediate postnatal period.

Heritability

It is unclear why NAFLD develops at varying ages and progresses to NASH in some but not all patients. Given the apparent clustering of NAFLD in families and higher prevalence in certain ethnicities, there is an increasing interest in genetic susceptibility to NAFLD [62,133]. In a familial aggregation study conducted at the authors' institution, higher rates of NAFLD were noted in the families of obese children with biopsy-proven NAFLD when compared with family members of obese children without evidence of NAFLD [134]. Parents and siblings of children with NAFLD had significantly higher fractions of MR-measured liver fat than those of children without NAFLD. When examined as a dichotomous variable with a 5% cut-off, heritability of NAFLD was estimated at 0.850, but increased to nearly 1.0 after controlling for age, sex, race, and BMI. When liver fat fraction was examined as a continuous variable, initial estimate of heritability was 0.581, but decreased to 0.386 when controlling for age, sex, race, and BMI. These data support a strong familial, and likely genetic, component in the development of NAFLD.

In the Insulin Resistance Atherosclerosis Family Study, 795 Hispanic American and 347 African American adults underwent CT scans of the abdomen to assess the presence or absence of fatty liver [135]. Heritability was estimated using a multipoint variance component procedure. The estimated prevalence of fatty liver disease based on CT imaging was 24% in Hispanic Americans and 10% in African Americans. When evaluating fatty liver using the liver to spleen density ratio, heritability was estimated to be 0.21 in Hispanic Americans and 0.19 in African Americans. When evaluating fatty liver using liver density, heritability estimates were estimated to be 0.35 in Hispanic Americans and 0.32 in African Americans.

Genetic Associations

The multiethnic population of subjects in the Dallas Heart Study (N = 2240) estimated hepatic triglyceride content by MRS. Investigators completed a genome-wide survey of nonsynonymous sequence variations of which one variant, a cytosine to guanine substitution in the rs738409 G allele in *PNPLA3*, was strongly associated with higher levels of intrahepatic fat [136]. No association was found between *PNPLA3* and measures of fasting glucose levels, insulin resistance, or BMI. This association was subsequently confirmed in 291 Finnish adults, in whom NAFLD was suspected based on MR findings [137] and in 172 Argentinean adults in whom the degree of liver steatosis on biopsy was strongly associated with the rs738409 G allele [138]. *PNPLA3* had been previously shown to encode adiponutrin, a 481-amino-acid protein of unknown function that belongs to the patatin-like phospholipase family [139]. In a study of 23,274 participants in 8 West-Eurasian study populations, a common variant of adiponutrin was associated with variations in lipoprotein concentrations, specifically in total cholesterol and low-density lipoprotein (LDL) levels, and researchers concluded that it may be involved in lipoprotein metabolism [140]. While much remains unknown about its ultimate function, the *PNPLA3* has been consistently associated with NAFLD across multiple ethnicities.

EPIDEMIOLOGY

Studies evaluating the prevalence of pediatric NAFLD are limited by lack of sensitive and specific biomarkers as well as the impracticality of conducting liver biopsies on all subjects enrolled in population-based studies. In light of this challenge, large population-based studies have used ALT elevation as a surrogate marker to estimate the prevalence of NAFLD. One such study, the National Health and Nutrition Examination Survey (NHANES) 1999–2004, found 8% of subjects aged 12 to 19 years to have an ALT level of greater than 30 U/L [141]. In the obese pediatric population, the reported rate of ALT elevation ranges between 14% and 52% [126,142–145] although the definition of elevated ALT is not consistent across studies. In a novel experimental design, the Study of Child and Adolescent Liver Epidemiology (SCALE) examined the histology of liver biopsies from children aged 2 to 19 years who had an autopsy in San Diego County between the years of 1993 and 2003 [133] (see Table 1). The standardized prevalence of NAFLD was 9.6% after adjusting for age, gender, race, and ethnicity. Tables 5 and 6 summarize studies that address the prevalence of NAFLD in the general and obese pediatric populations, respectively.

Age

The prevalence of NAFLD increases with age. In the Viva La Familia study of 475 normal-weight and 517 overweight Hispanic children, suspected NAFLD (defined by ALT >35 U/L) was present in 15% of 4- to 5-year-olds, 21% of 6- to 11-year-olds, and 30% of 12- to 19-year-olds [146]. In SCALE, the prevalence of NAFLD was found to be 0.7% among children aged 2 to 4 years old, 3.3% among children age 5 to 9 years old, 11.3% among children aged 10 to 14 years old, and 17.3% among adolescents aged 15 to 19 years old [133].

Gender

The literature on pediatric NAFLD almost universally finds a greater prevalence among boys than girls. Studies using elevated ALT as a surrogate marker for NAFLD find ALT elevation to be more common among males than females [141,145]. Likewise, in studies evaluating obese children for suspected NAFLD by ultrasonography, suspected NAFLD was significantly more common among males than females [144,147]. SCALE demonstrated NAFLD to be present in 11.1% of boys and 7.9% of girls between the ages of 2 and 19 [133].

Race and Ethnicity

The prevalence of pediatric NAFLD varies greatly by race and ethnicity. SCALE demonstrated NAFLD to be more common among Hispanic (11.8%), Asian (10.2%) and white children (8.6%), and less common among black children (1.5%) [133]. Among 150 obese 12th graders in the Children and Adolescent Trial for Cardiovascular Health (CATCH), unexplained ALT elevation was present in 66% of Hispanic adolescents, 20% of white adolescents, and 4% of black adolescents [145] (see Table 1). Similar differences by race were found when comparing ALT elevation (>40 U/L) among black and white children in a hospital clinic, where ALT elevation was 4 times more likely in white than black children after adjusting for BMI, age, and insurance type [148]. In NHANES 1999–2004, elevated ALT was found to be highest in Mexican Americans (11.5%); however, the prevalence of elevated ALT

Table 5
Prevalence rates of NAFLD in the general pediatric population

Study	Country	Study design & setting	Period of data collection	N	Age (years)	Presence of NAFLD assessed by	Prevalence (%)
Biopsy-proven NAFLD							
Schwimmer et al [133]	USA	Retrospective, population-based study of pediatric autopsies in San Diego County	1993–2003	742	2–19	Liver biopsy	9.6
NAFLD suspected by elevated ALT or ultrasonography							
Park et al [227]	Korea	Korean National Health and Nutrition Examination Survey	1998	1594	10–19	ALT >40 U/L	3.6 boys 2.8 girls
Fraser et al [141]	USA	US National Health and Nutrition Examination Survey	1999–2004	5586	12–19	ALT >30 U/L	8
Imhof et al [228]	Germany	Random subset of participants in cross-sectional health survey in southern Germany	2002	378	12–20	Ultrasonography	2.1
Zhou et al [229]	China	Stratified cluster and random sampling from large cross-sectional survey in Quangdong Province, China	2005	379	7–17	Ultrasonography	1.3
Tominaga et al [230]	Japan	Population-cased, cross-sectional, case-controlled study in public primary and junior high school in Northern Japan	1994	288	6–15	Ultrasonography	4.4

Table 6
Prevalence rates of NAFLD in the obese pediatric population

Study	Country	Setting	Period of data collection	N	Age (yrs)	Mean BMI (kg/m²)	NAFLD proven or suspected by	Prevalence (%)
Biopsy-Proven NAFLD								
Xanthakos et al [16]	USA	Morbidly obese bariatric surgery patients at surgery clinic in Cincinnati	–	41	13–19	59	Intraoperative biopsy	83
NAFLD Suspected by Elevated ALT or Ultrasonography								
Kawasaki et al [142]	Japan	Participants in school-based intervention	–	228	6–15	Not reported	ALT >35 U/L	24
Schwimmer et al [145]	USA	Obese subset of children enrolled in large school-based randomized trial	2000–2001	127	17.3 ± 0.2	35.2	ALT >40 U/L	23
Burgert et al [126]	USA	Pediatric obesity clinic	–	392	10–21	36.7	ALT >35 U/L	14
Quirós-Tejeira et al [146]	USA	Overweight subset of subjects enrolled in Viva La Familia study in Texas	2000–2005	517	4–19	Not reported	ALT >97.5th percentile for age and sex-specific reference values	24
Sagi et al [143]	Israel	Pediatric obesity clinic	2004	58	8–18	34.2[a]	ALT >40 U/L	25
Sartorio et al [147]	Italy	Consecutive obese patients seen at general health clinic	–	268	6–20	35.8[a]	Ultrasonography	44
Nadeau et al [144]	USA	Obese adolescents from urban and school based health care clinics in underserved Colorado	–	50	12–18	39.8	ALT >40 U/L / ALT >65 U/L / Ultrasonography	52 / 14 / 74

[a]Extrapolated from published data.

was found to be similar among white and black children, 7.4% and 6.9% respectively [141].

Prevalence of NASH

Studies evaluating the prevalence of NASH vary greatly by setting, and are summarized in Tables 5 and 6. In hepatology clinics in San Diego 84% of children, and in Italy 86% with biopsy-proven NAFLD were reported as having NASH [13,23]. However, in the SCALE study based in San Diego, only 23% of children with NAFLD showed evidence of NASH [133]. In the NASH CRN study, including American children from various geographic locations, 38% had borderline steatohepatitis and 39% were found to have definite NASH [149]. Among morbidly obese American adolescents undergoing bariatric surgery, intraoperative biopsy revealed 83% had NAFLD whereas only 20% had steatohepatitis [16].

International Perspective

The prevalence of pediatric NAFLD varies widely by world region. Unfortunately, vast methodological differences exist between studies, including differing definitions of obesity as well as nonstandard cut-offs for elevated serum markers and US echogenicity. To accurately assess the prevalence of NAFLD worldwide, a consensus must be reached regarding acceptable biomarkers and standard threshold values for these tests.

CLINICAL PRESENTATION

Symptoms

Symptoms have not been rigorously assessed in the majority of studies of children with biopsy-proven NAFLD; as a result the range of symptoms in children with NAFLD is not widely characterized. However, from 3 retrospective studies of children with biopsy-proven NAFLD, the most commonly reported symptom was abdominal pain. Abdominal pain was noted in 18 of 43 children at the authors' center [23]. Of note, abdominal pain was associated with the presence of portal fibrosis [23]. In a larger single-center study (N = 106), vague abdominal pain was cited as the reason for referral in 6% of the cases [150]. Finally, in a multicenter study of 130 children with NAFLD, abdominal pain was noted to be present in 18% of children and was the most common presenting symptom [14]. Estimating the true frequency of abdominal pain (as well as other symptoms) is difficult because symptoms may be the impetus for evaluation of NAFLD or alternatively, symptoms may be uncovered in the evaluation of NAFLD.

To address the knowledge gap in the frequency and severity of symptoms, the authors recently performed a prospective study using the National Institute of Diabetes and Digestive and Kidney Diseases liver symptoms questionnaire, administered to children and adolescents participating in the NASH CRN. Results from the survey revealed that symptoms are highly prevalent in children and adolescents with NAFLD [149]. In addition, the presence of multiple symptoms was common with 50% of participants reporting having 5 or more symptoms. Common symptoms were irritability, fatigue, headache, and trouble concentrating. Moreover, 17% of children reported severe fatigue. Fatigue may be a particularly important symptom in children with NAFLD, due to it being common and related to other symptoms. Fatigue appears to occur more frequently in children with NAFLD [149] than in healthy children [151]. To what extent symptoms are a direct result of NAFLD is unclear; however, the evaluation of symptoms should be an important area of research going forward.

Quality of Life

Quality of life (QOL) is an important component to the complete understanding of disease burden in children with NAFLD. Two studies have reported the QOL in children with biopsy-proven NAFLD. Initially the authors' group reported QOL in a pilot study of 10 children with NASH [67]. Recently, in a study of 239 children with NAFLD [149], the authors found that QOL for children with NAFLD was significantly lower compared with a reference population of healthy children (see Table 1). Although physical and psychosocial health were both lower, the greatest discrepancy was in psychosocial health. In addition, 39% of children had impaired QOL. In a multivariable analysis, symptoms were the only significant predictor of lower QOL score. In particular, fatigue was associated with both QOL score and impaired QOL. Other symptoms such as trouble sleeping, trouble concentrating, and sadness that were associated with impaired QOL may represent neuropsychological or physical (nausea) symptoms associated with fatigue.

Physical Examination

Certain physical examination findings, such as obesity, hepatomegaly, and acanthosis nigricans, may lead the general pediatrician or gastroenterologist to suspect NAFLD. Despite this, pediatric NAFLD often goes undiagnosed, due in large part to poor screening practices. In a recent retrospective report from 2 academic medical centers, screening for NAFLD was performed in 23%, 10%, and 2% of obese children seen by gastroenterologists, endocrinologists, and general pediatricians, respectively [152]. Clinical practice may change rapidly, however, because of recent expert committee recommendations. In 2007, the expert committee on childhood obesity issued a screening recommendation for pediatric NAFLD [153]. This recommendation includes screening AST and ALT levels for obese children (≥95th percentile BMI) as well as for overweight children (85th to 94th percentile) with additional risk factors. The committee also recommended that those children found to have AST or ALT greater than 2 times the upper limit of normal should be referred to a gastroenterologist for further evaluation. Of importance, new data clarify the appropriate threshold value of the upper limit of normal for ALT in children for detection of chronic liver disease [154].

Obesity

Unlike in adults, obesity and overweight in the pediatric population are defined by BMI percentile. To determine if a child is overweight or obese, it is necessary to measure their weight and height, and then use the mathematical formula to determine BMI, where BMI = [weight (kg)]/[height (m)]^2. Once the BMI is calculated, this value may be compared with standard BMI curves for age and gender to determine the child's BMI percentile. Those with a BMI at or above the 95th percentile are considered obese while those with a BMI at the 85th to 94th percentile are overweight [153].

Children with central obesity, as reflected by increased waist circumference, may be at additional risk of advanced NAFLD, specifically fibrosis [155] (see Table 1). There are many different methods for measuring waist circumference, which vary by placement of the tape measure around the child's torso. This variation becomes problematic when attempting to compare outcomes between studies. In the clinical setting, measurements of waist circumference may be used to monitor clinical change over time and in this setting, the most important factor is maintaining a consistent technique. The technique outlined by the NHANES anthropometry procedures manual instructs the clinician to locate the uppermost lateral border of the right ileum, place the tape measure in the horizontal plane around the torso, and then record the measurement at the end of a normal expiration [156].

Acanthosis Nigricans

Acanthosis nigricans is a clinical finding characterized by hyperpigmentation and velvety thickening of the skin occurring on the neck, axillae, and skin folds. Acanthosis nigricans is a marker of hyperinsulinemia, and has been observed in one-third to one-half of children with biopsy-proven NAFLD [23,157].

Acanthosis nigricans may be missed by clinicians without a systematic approach to examination. It is usually assessed at the neck, and has a standardized scoring system from 0 to 4, based on severity [158]. A score of 0 corresponds to undetectable skin changes, whereas a score of 1 indicates acanthosis nigricans that is very mild and detectable only on close inspection. A score of 2 indicates acanthosis nigricans confined to the posterior portion of the neck, and a score of 3 indicates moderate acanthosis nigricans where hyperpigmentation is present to the posterior border of sternocleidomastoid. Severe acanthosis nigricans (score of 4) extends the entire circumference of the neck and is visible when viewing the patient from the front. Becoming comfortable using this standardized scoring system takes time and practice, but proves useful in quantifying clinical change over time.

Hepatomegaly

Assessment of liver size is one of the most important tasks when evaluating a child for NAFLD, given that approximately half the children with biopsy-proven NAFLD have hepatomegaly [23,157]. When assessing liver size, it is important to have the child in a supine position on the examination table, and it may be useful to have the child bend his or her knees toward the ceiling to assist with abdominal muscle relaxation. A child who is initially sensitive and voluntarily guarding will prevent palpation of the liver edge, so it is important to be patient and methodical, using slow gentle pressure. Begin palpation in the right lower quadrant, near the anterior superior iliac spine, so as not to miss a severely enlarged liver.

Hypertension

Elevated blood pressure is a common finding among children with NAFLD [147,159], and the renin-angiotensin system is thought to play a role in the development of hepatic fibrosis [160]. When measuring blood pressure it is important to pay careful attention to technique, including proper position of the arm cuff, as well as appropriate cuff size, which in obese children and adolescents may mean using a larger cuff. Given that NAFLD and hypertension are commonly comorbid, it is important to be thoughtful about medication side effects when choosing antihypertensive therapy. For example, angiotensin-converting enzyme inhibitors and angiotensin receptor blockers may be more appropriate choices than either a thiazide or β-blocker, given these drugs may worsen insulin resistance [161].

Because many cases of pediatric NAFLD are asymptomatic and go unrecognized, pediatricians must have a high index of suspicion for NAFLD when examining overweight or obese children. If a child is overweight and found to have risk factors such as acanthosis nigricans, hepatomegaly, or hypertension, it is reasonable to consider the potential for NAFLD and to proceed with additional testing.

OBESITY AS A RISK FACTOR FOR PEDIATRIC NAFLD

According to data from the most recent NHANES, as of 2006 17% of children and adolescents are obese [162]. Multiple studies have identified obesity as a major risk factor for NAFLD, and most children with fatty liver are obese [23,157,163,164]. In SCALE, no cases of NAFLD were observed in underweight children, whereas 5% of normal weight, 16% of overweight, and 38% of obese children were found to have biopsy-proven NAFLD [133]. While subsequent studies support the association between obesity and NAFLD, rates of obesity and overweight among children with a clinical diagnosis of NAFLD remain variable. For example, no children were normal weight in a study from a Hepatology clinic in Korea [15], whereas between 2% and 20% of children were normal weight from studies in the United States [14,25] and as many as 50% of children were normal weight from studies in Italy [13,155]. To what extent these differences are due to the age or race-specific biology of fatty liver versus local practice of screening and/or referral is unknown. However, one should keep in mind this major difference in rate of obesity among clinical series when comparing data between countries.

While the precise relationship between obesity and NAFLD histology remains ill defined, the degree of obesity has been observed to correlate with fatty liver severity. Children with NASH tend to have higher BMI than children who have NAFLD without NASH [133]. In addition, obese children with NAFLD are 3 times more likely to develop fibrosis than nonobese children [23]. Italian data suggest that higher BMI may be a predictor of fibrosis in children with NAFLD [24]. While the NASH CRN study found no significant association between BMI and fibrosis severity, those patients with fibrosis did have a higher percentage of body fat than those without fibrosis [25].

OUTCOMES ASSOCIATED WITH PEDIATRIC NAFLD
Hepatic Outcomes
Determination of hepatic outcomes by NAFLD subtype is challenging in that it is dependent on integrative assessment of histologic features and clinical longitudinal monitoring. These challenges must be overcome to develop better pediatric data regarding the risk for disease progression. The natural course of NAFLD has largely been described in the adult population, for which approximately one-third of patients with NAFLD have demonstrated histologic evidence of disease progression over a period of 5 years [165,166]. Baseline histologic evaluation and its repeated assessment over time are essential to monitor disease activity and response to interventions.

In studies of children undergoing liver biopsy for suspected NAFLD, rates of cirrhosis have been reported to range from 2% to 10% [12,23,157]. Of those patients without evidence of cirrhosis in their initial biopsy, the risk for developing cirrhosis may vary by histology and subtype. In adults with steatohepatitis, Matteoni and colleagues [2] reported that 1 in 4 patients went on to develop cirrhosis. Longitudinal studies are warranted to further elucidate the risk disease progression in pediatric NAFLD. Of note, an association between endocrine dysfunction and severe disease has been reported. Children with hypothalamic pituitary axis disorders leading to extreme weight gain have demonstrated rapid progression to cirrhosis [167–169].

Multiple cross-sectional studies suggest that NAFLD is a significant risk factor for the development of HCC [170–172]. It is estimated that roughly 1000 cases of HCC in the United States each year can be attributed to NAFLD [173]. One prospective study of adult patients with NASH cirrhosis found HCC to develop in roughly 7% of patients over a 10-year period [174]. Less is known about the risk for HCC in children. While it is suspected that the majority of patients with NAFLD who develop HCC demonstrate cirrhotic features at some time during the course of their disease, there have also been cases of HCC developing in the setting of NASH without evidence of cirrhosis [171,172,175,176]. Duration of NASH may also strongly affect the development HCC for those who have NAFLD as children.

Over the past 2 decades, the frequency of NAFLD in hospitalized children has increased substantially [177]. This result may reflect the increased prevalence of childhood obesity and its comorbidities but also may reflect heightened awareness about pediatric NAFLD. Few data exist regarding mortality rates in children with NAFLD. The first, second, and third most common causes of mortality among adults with NAFLD are cardiovascular disease, cancer, and liver disease, respectively. Without long-term data to describe the course of the disease, estimation of survival in NAFLD remains difficult. A retrospective study in Minnesota found children with NAFLD to be at a higher risk of mortality than the general population [178]. Despite the limited data on clinical outcomes in children with NAFLD, these findings suggest that fatty liver is associated with significant morbidity and mortality in children with NAFLD.

Cardiometabolic Outcomes

Current data suggest that NAFLD confers an increased risk for the development of cardiovascular disease, particularly through its association with metabolic syndrome. The key components of metabolic syndrome include central obesity, impaired glucose tolerance, elevated blood pressure, and dyslipidemia [179]. A study performed by the authors' research group demonstrated NAFLD to be more frequent among children with metabolic syndrome than in children without metabolic syndrome [159] (see Table 1). Of the 300 children evaluated, those with biopsy-proven NAFLD had a significantly greater cardiovascular risk profile. Higher values for fasting glucose, insulin, LDL cholesterol, triglycerides, and systolic blood pressure were observed in the NAFLD group. In a Swedish cohort study, patients with a history of steatohepatitis had significantly higher rates of cardiovascular disease and mortality when compared with patients with isolated steatosis [180]. Identification of NAFLD should prompt consideration of cardiovascular health and relative risk reduction through lifestyle changes. In a subsequent substudy of 72 obese adolescents, those with fatty liver detected by MRI were nearly 3 times as likely to have metabolic syndrome as those without MRI evidence of fatty liver [126].

Recent data have demonstrated NAFLD to be associated with quantifiable markers of cardiovascular disease risk. Increased carotid intima-media thickness has been identified as an intermediate phenotype of cardiovascular disease. A study of Turkish children demonstrated obese children with ultrasonographic evidence of fatty liver to have greater carotid artery intima-media thickness than those children without evidence of fatty liver [181]. Similarly, Pacifico and colleagues [182] reported carotid artery intima-media thickness to be highest in obese children with evidence of hepatic fat on ultrasonography.

Children with NAFLD may have an increased risk for developing type 2 diabetes. In large studies of children with biopsy-proven NAFLD, 8% to 10% of children have type 2 diabetes at the time of diagnosis [23,183]. In addition, nearly 50% of children diagnosed with type 2 diabetes have suspected fatty liver based on ALT elevation [184]. It is important to understand progression to diabetes from both preventive and therapeutic standpoints. In adults, the risk for development of diabetes may be as high as 20% to 25% over 5 years [185,186]. Ekstedt and colleagues [180] reported an even higher incidence of diabetes over time in adults with NAFLD. In this cohort, the prevalence of diabetes increased from 9% to 78% over a 14-year period. Future research including longitudinal studies will be necessary to more precisely define the risk for diabetes at various stages of pediatric NAFLD.

TREATMENT

To date, treatment strategies have focused on addressing obesity, insulin resistance, and oxidative damage. There have been relatively few studies evaluating the treatment of pediatric NAFLD; those discussed here are presented in Table 7. Given that NAFLD is the most common chronic liver disease in children and has potential for significant morbidity and mortality, there is great interest in finding effective therapies. Table 8 presents currently active clinical treatment trials for pediatric NAFLD.

Lifestyle

Because NAFLD is associated with obesity and insulin resistance, diet and exercise therapy are universally recommended. In the only lifestyle intervention study to date, Nobili and colleagues [13] reported the findings from 12 months of lifestyle advice and weight loss on the outcome of liver ultrasonography. The lifestyle intervention involved individually tailored low-calorie diets and physical activity recommendations. In this uncontrolled study, of the 84 enrolled children, 52 overweight or obese children (62%) completed the trial. Seventeen children lost greater than 10% of their body weight; of these, 5 had a normal liver ultrasound at the end of the study. ALT was significantly reduced in most subjects, with the greatest reduction in those who lost the most weight.

Several studies have evaluated the appearance of the liver by ultrasonography in children being treated for obesity with a lifestyle intervention. As discussed in the Radiology section, ultrasonography is not a diagnostic tool for NAFLD and cannot be used to grade NAFLD disease severity. Thus, these studies provide preliminary data on the potential effects of lifestyle intervention, but do not directly target a population with the diagnosis of NAFLD. Table 9 describes a series of such studies performed in Germany, Brazil, and China. These studies have shown that children can lose significant weight when enrolled in intensive lifestyle intervention programs [187–190]. Furthermore, some studies have shown that children who lose weight may have a significant reduction in serum aminotransferases [188,190]. However, even with an intensive intervention, half or more of these children did not show convincing evidence of disease improvement.

Recent research has suggested a role for increased fructose consumption as a risk factor for NAFLD [191]. A 6-month pilot study evaluated the effect of a low fructose diet on aminotransferase levels and oxidized LDL [192]. Ten overweight children with a mean age of 13 years and biopsy-proven (n = 7) or suspected (n = 3) NAFLD based on ultrasonography participated in the study. Of these, 6 consumed a low-fructose diet and 4 consumed a low-fat diet. Although a significant decrease in oxidized LDL was shown, the low fructose diet did not have an effect on serum aminotransferases. Despite heightened

Table 7
Studies evaluating potential therapies for NAFLD in children

Study	Year	Location	N[a]	Duration	Biopsy-proven NAFLD	Baseline ALT (U/L)	Study population	Study design	Study intervention	Results
Diet and Lifestyle Intervention Studies										
Nobili et al [13]	2006	Italy	52/84	1 year	Yes	76 ± 63 range, 10–407	3–18.8 years (mean 11.7) 40% obese, 51% overweight 9% normal weight	Uncontrolled prospective trial	Lifestyle intervention	1. 33% lost >10% body weight 33% lost between 5% and 10% 33% lost <5% 2. ↓ALT from mean 62 U/L to 33 U/L
Vos et al [192]	2009	USA	10/10	6 months	Yes, in 7/10	125 ± 22 (low fructose) 103 ± 93 (low fat)	Mean 13.3 years All overweight or obese	Randomized controlled, open label	Low fructose diet versus low fat diet	1. Significantly ↓ oxidized LDL in low fructose group 2. No significant change in ALT in either group

Metformin Studies

Study	Year	Country	N	Duration	Biopsy	ALT/AST	Age/BMI	Design	Intervention	Results
Schwimmer et al [67]	2005	USA	10/10	6 months	Yes; NASH	219 ± 194	8–17 years (mean 11.2) All obese, mean BMI 30.4 kg/m²	Single-arm, open-label pilot	Metformin	1. Mean change −86 U/L in ALT, −46 U/L AST 2. Decreased liver fat on MRS
Nobili et al [193]	2008	Italy	57/60	2 years	Yes	Metformin group: mean 35 range, 21–43 Control group: mean 66, range 28–121	9–18 years All obese or overweight	Observational, open-label study; shared control group with other study	Treatment group: metformin daily and lifestyle intervention Control: lifestyle intervention and placebo	1. ALT decreased, but no significant difference between 2 groups 2. Several histologic features improved in both groups, but no difference between groups

Antioxidant Studies

Study	Year	Country	N	Duration	Biopsy	ALT/AST	Age/BMI	Design	Intervention	Results
Lavine [200]	2000	USA	11/11	4–10 months	No; ↑ ALT + US	175 ± 106	Mean 12.4 years Mean BMI 32.8 kg/m²	Single-arm, open-label pilot	400–1200 IU vitamin E daily	Significant decrease in ALT and AST

(continued on next page)

Table 7
(continued)

Study	Year	Location	N[a]	Duration	Biopsy-proven NAFLD	Baseline ALT (U/L)	Study population	Study design	Study intervention	Results
Nobili et al [201]	2006	Italy	88/90	1 year	Yes	57 ± 24	Mean 12.3 years Treatment group: 8 normal weight, 19 overweight, 18 obese	Randomized double-blind, reallocation of patients	Vitamin E + vitamin C and lifestyle intervention OR placebo + lifestyle intervention	Decreased serum ALT in both groups, no significant difference between the 2
Nobili et al [202]	2008	Italy	53/88	1 year continuation of above	Yes	Mean 71 (14–192)	Mean age 12 years BMI z-score mean 1.7, range 0.1–2.9	Randomized, open-label, controlled continuation	Vitamin E + vitamin C and lifestyle intervention (n = 25) OR placebo + lifestyle intervention (n = 28)	ALT and AST improved in both groups, but no significant difference between groups No difference between groups in degree of histologic improvement

Abbreviations: AA, African American; ALT, alanine aminotransferase; BMI, body mass index; CT, computed tomography; H, Hispanic
[a] Children completing the study/children initially enrolled in the study.

interest in determining the role of fructose consumption in the development of NAFLD, current data are inconclusive. Foods containing high-fructose corn syrup tend to be highly processed and have lower nutritional value. For this reason, measuring fructose consumption among patients with NAFLD may be confounded by a correlation between fructose consumption and poor general nutrition.

The amount of weight loss required to improve abnormalities of aminotransferases, imaging, or more importantly, histology in obese children with NAFLD is unclear. Whether particular diets or dietary modifications play a role in treatment remains to be determined. Given the benefits of a healthy lifestyle for all children, physical activity and a balanced diet should continue to be recommended. Weight loss should also be recommended for those children who are overweight, but specific targets are difficult to stipulate from the evidence base.

Pharmacologic

Drugs targeting insulin resistance

Insulin resistance is believed to be central to the development of NAFLD. Therefore, several studies have evaluated metformin as a potential treatment for NAFLD in children. In a study using MRS as a measure of hepatic steatosis, 10 nondiabetic children with biopsy-proven NASH received 500 mg of metformin by mouth twice daily for 6 months in an open-label pilot trial [67]. At the completion of the study, ALT normalized in 40% and AST normalized in 50%. Hepatic fat fraction was significantly reduced in 9 of 10 subjects, decreasing from a baseline mean of 30% ± 11% to 23% ± 9% after 24 weeks of treatment.

An open-label, 2-year observational pilot study from Rome evaluated the effect of metformin on NAFLD in children [193]. Thirty children with biopsy-proven NAFLD and mildly elevated ALT were enrolled and treated with 1500 mg of metformin daily. All subjects also received lifestyle advice, including an individually tailored hypocaloric or isocaloric diet, physical activity recommendations, and monthly 1-hour sessions with a dietitian. Of those enrolled, 40% had a follow-up biopsy. In this subset, several histologic features, including steatosis, ballooning, and lobular inflammation were noted to have improved. However, there was no change in fibrosis. The investigators compared this group to a group of 30 children from another of their studies who had only ongoing lifestyle intervention without pharmacotherapy. Of this group, 50% had a follow-up biopsy. The investigators reported no meaningful differences in outcomes between these 2 study groups. However, they acknowledged the very small sample size, open-label design, and lack of an appropriate control group, citing the need for further studies to evaluate the efficacy of metformin in treating pediatric NAFLD.

The Treatment Of NAFLD In Children (TONIC) trial is a large National Institutes of Health NASH-CRN multicenter, randomized, double-blind, placebo-controlled treatment trial recently completed. A total of 173 children ages 7 to 17 years with biopsy-proven NAFLD were randomized to receive

Table 8
Currently active or recruiting clinical trials for the treatment of NAFLD in children

Clinical trial name: number	Location and length of study	N	Study population	Study design	Study intervention	Outcome measures (1, primary; 2, secondary)	End date
A Pilot Study of Acarbose as Treatment for Pediatric Non-Alcoholic Fatty Liver Disease (NAFLD): NCT00677521	Toronto, Canada 12 weeks	12	10–18 years biopsy-proven NAFLD	Open-label pilot	Acarbose 50 mg 3 times daily	Percent hepatic steatosis determined by MRS	2/2009
Study of Fish Oil to Reduce ALT Levels in Adolescents: NCT00694746	Boston, MA 6 months	8	13–17 years hepatic fat on abdominal CT	Randomized, placebo-controlled, double-blind	2 capsules of 1 g fish oil twice daily, or placebo	Serum ALT at 3 and 6 months	7/2009
Effects of a Low Glycemic Load Diet on Fatty Liver in Children (DELIVER): NCT00480922	Boston, MA 6 months	40	8–17 years >10% hepatic steatosis on MRS	Randomized, open label	Low glycemic load diet with behavioral counseling or low fat diet with behavioral counseling (control)	Percent liver fat determined by MRS	12/2009

Study	Location / Duration	N	Inclusion	Design	Intervention	Outcome	Completion
A Preliminary Study to Evaluate Cysteamine Therapy in Human Subjects With Nonalcoholic Steatohepatitis (NASH): NCT00799578	San Diego, CA 3–6 months	12	10+ years biopsy-proven NASH ALT >60 U/L	Open-label efficacy trial	Cysteamine up to 1 g twice daily	Normalization or >50% reduction of serum ALT	12/2009
Treatment of Nonalcoholic Fatty Liver Disease in Children (TONIC): NCT00063635	Multicenter USA 96 weeks	180	7–17 years biopsy-proven NAFLD and ALT >60 U/L at least once in past 6 months	Randomized, placebo-controlled, double-blind	Metformin 500 mg twice daily OR vitamin E 400 IU twice daily OR placebo twice daily	1. Sustained reduction in ALT to <50% baseline 2. Change in liver fibrosis, steatosis, and inflammation	4/2010
Effects of Docosahexaenoic Acid on Children With Nonalcoholic Fatty Liver Disease (EDACN): NCT00885313	Rome, Italy 24 months	45	4–16 years biopsy-proven NAFLD	Randomized, placebo-controlled, double-blind	DHA 250 mg/kg/d + lifestyle OR DHA 500 mg/kg/d + lifestyle OR placebo + lifestyle intervention	1. Serum aminotransferases at 1 and 2 years 2. 2-year follow-up liver biopsy	3/2011

Abbreviations: ALT, alanine aminotransferase; DHA, docosahexaenoic acid; MRS, magnetic resonance spectroscopy; NAFLD, nonalcoholic fatty liver disease.

Table 9
International studies of lifestyle intervention on obese children with suspected NAFLD determined by ultrasound

Study	Year	Location	Nᵃ	Duration	Study population	Intensity of intervention	Amount of weight lost	Results
Reinehr et al [188]	2009	Germany	152/160	2 years	Ages 6–16 years All obese NAFLD suspected based on US, ↑ ALT, exclusion other causes	1-year outpatient intervention program including group exercise 1×/week nutritional course 2×/month for 3 months behavior therapy 2×/month for 3 months individual psychological counseling for 6 months parent counseling 1–2×/month for 6 months	82/109 (75%) in intervention ↓ BMI Z-score at 1 and 2 years (−0.23 year 1, −0.3 year 2)	↓ ALT by mean 9 U/L from baseline in intervention group Greatest degree of improvement seen in those children with greatest amount of weight loss (↓ BMI Z-score >0.5, or approximately 5 kg)

Study	Year	Country	n[a]	Duration	Population	Intervention	BMI Results	Liver Results
Wang et al [190]	2008	China	76/76	1 month	Ages 10–17 years (mean 13.7) All obese NAFLD suspected based on US, ↑ ALT	Summer camp intervention (n = 19): 3 hours of aerobic exercise daily 1300–1600 kcal, individualized, low fat diet daily Control group (n = 38) no intervention Vitamin E group + lifestyle advice (n = 19)	Summer camp group: ↓ mean BMI Z-score from 3.02 to 2.15 (approx 7 kg weight loss)	Summer camp: ↓ ALT from mean 153 ± 49 to 64 ± 24 U/L ↓ AST from mean 93 ± 39 to 45 ± 19 Significantly greater decrease in ALT and BMI versus vitamin E/lifestyle group No change in ALT, AST, BMI control group
de Piano et al [187]	2007	Brazil	34/43	12 weeks	Ages 15 to 19 years BMI 34.2 ± 2.9 kg/m^2 13 patients with suspected NAFLD based on US	Monthly endocrine consults Weekly nutrition classes Weekly behavior modification classes 1 hour personalized aerobic exercise 3×/week	With NAFLD: BMI ↓ BMI 35.8 to 33.9 (NS) Without NAFLD: ↓ BMI from 33.5 to 32.5 ($P = .01$)	10 subjects with suspected NAFLD completed study, 24 without Ultrasound normalized in 4/10 with NAFLD
Tock et al [189]	2006	Brazil	73/73	12 weeks	Ages 15–19, mean 17 years BMI 36.5 ± 2.9	Nutritional training every 3 weeks Telephone access to dietitian 2 group 1-hour aerobic exercise sessions/week	48% lost weight, 48% maintained weight, 4% gained weight ↓ BMI from 36.5 to 34.4	Unclear how many children had normalization of liver US at the end of the study

Abbreviations: ALT, alanine aminotransferase; AST, aspartate aminotransferase; BMI, body mass index; NAFLD, nonalcoholic fatty liver disease; NS, not significant; US, ultrasonography.

[a]Children completing study/children initially enrolled in study.

either metformin or vitamin E or placebo for 96 weeks. The trial will assess the change in serum ALT and histology. A detailed description of the trial design was recently published [194]. The outcomes from the trial are anticipated in 2010.

Several adult trials have evaluated the efficacy of thiazolinediones for the treatment of NAFLD, and have produced conflicting results. Most trials showed improvement in hepatic steatosis [195–197] and inflammation [195,196]. However, only one trial to date showed improvement in fibrosis compared with placebo [195]. The Pioglitazone versus Vitamin E versus Placebo for the Treatment of Nondiabetic Patients with Nonalcoholic Steatohepatitis trial was recently completed. This multicenter, 96-week study with 247 subjects assessed the response to pioglitazone or vitamin E on liver histology with pre- and posttreatment liver biopsies. Subjects receiving vitamin E and pioglitazone both had improved serum ALT, steatosis, inflammation, and ballooning compared with placebo. However, only vitamin E met the primary end point of the study, a decrease in NAS of 2 points or more. Neither drug resulted in a change in fibrosis [198,199]. Of note, the safety of these medications has not been established in children.

Hepatoprotective agents

Several studies have or are currently investigating the effects of hepatoprotective agents on NAFLD in children. An open-label pilot study of vitamin E in 11 children with suspected NAFLD based on ultrasonography showed improvement in serum aminotransferases in all subjects, without concomitant weight loss [200]. Further studies have shown conflicting results. In a 1-year trial of 88 children with biopsy-proven NAFLD, Nobili and colleagues [201] evaluated the effect of 600 IU/d of vitamin E and 500 IU/d of vitamin C or placebo on serum aminotransferases and prevalence of NAFLD by ultrasonography. Both the treatment group and the control group also received nutritional and physical activity counseling, with monthly 1-hour sessions with a dietitian. Serum ALT decreased in both the treatment and placebo groups, but was not significantly different between groups. In a 1-year open-label continuation of the same trial, the investigators reported the effect of vitamins E and C on liver histology, among the 60% of children who chose to continue the study and undergo a repeat liver biopsy [202]. All 25 children in the vitamin group and 28 children in the placebo group were also enrolled in the same lifestyle intervention program as described for the first year of the trial. ALT and AST improved in both treatment and placebo groups, but there was no significant difference between the 2 groups. Investigators reported significant improvement in steatosis, ballooning, and lobular inflammation in both groups, but no significant difference between the groups. There was no change in fibrosis or portal inflammation.

There has been great interest in the potential hepatoprotective properties of bile acids and bile acid–like compounds. In the first study to evaluate pharmacologic treatment of NAFLD in children, Obinata and colleagues [203] evaluated taurine, a major constituent of bile, in 10 obese children with suspected NAFLD based on CT and elevated aminotransferases. Subjects received 2 to 6 g of taurine powder daily for 6 months, as well as a dietary modification. A decrease in the degree of hepatic fat on CT and improvement in serum ALT was found, irrespective of the amount of weight lost. Despite this finding, there have been no subsequent studies on the potential therapeutic value of taurine on NAFLD.

Ursodeoxycholic acid (UDCA), a secondary bile acid formed by intestinal bacteria, has been evaluated in several randomized, controlled treatment trials of NAFLD in adults. UDCA alone or in combination with vitamin E or C has not been shown to significantly decrease serum ALT compared with placebo [204,205]. An adult trial with end-of-treatment biopsy also did not find a difference in histology between subjects taking UDCA versus those taking placebo [166]. However, this study did not meet statistical power, and thus the question of whether UDCA improves histology in NAFLD remains controversial. A 12-month trial of 98 adults with NAFLD assessing the effect of high-dose UDCA on serum ALT was recently completed in Europe [206]. The results of this trial are pending. There have been no randomized controlled trials on the effect of UDCA in children with NAFLD.

A novel application of the hepatoprotective concept under investigation is bile acid activation of the nuclear hormone receptor Farnesoid X. In a preliminary double-blind, randomized, placebo-controlled study of INT-747, a synthetic agonist of the Farnesoid X receptor, 63 adults with diabetes and NAFLD received either INT-747 or placebo for 6 weeks. Compared with placebo, INT-747 led to improved glucose disposal rate, markers of fibrosis, and weight loss [207]. A second nonrandomized, placebo-controlled, double-blind, crossover trial of 48 patients is currently under way in Europe to evaluate the effects of activation of this receptor on hepatic lipid and glucose metabolism [208].

Other antioxidants, such as low-dose carnitine, probucol, and N-acetylcysteine, have been tested in adult treatment trials; none of these were found to significantly decrease ALT compared with placebo [209–211]. However, one 6-month controlled trial did show a significant reduction in ALT levels in subjects taking high-dose (3 g per day) L-carnitine versus placebo [211]. However, this was not associated with a significant change in the degree of steatosis in the 50 subjects who received an end-of-study biopsy.

Other pharmacologic treatments

Other pharmacologic treatments have been explored in adults with NAFLD. Several very small studies have evaluated the effect of 3-hydroxy-3-methyl-glutaryl-CoA (HMG-CoA) reductase inhibitors on liver histology, with conflicting results [212,213]. Whether these agents result in improvement in adult NAFLD remains to be determined by adequately powered treatment trials. No data exist as to whether HMG-CoA reductase inhibitors have a therapeutic effect on pediatric NAFLD. The American Association of Pediatrics currently endorses these drugs as first-line therapy in children aged 8 years and older with hypercholesterolemia [214]. Though most treatment trials to date do not report significant side effects [215], the long-term safety of these drugs has not been definitively established in children [216]. Serum aminotransferases should be followed in children with NAFLD who are prescribed a statin for treatment of hypercholesterolemia.

The gastric and pancreatic lipase inhibitor orlistat has been evaluated in adult studies. In a randomized controlled trial, 40 patients with biopsy-proven NAFLD completed the study, which included orlistat or placebo plus behavioral modification. Of these, 22 underwent repeat liver biopsy. There was no difference in the degree of improvement of fibrosis or steatosis between the treatment and placebo groups. However, serum ALT was reduced by nearly 50% in the orlistat group, versus 26% in the control group. The amount of weight lost was not significantly different between groups [217]. Although orlistat is approved for the treatment of obesity in children aged 12 years and older, whether it has a therapeutic effect on NAFLD is unknown.

Surgery

Given the role of obesity in the pathogenesis of NAFLD, bariatric surgery has been proposed as a potential treatment strategy. Bariatric surgery in adults has been shown to improve several metabolic abnormalities associated with NAFLD, including markers of inflammation and fibrogenesis, even in the absence of a concomitant decrease in the degree of hepatic inflammation or fibrosis [218]. In adults, weight loss surgery has also been shown to resolve hepatic steatosis and, in most studies, inflammation. NASH was improved in the majority of affected patients [219–221]. The degree of improvement in steatosis may be related to the degree of improvement in insulin resistance [221]. Furthermore, some studies report a decrease in hepatic fibrosis after surgery [220,222]. However, one prospective study of 267 patients found a slight increase in fibrosis [221].

The issue of NAFLD and bariatric surgery in children is complex, as children with a clinical diagnosis of NAFLD are different to those typically undergoing bariatric surgery. Children with a clinical diagnosis of NAFLD tend to be younger, less obese, and with more severe disease than adolescents undergoing surgical treatment of obesity. Whether requirements for bariatric surgery should be modified in the context of NAFLD needs to be determined [110]. Though several studies report comorbidity resolution after bariatric surgery in adolescents [223–225], none comment on the resolution of NAFLD. Only one study reports reduced ALT and AST 1 to 2 years after surgery [224]. Despite the lack of pediatric data regarding bariatric surgery and NAFLD, current best practice guidelines for adolescent weight-loss surgery state that severe or progressive NASH is a "strong indication" for early surgical intervention. These guidelines also recommend a BMI cut-point for surgery in affected adolescents of greater than 35 kg/m^2. Roux-en-Y gastric bypass is considered safe and effective in very obese adolescents. Adjustable gastric banding is not currently approved by the Food and Drug Administration for patients younger than 18 years [226]. Future studies with follow-up liver biopsies are needed to identify whether bariatric surgery improves NAFLD in adolescents.

No definitive treatment for NAFLD yet exists. Only 2 studies to date have assessed histologic response to treatment with an end-of-study biopsy; thus, the effect of treatment on pediatric NAFLD is largely unknown. Furthermore, many studies to date have been limited by small sample size and significant dropout rates, illustrating the need for adequate enrollment and follow-up. In addition, most studies have targeted the broader spectrum of NAFLD, rather than focusing on NASH, which is associated with the most morbidity and mortality. Adequately powered, controlled clinical trials with appropriate end points are needed to guide treatment protocols.

SUMMARY

Our understanding of pediatric NAFLD has progressed substantially over the past 20 years. Symptoms of NAFLD appear to be more frequent than previously recognized, suggesting that physicians should give consideration to a broader range of symptoms than those traditionally thought to be related to liver disease. Children with NAFLD are at risk for cirrhosis and end-stage liver disease. This risk varies greatly by the histologic severity of disease at diagnosis. For noninvasive biomarkers to be clinically useful for risk stratification, large well-designed discovery and validation studies are needed. Major advancements have been made in the radiologic evaluation of NAFLD, especially with MRI, which is an attractive candidate for noninvasive diagnosis and monitoring of disease severity. This technology has been for fundamental for studies on the heritability and genetics of NAFLD.

Children with NAFLD are also at risk for diabetes and cardiovascular disease, and screening for such diseases should be incorporated into diagnostic and therapeutic strategies. Numerous clinical trials are ongoing. The results of such work are eagerly anticipated and will allow for refinement of treatment. The worldwide prevalence of NAFLD remains high, and warrants a campaign for greater awareness as well as collaboration between physicians in both primary and subspecialty care to optimize clinical outcomes.

References

[1] Brunt EM. Pathology of fatty liver disease. Mod Pathol 2007;20(Suppl 1):S40–8.

[2] Matteoni CA, Younossi ZM, Gramlich T, et al. Nonalcoholic fatty liver disease: a spectrum of clinical and pathological severity. Gastroenterology 1999;116:1413–9.

[3] Brunt EM. Nonalcoholic steatohepatitis: definition and pathology. Semin Liver Dis 2001;21:3–16.

[4] Brunt EM, Janney CG, Di Bisceglie AM, et al. Nonalcoholic steatohepatitis: a proposal for grading and staging the histological lesions. Am J Gastroenterol 1999;94:2467–74.

[5] Kleiner DE, Brunt EM, Van Natta M, et al. Design and validation of a histological scoring system for nonalcoholic fatty liver disease. Hepatology 2005;41:1313–21.

[6] Mendler MH, Kanel G, Govindarajan S. Proposal for a histological scoring and grading system for non-alcoholic fatty liver disease. Liver Int 2005;25:294–304.

[7] Promrat K, Lutchman G, Uwaifo GI, et al. A pilot study of pioglitazone treatment for nonalcoholic steatohepatitis. Hepatology 2004;39:188–96.

[8] Brunt EM. Nonalcoholic steatohepatitis. Semin Liver Dis 2004;24:3–20.

[9] Chalasani N, Wilson L, Kleiner DE, et al. Relationship of steatosis grade and zonal location to histological features of steatohepatitis in adult patients with non-alcoholic fatty liver disease. J Hepatol 2008;48:829–34.

[10] Schaff Z, Lapis K. Fine structure of hepatocytes during the etiology of several common pathologies. J Electron Microsc Tech 1990;14:179–207.

[11] Lackner C, Gogg-Kamerer M, Zatloukal K, et al. Ballooned hepatocytes in steatohepatitis: the value of keratin immunohistochemistry for diagnosis. J Hepatol 2008;48:821–8.

[12] Schwimmer JB, Behling C, Newbury R, et al. Histopathology of pediatric nonalcoholic fatty liver disease. Hepatology 2005;42:641–9.

[13] Nobili V, Marcellini M, Devito R, et al. NAFLD in children: a prospective clinical-pathological study and effect of lifestyle advice. Hepatology 2006;44:458–65.

[14] Carter-Kent C, Yerian LM, Brunt EM, et al. Nonalcoholic steatohepatitis in children: a multicenter clinicopathological study. Hepatology 2009;50:1113–20.

[15] Ko JS, Yoon JM, Yang HR, et al. Clinical and histological features of nonalcoholic fatty liver disease in children. Dig Dis Sci 2009;54:2225–30.

[16] Xanthakos S, Miles L, Bucuvalas J, et al. Histologic spectrum of nonalcoholic fatty liver disease in morbidly obese adolescents. Clin Gastroenterol Hepatol 2006;4: 226–32.

[17] Brunt EM, Kleiner DE, Wilson LA, et al. Portal chronic inflammation in nonalcoholic fatty liver disease (NAFLD): a histologic marker of advanced NAFLD-Clinicopathologic correlations from the nonalcoholic steatohepatitis clinical research network. Hepatology 2009;49:809–20.

[18] Adani GL, Baccarani U, Sainz-Barriga M, et al. The role of hepatic biopsy to detect macrovacuolar steatosis during liver procurement. Transplant Proc 2006;38:1404–6.

[19] Joy D, Thava VR, Scott BB. Diagnosis of fatty liver disease: is biopsy necessary? Eur J Gastroenterol Hepatol 2003;15:539–43.

[20] Longo R, Pollesello P, Ricci C, et al. Proton MR spectroscopy in quantitative in vivo determination of fat content in human liver steatosis. J Magn Reson Imaging 1995;5:281–5.

[21] Lupsor M, Badea R. Imaging diagnosis and quantification of hepatic steatosis: is it an accepted alternative to needle biopsy? Rom J Gastroenterol 2005;14:419–25.

[22] Smith EH. Complications of percutaneous abdominal fine-needle biopsy. Radiology 1991;178:253–8 [review].

[23] Schwimmer JB, Deutsch R, Rauch JB, et al. Obesity, insulin resistance, and other clinicopathological correlates of pediatric nonalcoholic fatty liver disease. J Pediatr 2003;143:500–5.

[24] Nobili V, Manco M, Ciampalini P, et al. Leptin, free leptin index, insulin resistance and liver fibrosis in children with non-alcoholic fatty liver disease. Eur J Endocrinol 2006;155: 735–43.

[25] Patton HM, Lavine JE, Van Natta ML, et al. Clinical correlates of histopathology in pediatric nonalcoholic steatohepatitis. Gastroenterology 2008;135:1961–71, e1962.

[26] Nobili V, Alkhouri N, Alisi A, et al. Retinol-binding protein 4: a promising circulating marker of liver damage in pediatric nonalcoholic fatty liver disease. Clin Gastroenterol Hepatol 2009;7:575–9.

[27] Poynard T, Ratziu V, Charlotte F, et al. Diagnostic value of biochemical markers (NashTest) for the prediction of non alcoholo steato hepatitis in patients with non-alcoholic fatty liver disease. BMC Gastroenterol 2006;6:34.

[28] Miele L, Forgione A, La Torre G, et al. Serum levels of hyaluronic acid and tissue metalloproteinase inhibitor-1 combined with age predict the presence of nonalcoholic steatohepatitis in a pilot cohort of subjects with nonalcoholic fatty liver disease. Transl Res 2009;154: 194–201.

[29] Feldstein AE, Canbay A, Angulo P, et al. Hepatocyte apoptosis and fas expression are prominent features of human nonalcoholic steatohepatitis. Gastroenterology 2003;125: 437–43.

[30] Danial NN, Korsmeyer SJ. Cell death: critical control points. Cell 2004;116:205–19.

[31] Wieckowska A, Zein NN, Yerian LM, et al. In vivo assessment of liver cell apoptosis as a novel biomarker of disease severity in nonalcoholic fatty liver disease. Hepatology 2006;44:27–33.

[32] Feldstein AE, Wieckowska A, Lopez AR, et al. Cytokeratin-18 fragment levels as noninvasive biomarkers for nonalcoholic steatohepatitis: a multicenter validation study. Hepatology 2009;50:1072–8.

[33] Mitry RR, De Bruyne R, Quaglia A, et al. Noninvasive diagnosis of nonalcoholic fatty liver disease using serum biomarkers. Hepatology 2007;46:2047–8, author reply 2048.

[34] Nobili V, Parkes J, Bottazzo G, et al. Performance of ELF serum markers in predicting fibrosis stage in pediatric non-alcoholic fatty liver disease. Gastroenterology 2009;136: 160–7.

[35] Yajima Y, Ohta K, Narui T, et al. Ultrasonographical diagnosis of fatty liver: significance of the liver-kidney contrast. Tohoku J Exp Med 1983;139:43–50.

[36] Zwiebel WJ. Sonographic diagnosis of diffuse liver disease. Semin Ultrasound CT MR 1995;16:8–15.

[37] Karcaaltincaba M, Akhan O. Imaging of hepatic steatosis and fatty sparing. Eur J Radiol 2007;61:33–43.

[38] Saadeh S, Younossi ZM, Remer EM, et al. The utility of radiological imaging in nonalcoholic fatty liver disease. Gastroenterology 2002;123:745–50.

[39] Pacifico L, Celestre M, Anania C, et al. MRI and ultrasound for hepatic fat quantification: relationships to clinical and metabolic characteristics of pediatric nonalcoholic fatty liver disease. Acta Paediatr 2007;96:542–7.

[40] Graif M, Yanuka M, Baraz M, et al. Quantitative estimation of attenuation in ultrasound video images: correlation with histology in diffuse liver disease. Invest Radiol 2000;35: 319–24.

[41] Joseph AE, Saverymuttu SH, al-Sam S, et al. Comparison of liver histology with ultrasonography in assessing diffuse parenchymal liver disease. Clin Radiol 1991;43:26–31.

[42] Mathiesen UL, Franzen LE, Aselius H, et al. Increased liver echogenicity at ultrasound examination reflects degree of steatosis but not of fibrosis in asymptomatic patients with mild/moderate abnormalities of liver transaminases. Dig Liver Dis 2002;34:516–22.

[43] Saverymuttu SH, Joseph AE, Maxwell JD. Ultrasound scanning in the detection of hepatic fibrosis and steatosis. Br Med J (Clin Res Ed) 1986;292:13–5.

[44] Ali R, Cusi K. New diagnostic and treatment approaches in non-alcoholic fatty liver disease (NAFLD). Ann Med 2009;41:265–78.

[45] Celle G, Savarino V, Picciotto A, et al. Is hepatic ultrasonography a valid alternative tool to liver biopsy? Report on 507 cases studied with both techniques. Dig Dis Sci 1988;33: 467–71.

[46] Hepburn MJ, Vos JA, Fillman EP, et al. The accuracy of the report of hepatic steatosis on ultrasonography in patients infected with hepatitis C in a clinical setting: a retrospective observational study. BMC Gastroenterol 2005;5:14.

[47] Needleman L, Kurtz AB, Rifkin MD, et al. Sonography of diffuse benign liver disease: accuracy of pattern recognition and grading. AJR Am J Roentgenol 1986;146:1011–5.

[48] Strauss S, Gavish E, Gottlieb P, et al. Interobserver and intraobserver variability in the sonographic assessment of fatty liver. AJR Am J Roentgenol 2007;189:W320–3.

[49] Bydder GM, Chapman RW, Harry D, et al. Computed tomography attenuation values in fatty liver. J Comput Tomogr 1981;5:33–5.

[50] Speliotes EK, Massaro JM, Hoffmann U, et al. Liver fat is reproducibly measured using computed tomography in the Framingham Heart Study. J Gastroenterol Hepatol 2008;23:894–9.

[51] Limanond P, Raman SS, Lassman C, et al. Macrovesicular hepatic steatosis in living related liver donors: correlation between CT and histologic findings. Radiology 2004;230: 276–80.

[52] Lee SW, Park SH, Kim KW, et al. Unenhanced CT for assessment of macrovesicular hepatic steatosis in living liver donors: comparison of visual grading with liver attenuation index. Radiology 2007;244:479–85.

[53] Schwimmer JB. Definitive diagnosis and assessment of risk for nonalcoholic fatty liver disease in children and adolescents. Semin Liver Dis 2007;27:312–8.

[54] Hamer OW, Aguirre DA, Casola G, et al. Fatty liver: imaging patterns and pitfalls. Radiographics 2006;26:1637–53.

[55] Siegelman ES, Rosen MA. Imaging of hepatic steatosis. Semin Liver Dis 2001;21:71–80.

[56] Mehta SR, Thomas EL, Bell JD, et al. Non-invasive means of measuring hepatic fat content. World J Gastroenterol 2008;14:3476–83.

[57] Cassidy FH, Yokoo T, Aganovic L, et al. Fatty liver disease: MR imaging techniques for the detection and quantification of liver steatosis. Radiographics 2009;29:231–60.

[58] Longo R, Ricci C, Masutti F, et al. Fatty infiltration of the liver. Quantification by 1H localized magnetic resonance spectroscopy and comparison with computed tomography. Invest Radiol 1993;28:297–302.

[59] Thomsen C, Becker U, Winkler K, et al. Quantification of liver fat using magnetic resonance spectroscopy. Magn Reson Imaging 1994;12:487–95.

[60] Kim H, Taksali SE, Dufour S, et al. Comparative MR study of hepatic fat quantification using single-voxel proton spectroscopy, two-point Dixon and three-point IDEAL. Magn Reson Med 2008;59:521–7.

[61] Thomas EL, Hamilton G, Patel N, et al. Hepatic triglyceride content and its relation to body adiposity: a magnetic resonance imaging and proton magnetic resonance spectroscopy study. Gut 2005;54:122–7.

[62] Browning JD, Szczepaniak LS, Dobbins R, et al. Prevalence of hepatic steatosis in an urban population in the United States: impact of ethnicity. Hepatology 2004;40: 1387–95.

[63] Szczepaniak LS, Nurenberg P, Leonard D, et al. Magnetic resonance spectroscopy to measure hepatic triglyceride content: prevalence of hepatic steatosis in the general population. Am J Physiol Endocrinol Metab 2005;288:E462–8.

[64] Vuppalanchi R, Cummings OW, Saxena R, et al. Relationship among histologic, radiologic, and biochemical assessments of hepatic steatosis: a study of human liver samples. J Clin Gastroenterol 2007;41:206–10.

[65] Bugianesi E, Gentilcore E, Manini R, et al. A randomized controlled trial of metformin versus vitamin E or prescriptive diet in nonalcoholic fatty liver disease. Am J Gastroenterol 2005;100:1082–90.

[66] Carey DG, Cowin GJ, Galloway GJ, et al. Effect of rosiglitazone on insulin sensitivity and body composition in type 2 diabetic patients. Obes Res 2002;10:1008–15.

[67] Schwimmer JB, Middleton MS, Deutsch R, et al. A phase 2 clinical trial of metformin as a treatment for non-diabetic paediatric non-alcoholic steatohepatitis. Aliment Pharmacol Ther 2005;21:871–9.

[68] Hamilton G, Middleton MS, Bydder M, et al. Effect of PRESS and STEAM sequences on magnetic resonance spectroscopic liver fat quantification. J Magn Reson Imaging 2009;30:145–52.

[69] Taouli B, Ehman RL, Reeder SB. Advanced MRI methods for assessment of chronic liver disease. AJR Am J Roentgenol 2009;193:14–27.

[70] Dixon WT. Simple proton spectroscopic imaging. Radiology 1984;153:189–94.

[71] Sirlin CB. Noninvasive imaging biomarkers for steatosis assessment. Liver Transpl 2009;15:1389–91.

[72] Mazhar SM, Shiehmorteza M, Sirlin CB. Noninvasive assessment of hepatic steatosis. Clin Gastroenterol Hepatol 2009;7:135–40.

[73] Fishbein M, Castro F, Cheruku S, et al. Hepatic MRI for fat quantitation: its relationship to fat morphology, diagnosis, and ultrasound. J Clin Gastroenterol 2005;39:619–25.

[74] Kim SH, Lee JM, Han JK, et al. Hepatic macrosteatosis: predicting appropriateness of liver donation by using MR imaging—correlation with histopathologic findings. Radiology 2006;240:116–29.

[75] Qayyum A, Goh JS, Kakar S, et al. Accuracy of liver fat quantification at MR imaging: comparison of out-of-phase gradient-echo and fat-saturated fast spin-echo techniques—initial experience. Radiology 2005;237:507–11.

[76] Borra RJ, Salo S, Dean K, et al. Nonalcoholic fatty liver disease: rapid evaluation of liver fat content with in-phase and out-of-phase MR imaging. Radiology 2009;250:130–6.

[77] Fishbein MH, Gardner KG, Potter CJ, et al. Introduction of fast MR imaging in the assessment of hepatic steatosis. Magn Reson Imaging 1997;15:287–93.

[78] Hussain HK, Chenevert TL, Londy FJ, et al. Hepatic fat fraction: MR imaging for quantitative measurement and display—early experience. Radiology 2005;237:1048–55.

[79] Bydder M, Yokoo T, Hamilton G, et al. Relaxation effects in the quantification of fat using gradient echo imaging. Magn Reson Imaging 2008;26:347–59.

[80] Liu CY, McKenzie CA, Yu H, et al. Fat quantification with IDEAL gradient echo imaging: correction of bias from T(1) and noise. Magn Reson Med 2007;58:354–64.

[81] Yokoo T, Bydder M, Hamilton G, et al. Nonalcoholic fatty liver disease: diagnostic and fat-grading accuracy of low-flip-angle multiecho gradient-recalled-echo MR imaging at 1.5 T. Radiology 2009;251:67–76.

[82] Brix G, Heiland S, Bellemann ME, et al. MR imaging of fat-containing tissues: valuation of two quantitative imaging techniques in comparison with localized proton spectroscopy. Magn Reson Imaging 1993;11:977–91.

[83] Reeder SB, Robson PM, Yu H, et al. Quantification of hepatic steatosis with MRI: the effects of accurate fat spectral modeling. J Magn Reson Imaging 2009;29:1332–9.

[84] Yu H, Shimakawa A, McKenzie CA, et al. Multiecho water-fat separation and simultaneous R2* estimation with multifrequency fat spectrum modeling. Magn Reson Med 2008;60:1122–34.

[85] Hines CD, Yu H, Shimakawa A, et al. T1 independent, T2* corrected MRI with accurate spectral modeling for quantification of fat: validation in a fat-water-SPIO phantom. J Magn Reson Imaging 2009;30:1215–22.

[86] Huwart L, Sempoux C, Vicaut E, et al. Magnetic resonance elastography for the noninvasive staging of liver fibrosis. Gastroenterology 2008;135:32–40.

[87] Sandrin L, Fourquet B, Hasquenoph JM, et al. Transient elastography: a new noninvasive method for assessment of hepatic fibrosis. Ultrasound Med Biol 2003;29:1705–13.

[88] Yeh WC, Li PC, Jeng YM, et al. Elastic modulus measurements of human liver and correlation with pathology. Ultrasound Med Biol 2002;28:467–74.

[89] Yoneda M, Yoneda M, Mawatari H, et al. Noninvasive assessment of liver fibrosis by measurement of stiffness in patients with nonalcoholic fatty liver disease (NAFLD). Dig Liver Dis 2008;40:371–8.

[90] Nobili V, Vizzutti F, Arena U, et al. Accuracy and reproducibility of transient elastography for the diagnosis of fibrosis in pediatric nonalcoholic steatohepatitis. Hepatology 2008;48:442–8.

[91] Fraquelli M, Rigamonti C, Casazza G, et al. Reproducibility of transient elastography in the evaluation of liver fibrosis in patients with chronic liver disease. Gut 2007;56:968–73.

[92] Coco B, Oliveri F, Maina AM, et al. Transient elastography: a new surrogate marker of liver fibrosis influenced by major changes of transaminases. J Viral Hepat 2007;14:360–9.

[93] Lebray P, Varnous S, Charlotte F, et al. Liver stiffness is an unreliable marker of liver fibrosis in patients with cardiac insufficiency. Hepatology 2008;48:2089.

[94] Ganne-Carrie N, Ziol M, de Ledinghen V, et al. Accuracy of liver stiffness measurement for the diagnosis of cirrhosis in patients with chronic liver diseases. Hepatology 2006;44:1511–7.

[95] Ito K, Mitchell DG, Siegelman ES. Cirrhosis: MR imaging features. Magn Reson Imaging Clin N Am 2002;10:75–92, vi.

[96] Martin DR. Magnetic resonance imaging of diffuse liver diseases. Top Magn Reson Imaging 2002;13:151–63.

[97] Brancatelli G, Federle MP, Ambrosini R, et al. Cirrhosis: CT and MR imaging evaluation. Eur J Radiol 2007;61:57–69.

[98] Aguirre DA, Behling CA, Alpert E, et al. Liver fibrosis: noninvasive diagnosis with double contrast material-enhanced MR imaging. Radiology 2006;239:425–37.

[99] Hughes-Cassidy F, Chavez AD, Schlang A, et al. Superparamagnetic iron oxides and low molecular weight gadolinium chelates are synergistic for direct visualization of advanced liver fibrosis. J Magn Reson Imaging 2007;26:728–37.

[100] Faria SC, Ganesan K, Mwangi I, et al. MR imaging of liver fibrosis: current state of the art. Radiographics 2009;29:1615–35.

[101] Semelka RC, Chung JJ, Hussain SM, et al. Chronic hepatitis: correlation of early patchy and late linear enhancement patterns on gadolinium-enhanced MR images with histopathology initial experience. J Magn Reson Imaging 2001;13:385–91.

[102] Ide M, Yamate J, Machida Y, et al. Emergence of different macrophage populations in hepatic fibrosis following thioacetamide-induced acute hepatocyte injury in rats. J Comp Pathol 2003;128:41–51.

[103] Lieber CS. Alcoholic fatty liver: its pathogenesis and mechanism of progression to inflammation and fibrosis. Alcohol 2004;34:9–19.

[104] Tanimoto A, Yuasa Y, Shinmoto H, et al. Superparamagnetic iron oxide-mediated hepatic signal intensity change in patients with and without cirrhosis: pulse sequence effects and Kupffer cell function. Radiology 2002;222:661–6.

[105] Hanna RF, Kased N, Kwan SW, et al. Double-contrast MRI for accurate staging of hepatocellular carcinoma in patients with cirrhosis. AJR Am J Roentgenol 2008;190:47–57.

[106] Bensamoun SF, Wang L, Robert L, et al. Measurement of liver stiffness with two imaging techniques: magnetic resonance elastography and ultrasound elastometry. J Magn Reson Imaging 2008;28:1287–92.

[107] Rouviere O, Yin M, Dresner MA, et al. MR elastography of the liver: preliminary results. Radiology 2006;240:440–8.

[108] Yin M, Talwalkar JA, Glaser KJ, et al. Assessment of hepatic fibrosis with magnetic resonance elastography. Clin Gastroenterol Hepatol 2007;5:1207–13, e1202.

[109] Talwalkar JA, Yin M, Fidler JL, et al. Magnetic resonance imaging of hepatic fibrosis: emerging clinical applications. Hepatology 2008;47:332–42.

[110] Pardee PE, Lavine JE, Schwimmer JB. Diagnosis and treatment of pediatric nonalcoholic steatohepatitis and the implications for bariatric surgery. Semin Pediatr Surg 2009;18: 144–51.

[111] Kahn CR, Flier JS, Bar RS, et al. The syndromes of insulin resistance and acanthosis nigricans. Insulin-receptor disorders in man. N Engl J Med 1976;294:739–45.

[112] Moller DE, Flier JS. Insulin resistance—mechanisms, syndromes, and implications. N Engl J Med 1991;325:938–48.

[113] Poretsky L, Piper B. Insulin resistance, hypersecretion of LH, and a dual-defect hypothesis for the pathogenesis of polycystic ovary syndrome. Obstet Gynecol 1994;84: 613–21.

[114] Jeanrenaud B. Hyperinsulinemia in obesity syndromes: its metabolic consequences and possible etiology. Metabolism 1978;27:1881–92.

[115] Barrows BR, Parks EJ. Contributions of different fatty acid sources to very low-density lipoprotein-triacylglycerol in the fasted and fed states. J Clin Endocrinol Metab 2006;91: 1446–52.

[116] Donnelly KL, Smith CI, Schwarzenberg SJ, et al. Sources of fatty acids stored in liver and secreted via lipoproteins in patients with nonalcoholic fatty liver disease. J Clin Invest 2005;115:1343–51.

[117] Fabbrini E, deHaseth D, Deivanayagam S, et al. Alterations in fatty acid kinetics in obese adolescents with increased intrahepatic triglyceride content. Obesity (Silver Spring) 2009;17:25–9.

[118] Boden G, She P, Mozzoli M, et al. Free fatty acids produce insulin resistance and activate the proinflammatory nuclear factor-kappaB pathway in rat liver. Diabetes 2005;54: 3458–65.

[119] Cai D, Yuan M, Frantz DF, et al. Local and systemic insulin resistance resulting from hepatic activation of IKK-beta and NF-kappaB. Nat Med 2005;11:183–90.

[120] Musso G, Gambino R, Cassader M. Non-alcoholic fatty liver disease from pathogenesis to management: an update. Obes Rev 2010;11:430–45.

[121] Li Z, Berk M, McIntyre TM, et al. The lysosomal-mitochondrial axis in free fatty acid-induced hepatic lipotoxicity. Hepatology 2008;47:1495–503.

[122] Connolly MK, Bedrosian AS, Mallen-St Clair J, et al. In liver fibrosis, dendritic cells govern hepatic inflammation in mice via TNF-alpha. J Clin Invest 2009;119:3213–25.

[123] Nieto N. Oxidative-stress and IL-6 mediate the fibrogenic effects of Kupffer cells on stellate cells. Hepatology 2006;44:1487–501.

[124] Wang J, Leclercq I, Brymora JM, et al. Kupffer cells mediate leptin-induced liver fibrosis. Gastroenterology 2009;137:713–23.

[125] Louthan MV, Barve S, McClain CJ, et al. Decreased serum adiponectin: an early event in pediatric nonalcoholic fatty liver disease. J Pediatr 2005;147:835–8.

[126] Burgert TS, Taksali SE, Dziura J, et al. Alanine aminotransferase levels and fatty liver in childhood obesity: associations with insulin resistance, adiponectin, and visceral fat. J Clin Endocrinol Metab 2006;91:4287–94.

[127] Asano T, Watanabe K, Kubota N, et al. Adiponectin knockout mice on high fat diet develop fibrosing steatohepatitis. J Gastroenterol Hepatol 2009;24:1669–76.

[128] Fukushima J, Kamada Y, Matsumoto H, et al. Adiponectin prevents progression of steato-hepatitis in mice by regulating oxidative stress and Kupffer cell phenotype polarization. Hepatol Res 2009;39:724–38.

[129] Yamaguchi K, Yang L, McCall S, et al. Inhibiting triglyceride synthesis improves hepatic steatosis but exacerbates liver damage and fibrosis in obese mice with nonalcoholic stea-tohepatitis. Hepatology 2007;45:1366–74.

[130] Rigazio S, Lehto HR, Tuunanen H, et al. The lowering of hepatic fatty acid uptake improves liver function and insulin sensitivity without affecting hepatic fat content in humans. Am J Physiol Endocrinol Metab 2008;295:E413–9.

[131] Bruce KD, Cagampang FR, Argenton M, et al. Maternal high-fat feeding primes steatohe-patitis in adult mice offspring, involving mitochondrial dysfunction and altered lipogenesis gene expression. Hepatology 2009;50:1796–808.

[132] McCurdy CE, Bishop JM, Williams SM, et al. Maternal high-fat diet triggers lipotoxicity in the fetal livers of nonhuman primates. J Clin Invest 2009;119:323–35.

[133] Schwimmer JB, Deutsch R, Kahen T, et al. Prevalence of fatty liver in children and adoles-cents. Pediatrics 2006;118:1388–93.

[134] Schwimmer JB, Celedon MA, Lavine JE, et al. Heritability of nonalcoholic fatty liver disease. Gastroenterology 2009;136:1585–92.

[135] Wagenknecht LE, Scherzinger AL, Stamm ER, et al. Correlates and heritability of nonalco-holic fatty liver disease in a minority cohort. Obesity (Silver Spring) 2009;17:1240–6.

[136] Romeo S, Kozlitina J, Xing C, et al. Genetic variation in PNPLA3 confers susceptibility to nonalcoholic fatty liver disease. Nat Genet 2008;40:1461–5.

[137] Kotronen A, Johansson LE, Johansson LM, et al. A common variant in PNPLA3, which encodes adiponutrin, is associated with liver fat content in humans. Diabetologia 2009;52:1056–60.

[138] Sookoian S, Castano GO, Burgueno AL, et al. A nonsynonymous gene variant in the adi-ponutrin gene is associated with nonalcoholic fatty liver disease severity. J Lipid Res 2009;50:2111–6.

[139] Wilson PA, Gardner SD, Lambie NM, et al. Characterization of the human patatin-like phospholipase family. J Lipid Res 2006;47:1940–9.

[140] Kollerits B, Coassin S, Beckmann ND, et al. Genetic evidence for a role of adiponutrin in the metabolism of apolipoprotein B-containing lipoproteins. Hum Mol Genet 2009;18: 4669–76.

[141] Fraser A, Longnecker MP, Lawlor DA. Prevalence of elevated alanine aminotransferase among US adolescents and associated factors: NHANES 1999-2004. Gastroenterology 2007;133:1814–20.

[142] Kawasaki T, Hashimoto N, Kikuchi T, et al. The relationship between fatty liver and hyperinsulinemia in obese Japanese children. J Pediatr Gastroenterol Nutr 1997;24:317–21.

[143] Sagi R, Reif S, Neuman G, et al. Nonalcoholic fatty liver disease in overweight children and adolescents. Acta Paediatr 2007;96:1209–13.

[144] Nadeau KJ, Ehlers LB, Zeitler PS, et al. Treatment of non-alcoholic fatty liver disease with metformin versus lifestyle intervention in insulin-resistant adolescents. Pediatr Diabetes 2009;10:5–13.

[145] Schwimmer JB, McGreal N, Deutsch R, et al. Influence of gender, race, and ethnicity on suspected fatty liver in obese adolescents. Pediatrics 2005;115:e561–5.

[146] Quirós-Tejeira RE, Rivera CA, Ziba TT, et al. Risk for nonalcoholic fatty liver disease in Hispanic youth with BMI > or =95th percentile. J Pediatr Gastroenterol Nutr 2007;44: 228–36.

[147] Sartorio A, Del Col A, Agosti F, et al. Predictors of non-alcoholic fatty liver disease in obese children. Eur J Clin Nutr 2007;61:877–83.

[148] Louthan MV, Theriot JA, Zimmerman E, et al. Decreased prevalence of nonalcoholic fatty liver disease in black obese children. J Pediatr Gastroenterol Nutr 2005;41:426–9.

[149] Kistler KD, Molleston J, Unalp A, et al. Symptoms and quality of life in obese children and adolescents with nonalcoholic fatty liver disease. Aliment Pharmacol Ther 2009;31: 396–406.

[150] Hh AK, Henderson J, Vanhoesen K, et al. Nonalcoholic fatty liver disease in children: a single center experience. Clin Gastroenterol Hepatol 2008;6:799–802.

[151] Rhee H, Miles MS, Halpern CT, et al. Prevalence of recurrent physical symptoms in U.S. adolescents. Pediatr Nurs 2005;31:314–9, 350.

[152] Riley MR, Bass NM, Rosenthal P, et al. Underdiagnosis of pediatric obesity and underscreening for fatty liver disease and metabolic syndrome by pediatricians and pediatric subspecialists. J Pediatr 2005;147:839–42.

[153] Barlow SE. Expert committee recommendations regarding the prevention, assessment, and treatment of child and adolescent overweight and obesity: summary report. Pediatrics 2007;120(Suppl 4):S164–92.

[154] Schwimmer JB, Dunn W, Norman GJ, et al. SAFETY study: alanine aminotransferase cutoff values are set too high for reliable detection of pediatric chronic liver disease. Gastroenterology 2010;138:1357–64.

[155] Manco M, Bedogni G, Marcellini M, et al. Waist circumference correlates with liver fibrosis in children with non-alcoholic steatohepatitis. Gut 2008;57:1283–7.

[156] Anthropometry procedures manual. National Health and Nutrition Examination Survey. Center for Disease Control; 2000. Available at: http://www.cdc.gov/nchs/data/ nhanes/bm.pdf. Accessed September 12, 2009.

[157] Rashid M, Roberts EA. Nonalcoholic steatohepatitis in children. J Pediatr Gastroenterol Nutr 2000;30:48–53.

[158] Burke JP, Hale DE, Hazuda HP, et al. A quantitative scale of acanthosis nigricans. Diabetes Care 1999;22:1655–9.

[159] Schwimmer JB, Pardee PE, Lavine JE, et al. Cardiovascular risk factors and the metabolic syndrome in pediatric nonalcoholic fatty liver disease. Circulation 2008;118:277–83.

[160] Moreno M, Bataller R. Cytokines and renin-angiotensin system signaling in hepatic fibrosis. Clin Liver Dis 2008;12:825–52, ix.

[161] Puri M, Flynn JT. Management of hypertension in children and adolescents with the metabolic syndrome. J Cardiometab Syndr 2006;1:259–68.

[162] Ogden CL, Carroll MD, Curtin LR, et al. Prevalence of overweight and obesity in the United States, 1999–2004. JAMA 2006;295:1549–55.

[163] Guzzaloni G, Grugni G, Minocci A, et al. Liver steatosis in juvenile obesity: correlations with lipid profile, hepatic biochemical parameters and glycemic and insulinemic responses to an oral glucose tolerance test. Int J Obes Relat Metab Disord 2000;24:772–6.

[164] Manton ND, Lipsett J, Moore DJ, et al. Non-alcoholic steatohepatitis in children and adolescents. Med J Aust 2000;173:476–9.

[165] Harrison SA, Torgerson S, Hayashi PH. The natural history of nonalcoholic fatty liver disease: a clinical histopathological study. Am J Gastroenterol 2003;98:2042–7.

[166] Lindor KD, Kowdley KV, Heathcote EJ, et al. Ursodeoxycholic acid for treatment of nonalcoholic steatohepatitis: results of a randomized trial. Hepatology 2004;39:770–8.

[167] Adams LA, Feldstein A, Lindor KD, et al. Nonalcoholic fatty liver disease among patients with hypothalamic and pituitary dysfunction. Hepatology 2004;39:909–14.

[168] Evans HM, Shaikh MG, McKiernan PJ, et al. Acute fatty liver disease after suprasellar tumor resection. J Pediatr Gastroenterol Nutr 2004;39:288–91.

[169] Nakajima K, Hashimoto E, Kaneda H, et al. Pediatric nonalcoholic steatohepatitis associated with hypopituitarism. J Gastroenterol 2005;40:312–5.

[170] Bugianesi E. Non-alcoholic steatohepatitis and cancer. Clin Liver Dis 2007;11:191–207, x–xi.

[171] Cuadrado A, Orive A, Garcia-Suarez C, et al. Non-alcoholic steatohepatitis (NASH) and hepatocellular carcinoma. Obes Surg 2005;15:442–6.

[172] Hashizume H, Sato K, Takagi H, et al. Primary liver cancers with nonalcoholic steatohepatitis. Eur J Gastroenterol Hepatol 2007;19:827–34.

[173] Rubinstein E, Lavine JE, Schwimmer JB. Hepatic, cardiovascular, and endocrine outcomes of the histological subphenotypes of nonalcoholic fatty liver disease. Semin Liver Dis 2008;28:380–5.

[174] Sanyal AJ, Banas C, Sargeant C, et al. Similarities and differences in outcomes of cirrhosis due to nonalcoholic steatohepatitis and hepatitis C. Hepatology 2006;43:682–9.

[175] Bullock RE, Zaitoun AM, Aithal GP, et al. Association of non-alcoholic steatohepatitis without significant fibrosis with hepatocellular carcinoma. J Hepatol 2004;41:685–6.

[176] Zen Y, Katayanagi K, Tsuneyama K, et al. Hepatocellular carcinoma arising in non-alcoholic steatohepatitis. Pathol Int 2001;51:127–31.

[177] Koebnick C, Getahun D, Reynolds K, et al. Trends in nonalcoholic fatty liver disease-related hospitalizations in US children, adolescents, and young adults. J Pediatr Gastroenterol Nutr 2009;48:597–603.

[178] Feldstein AE, Charatcharoenwitthaya P, Treeprasertsuk S, et al. The natural history of nonalcoholic fatty liver disease in children: a follow-up study for up to 20 years. Gut 2009;58:1538–44.

[179] National Cholesterol Education Program (NCEP) Expert Panel on Detection, Evaluation, and Treatment of High Blood Cholesterol in Adults (Adult Treatment Panel III). Third Report of the National Cholesterol Education Program (NCEP) Expert Panel on Detection, Evaluation, and Treatment of High Blood Cholesterol in Adults (Adult Treatment Panel III) final report. Circulation 2002;106:3143–421.

[180] Ekstedt M, Franzen LE, Mathiesen UL, et al. Long-term follow-up of patients with NAFLD and elevated liver enzymes. Hepatology 2006;44:865–73.

[181] Demircioglu F, Kocyigit A, Arslan N, et al. Intima-media thickness of carotid artery and susceptibility to atherosclerosis in obese children with nonalcoholic fatty liver disease. J Pediatr Gastroenterol Nutr 2008;47:68–75.

[182] Pacifico L, Cantisani V, Ricci P, et al. Nonalcoholic fatty liver disease and carotid atherosclerosis in children. Pediatr Res 2008;63:423–7.

[183] Aygun C, Kocaman O, Sahin T, et al. Evaluation of metabolic syndrome frequency and carotid artery intima-media thickness as risk factors for atherosclerosis in patients with nonalcoholic fatty liver disease. Dig Dis Sci 2008;53:1352–7.

[184] Nadeau KJ, Klingensmith G, Zeitler P. Type 2 diabetes in children is frequently associated with elevated alanine aminotransferase. J Pediatr Gastroenterol Nutr 2005;41:94–8.

[185] Adams LA, Lymp JF, St Sauver J, et al. The natural history of nonalcoholic fatty liver disease: a population-based cohort study. Gastroenterology 2005;129:113–21.

[186] Fan JG, Li F, Cai XB, et al. Effects of nonalcoholic fatty liver disease on the development of metabolic disorders. J Gastroenterol Hepatol 2007;22:1086–91.

[187] de Piano A, Prado WL, Caranti DA, et al. Metabolic and nutritional profile of obese adolescents with nonalcoholic fatty liver disease. J Pediatr Gastroenterol Nutr 2007;44:446–52.

[188] Reinehr T, Schmidt C, Toschke AM, et al. Lifestyle intervention in obese children with nonalcoholic fatty liver disease: 2-year follow-up study. Arch Dis Child 2009;94:437–42.

[189] Tock L, Prado WL, Caranti DA, et al. Nonalcoholic fatty liver disease decrease in obese adolescents after multidisciplinary therapy. Eur J Gastroenterol Hepatol 2006;18:1241–5.

[190] Wang CL, Liang L, Fu JF, et al. Effect of lifestyle intervention on non-alcoholic fatty liver disease in Chinese obese children. World J Gastroenterol 2008;14:1598–602.

[191] Ouyang X, Cirillo P, Sautin Y, et al. Fructose consumption as a risk factor for non-alcoholic fatty liver disease. J Hepatol 2008;48:993–9.

[192] Vos MB, Weber MB, Welsh J, et al. Fructose and oxidized low-density lipoprotein in pediatric nonalcoholic fatty liver disease: a pilot study. Arch Pediatr Adolesc Med 2009;163:674–5.

[193] Nobili V, Manco M, Ciampalini P, et al. Metformin use in children with nonalcoholic fatty liver disease: an open-label, 24-month, observational pilot study. Clin Ther 2008;30:1168–76.

[194] Lavine JE, Schwimmer JB, Molleston JP, et al. Treatment of nonalcoholic fatty liver disease in children: TONIC trial design. Contemp Clin Trials 2010;31:62–70.

[195] Aithal GP, Thomas JA, Kaye PV, et al. Randomized, placebo-controlled trial of pioglitazone in nondiabetic subjects with nonalcoholic steatohepatitis. Gastroenterology 2008;135:1176–84.

[196] Belfort R, Harrison SA, Brown K, et al. A placebo-controlled trial of pioglitazone in subjects with nonalcoholic steatohepatitis. N Engl J Med 2006;355:2297–307.

[197] Ratziu V, Giral P, Jacqueminet S, et al. Rosiglitazone for nonalcoholic steatohepatitis: one-year results of the randomized placebo-controlled Fatty Liver Improvement with Rosiglitazone Therapy (FLIRT) Trial. Gastroenterology 2008;135:100–10.

[198] Chalasani NP, Sanyal AJ, Kowdley KV, et al. Pioglitazone versus vitamin E versus placebo for the treatment of non-diabetic patients with non-alcoholic steatohepatitis: PIVENS trial design. Contemp Clin Trials 2009;30:88–96.

[199] Sanjay A. A randomized controlled trial of pioglitazone or vitamin E for nonalcoholic steatohepatitis (PIVENS). Hepatology 2009;50(Suppl 4):90A.

[200] Lavine JE. Vitamin E treatment of nonalcoholic steatohepatitis in children: a pilot study. J Pediatr 2000;136:734–8.

[201] Nobili V, Manco M, Devito R, et al. Effect of vitamin E on aminotransferase levels and insulin resistance in children with non-alcoholic fatty liver disease. Aliment Pharmacol Ther 2006;24:1553–61.

[202] Nobili V, Manco M, Devito R, et al. Lifestyle intervention and antioxidant therapy in children with nonalcoholic fatty liver disease: a randomized, controlled trial. Hepatology 2008;48:119–28.

[203] Obinata K, Maruyama T, Hayashi M, et al. Effect of taurine on the fatty liver of children with simple obesity. Adv Exp Med Biol 1996;403:607–13.

[204] Dufour JF, Oneta CM, Gonvers JJ, et al. Randomized placebo-controlled trial of ursodeoxycholic acid with vitamin e in nonalcoholic steatohepatitis. Clin Gastroenterol Hepatol 2006;4:1537–43.

[205] Ersoz G, Gunsar F, Karasu Z, et al. Management of fatty liver disease with vitamin E and C compared to ursodeoxycholic acid treatment. Turk J Gastroenterol 2005;16:124–8.

[206] ClinicalTrials.gov. Pilot Study of Ursodeoxycholic Acid in Non-Alcoholic Steatohepatitis (URSONASH) Identifier: NCT00470171. Available at: http://clinicaltrials.gov/ct2/show/NCT00470171. Accessed February 2, 2009.

[207] Sanyal A, Mudaliar S, Henry R. A new therapy for nonalcoholic fatty liver disease and diabetes? INT-747—the first FXR hepatic therapeutic study. Hepatology 2009;50(Suppl 4): 389A.

[208] ClinicalTrials.gov. Effects of FXR activation on hepatic lipid and glucose metabolism Identifier: NCT00465751. Available at: http://clinicaltrials.gov/ct2/show/NCT00465751. Accessed October 31, 2007.

[209] Merat S, Malekzadeh R, Sohrabi MR, et al. Probucol in the treatment of non-alcoholic steatohepatitis: a double-blind randomized controlled study. J Hepatol 2003;38:414–8.

[210] Pamuk GE, Sonsuz A. N-acetylcysteine in the treatment of non-alcoholic steatohepatitis. J Gastroenterol Hepatol 2003;18:1220–1.

[211] Uygun A, Kadayıfcı A, Bağcı S, et al. L-Carnitine therapy in non-alcoholic steatohepatitis. Turk J Gastroenterol 2000;11:196–201.

[212] Hyogo H, Tazuma S, Arihiro K, et al. Efficacy of atorvastatin for the treatment of nonalcoholic steatohepatitis with dyslipidemia. Metabolism 2008;57:1711–8.

[213] Nelson A, Torres DM, Morgan AE, et al. A pilot study using simvastatin in the treatment of nonalcoholic steatohepatitis: a randomized placebo-controlled trial. J Clin Gastroenterol 2009;43:990–4.

[214] Daniels SR, Greer FR. Lipid screening and cardiovascular health in childhood. Pediatrics 2008;122:198–208.

[215] O'Gorman CS, Higgins MF, O'Neill MB. Systematic review and metaanalysis of statins for heterozygous familial hypercholesterolemia in children: evaluation of cholesterol changes and side effects. Pediatr Cardiol 2009;30:482–9.

[216] de Ferranti S, Ludwig DS. Storm over statins—the controversy surrounding pharmacologic treatment of children. N Engl J Med 2008;359:1309–12.

[217] Zelber-Sagi S, Kessler A, Brazowsky E, et al. A double-blind randomized placebo-controlled trial of orlistat for the treatment of nonalcoholic fatty liver disease. Clin Gastroenterol Hepatol 2006;4:639–44.

[218] Klein S, Mittendorfer B, Eagon JC, et al. Gastric bypass surgery improves metabolic and hepatic abnormalities associated with nonalcoholic fatty liver disease. Gastroenterology 2006;130:1564–72.

[219] Barker KB, Palekar NA, Bowers SP, et al. Non-alcoholic steatohepatitis: effect of Roux-en-Y gastric bypass surgery. Am J Gastroenterol 2006;101:368–73.

[220] Dixon JB, Bhathal PS, O'Brien PE. Weight loss and non-alcoholic fatty liver disease: falls in gamma-glutamyl transferase concentrations are associated with histologic improvement. Obes Surg 2006;16:1278–86.

[221] Mathurin P, Hollebecque A, Arnalsteen L, et al. Prospective study of the long-term effects of bariatric surgery on liver injury in patients without advanced disease. Gastroenterology 2009;137:532–40.

[222] Mattar SG, Velcu LM, Rabinovitz M, et al. Surgically-induced weight loss significantly improves nonalcoholic fatty liver disease and the metabolic syndrome. Ann Surg 2005;242:610–7 [discussion: 618–20].

[223] Holterman AX, Browne A, Dillard BE 3rd, et al. Short-term outcome in the first 10 morbidly obese adolescent patients in the FDA-approved trial for laparoscopic adjustable gastric banding. J Pediatr Gastroenterol Nutr 2007;45:465–73.

[224] Nadler EP, Reddy S, Isenalumhe A, et al. Laparoscopic adjustable gastric banding for morbidly obese adolescents affects android fat loss, resolution of comorbidities, and improved metabolic status. J Am Coll Surg 2009;209:638–44.

[225] Nadler EP, Youn HA, Ren CJ, et al. An update on 73 US obese pediatric patients treated with laparoscopic adjustable gastric banding: comorbidity resolution and compliance data. J Pediatr Surg 2008;43:141–6.

[226] Pratt JS, Lenders CM, Dionne EA, et al. Best practice updates for pediatric/adolescent weight loss surgery. Obesity (Silver Spring) 2009;17:901–10.

[227] Park HS, Han JH, Choi KM, et al. Relation between elevated serum alanine aminotransferase and metabolic syndrome in Korean adolescents. Am J Clin Nutr 2005;82:1046–51.

[228] Imhof A, Kratzer W, Boehm B, et al. Prevalence of non-alcoholic fatty liver and characteristics in overweight adolescents in the general population. Eur J Epidemiol 2007;22:889–97.

[229] Zhou YJ, Li YY, Nie YQ, et al. Prevalence of fatty liver disease and its risk factors in the population of South China. World J Gastroenterol 2007;13:6419–24.

[230] Tominaga K, Fujimoto E, Suzuki K, et al. Prevalence of non-alcoholic fatty liver disease in children and relationship to metabolic syndrome, insulin resistance, and waist circumference. Environ Health Prev Med 2009;14:142–9.

Advances in Pediatrics 57 (2010) 141–162

ADVANCES IN PEDIATRICS

ELSEVIER
MOSBY

Chronic Pediatric Pain

Robin Slover, MD[a,b,*], Gail L. Neuenkirchen, MS, RN, CPNP[a,b], Sola Olamikan, MD[b], Sheryl Kent, PhD[a,b]

[a]Department of Anesthaseology, University of Colorado Denver, 12401 East 17th Avenue, Aurora, CO 80045, USA
[b]Chronic Pain Consultative Service, The Children's Hospital, 13123 East 16th Avenue, Aurora, CO 80045, USA

P ediatric chronic pain has been an increasingly significant problem over the last 5 years. It is estimated to occur in 15% to 30% of school-age children [1]. Pain is not only a significant emotional stressor for the family unit but also an expensive one. Lost work from parental absences to care for the child as well as increasing costs of health care use are significant. There is increasing evidence that the development of chronic pain in childhood may lead to chronic pain as an adult. The behavioral consequences of school absences, changed peer relationships, effects on social activities, and effects on family interactions affect the child, his siblings, and his future.

It is important to recognize that in the pediatric population, nonorganic factors may be as important as organic factors in maintaining pain and that both need to be addressed. Because all pain involves neurosensory changes and may involve altered pain processing, the use of "organic" or "medical" versus "nonorganic" is probably artificial. While most parents prefer a biologic explanation for pain, a multifactorial approach to pain management usually leads to the best results.

Each pediatric age seems to have a significant area of pain during specific ages. Infants frequently have colic. Stomach ache and headache are frequent chronic complaints in young children who do not wish to leave the home and go to school, and can usually be handled by the pediatrician. Headaches and musculoskeletal pains are commonly seen in adolescents [2]. The authors discuss problems that frequently occur in preteens and adolescents. Frequent presenting chronic complaints include headache, abdominal pain, musculoskeletal pain (including back pain), and limb pain thought to be complex regional pain syndrome. Cancer survivors with ongoing neuropathic pain are an increasingly large group, a result of the improved cancer cure rates. A few patients have genetic illnesses

*Corresponding author. Chronic Pain Consultative Service, The Children's Hospital, 13123 East 16th Avenue, Aurora, CO 80045. E-mail address: robin.slover@ucdenver.edu

0065-3101/10/$ – see front matter
doi:10.1016/j.yapd.2010.08.009

responsible for their pain (such as sickle cell anemia or neurofibromatosis). A multimodal combination of medications, physical therapy, and psychological interventions are usually required for the effective treatment of chronic pain. Specific injections may be helpful in combination with the other modalities. Alternative therapies such as acupuncture and massage therapy may also be helpful.

PAIN PROCESSING

Injuries in normal patients produce release of neurotransmitters that stimulate free nerve endings. These impulses are transmitted to the spinal cord on A-delta or C fibers, which synapse in the substantia gelatinosa and in lamina 5 of the dorsal horn. From these synapses, information is carried to the cortex. Lamina 5 has been shown to contain wide dynamic range neurons, which can be activated or "turned on." These neurons can sensitize, releasing increasing amounts of transmitters in response to a repetitive stimulation, which can cause nonpainful stimuli to be interpreted as painful. In addition, wide dynamic neurons can increase the area of the body, contiguously, from which they receive input. Interneurons can affect pain transmission at multiple levels along the pathway. Pain processing is not just a relay of signals from the periphery to the cortex, but a dynamic redundant system composed of multiple synaptic pathways using multiple types of signals [3]. Chronic pain etiology includes not just peripheral dysfunctions (peripheral neuropathies) but also changes in receptors that involve heat, cold, touch, and chemical responses. As a result of peripheral nociceptor hyperactivity, dramatic secondary changes involving up-regulation of sodium channels and receptor molecules occur in the spinal cord. There is also evidence of neuronal sensitization in the brain.

Microglia and astrocytes are now recognized as modulators of pain [4]. Glia were traditionally associated with "housekeeping" functions that kept nerves healthy and helped them communicate. Recently it has been shown that microglia can release glial and neuronal signaling molecules such as cytokines and leukotrienes; these can affect neuropathic pain processing. Release of cytokines and leukotrienes can lead to proinflammatory changes such as neuronal hyperexcitation, neurotoxicity, and chronic inflammation. In addition, glia may be responsible for releasing anti-inflammatory factors, helping to restore normal pain signaling and protect against neurotoxicity [5]. Microglial activation may help explain conditions such as functional abdominal pain, in which pain sensation persists despite absence of identifiable causes. Glial cells enclose nerve endings, so it is easy to see how they can release substances that modulate signal processing at multiple levels.

Recently, opioids (specifically morphine and methadone) have been shown to cause release of proinflammatory cytokines and leukotrienes from glial cells. Naloxone helps prevent this release [6].

NEUROPATHIC PAIN MEDICATIONS

There are several medications that are useful for treating neuropathic pain (Tables 1 and 2). Most chronic pain conditions involve neuropathic pain: visceral pain, headaches, myofascial pain, and neuropathies. The major groups are reviewed here.

Anticonvulsants

Anticonvulsants are the mainstay for treatment of neuropathic pain, which also includes headaches, myofascial pain, abdominal visceral pain, pelvic pain, and back pain as well as known nerve entrapment or injury syndromes. Most cancer survivors also have neuropathic pain. Pregabalin (Lyrica) is helpful in adults, but has no pediatric dosing as yet. Gabapentin has been used more often in pediatric patients. Topiramate (Topamax) is particularly helpful for pelvic pain and headaches. Topiramate has been shown to be helpful in vinca alkaloid–induced neuropathies. Topiramate can cause weight loss as well as significant sedation; Pregabalin can cause weight gain and fluid retention in addition to sedation, as can gabapentin, in up to 10% of patients using them. Lamotrigine causes less weight gain and can be helpful in neuropathic pain as well as potentiating antidepressants. Carbamazepine (Tegretol), valproic acid (Depakote), oxcarbazepine (Trileptal), and clonazepam have been helpful in some patients. Clonazepam is usually used for patients who have an anxiety component to their pain, because it may be safer than long-term use of other benzodiazepines.

Monotherapy with anticonvulsants helps many patients. Dual therapy can be used; the seizure literature shows that only 30% of patients can be controlled by monotherapy. Topiramate and pregabalin (or gabapentin) are a good combination because they block different receptors.

Tricyclic Antidepressants

The tricyclic antidepressants (TCAs) are still effective but sometimes overlooked. Amitriptyline has been the most studied but also has the most side effects. Nortriptyline or desipramine are better tolerated. These agents are given at bedtime. The antidepressant dose is usually 200 mg. Pain doses vary from 5 to 75 mg, depending on the age and size of the child. The antidepressant dose is around 200 mg in a full-sized patient. Dry mouth, sedation, and sometimes urinary retention are common side effects. Antidepressants can be combined with anticonvulsants or other types of antidepressants in full-sized patients.

Muscle Relaxants

Muscle relaxants are useful because most teenagers have "head-forward syndrome," causing muscle spasms in the neck, trapezius, and paraspinal muscles. This syndrome can be a primary pain generator or exist in addition to other pain issues. Even if the patient does not appreciate any change, often an examiner will appreciate decreased resting muscle tension in these muscles after starting the drug for a week or so. Sedation is the major side effect. Although most patients get used to the sedation, Flexeril can affect some people so severely that they never accommodate. In addition, Flexeril is structurally similar to TCAs and should not be used in bipolar patients.

Table 1
Proposed neuropathic pain mechanisms

Symptom	Proposed mechanism	Targets	Available compounds
Shooting spontaneous pain	*Peripheral nociceptor hyperexcitability*	Na channels	Lidocaine
	Ectopic impulse generation		Carbamazepine
			Lamotrigine
			Amitriptyline
			Oxycarbamazepine
Ongoing spontaneous pain	*Peripheral nociceptor sensitization*	Cytokines	NSAIDs?
	Inflammation within nerves (cytokine release)		TNF-α agonist
	Central dorsal horn hyperexcitability [see below]	mu receptors	Opioids
	Changes in the supraspinal descending modulation	Ca channels	Gabapentin
		NMDA	Pregabalin
		NK-1	Ketamine
		Sodium channels	Dextromethorphan?
			Carbamazepine?
	Effect on GABAergic inhibitory neurons	GABAB receptors	Baclofen
			Opioids
Heat allodynia	Reduced activation threshold to heat	TRPV1 receptor	Capsaicin cream
Cold allodynia	Reduced activation threshold to cold	TRPM8 receptor	Menthol
Static mechanical allodynia	Reduced activation threshold to mechanical stimuli	ASIC receptor?	?
Sympathetic pain	Reduced activation threshold to noradrenaline	α receptor	Sympathetic block TCAs
	Histamine	Histamine H1 receptor	TCA

Dynamic mechanical allodynia and punctate mechanical hyperalgesia	*Central dorsal horn excitability*		
	Central sensitization on spinal level, ongoing	Mu receptors	Opioids
	C-fiber input increases synaptic transmission	Calcium channels	Gabapentin Pregabalin
	Amplification of C-fiber input		
	Gating of Aβ fiber input (mechanical dynamic hyperalgesia)	NMDA antagonists	Ketamine
	Gating of Aβ fiber input (mechanical punctuate hyperalgesia)	NK-1 antagonists	Dextromethorphan?
	Intraspinal inhibitory interneurons (functional, degeneration)	Na channels	Carbamazepine?
	GABAergic	GABA$_B$ receptors	Baclofen
	Opioidergic	mu receptors	Opioids
	Changes in supraspinal descending modulation		
	Inhibitory control (noradrenaline, 5-HT)	α2 receptors 5-HT receptors	Clonidine TCA antidepressants Venlafaxine Duloxetine
	Facilitatory control	?	?

Abbreviations: ASIC, acid-sensing ion channel; GABA, γ-aminobutyric acid; 5-HT, 5-hydroxytryptamine; NK, neurokinin; NMDA, N-methyl-D-aspartic acid; NSAID, nonsteroidal anti-inflammatory drug; TCA, tricyclic antidepressant; TNF, tumor necrosis factor; TRPM, transient receptor potential melastatin; TRPV, transient receptor potential vanilloid.
Data from Baron R. Mechanisms of disease: neuropathic pain—a clinical perspective. Vol. 2 No. 2. Available at: www.nature.com. Accessed February 2006.

Table 2
Neuropathic pain medications

Name	Dose	Common side effects
Anticonvulsants		
Gabapentin (Neurontin)	Children 12 y or younger: Begin 5 mg/kg/d at bedtime and increase as tolerated to 8–35 mg/kg/d in 3 doses Children older than 12 y: 100 mg at bedtime and increase as tolerated to a maximum of 3600 mg Older adolescents: Minimum effective dose is 900 mg with the usual range 1500–2400 mg	Sedation Weight gain 10% Hostility/aggression 5% Hyperactivity 4% Thought disorders 1.7% Peripheral edema Constipation Back pain
Pregabalin (Lyrica)	Not approved for children: no doses available In adults, can switch from gabapentin without titrating off. Authors' center uses a proportion dose adjustment in full sized older adolescents 300 mg pregabalin = 3600 mg gabapentin; ie, if patient is on 2400 mg gabapentin, would switch to 200 mg pregabalin Initial dose 25–50 mg at bedtime and increase as tolerated to 300–450 mg In adults, doses of 600 mg were tested with no additional benefits and increasing side effects	Sedation Weight gain 16% Neuromuscular or skeletal tremor 11% Peripheral edema 16% Neuropathy 9% Balance disorders 9% Constipation
Topiramate (Topamax)	2–12 y: start 0.5–3 mg/kg/d at bedtime. Increase as tolerated to a 6–8 mg/kg/d in 2 doses. Maximum 200 mg >12 y: start at 12.5 mg at bedtime. Increase as tolerated to 100 mg at bedtime or 200 mg twice a day. Slow titration every 7–14 days is necessary due to sedation Very helpful for headaches, chemotherapy-induced neuropathic pain, and abdominal pain	Somnolence Ataxia Fatigue Memory problems Depression or mood issues Weight loss (dose related) Paresthesia Tremor Metabolic acidosis Decreased sodium channels

Lamotrigine (Lamictal)	2–12 y: start at 0.15 mg/kg/d at night. Increase as tolerated to 1–3 mg/kg/d in 2 doses. Use whole tablets. Maximum 300 mg/d >12 y: 25 mg at bedtime. Increase as tolerated to 400 mg/d in 2 doses	Ocular syndrome (blurred vision or pain); can be serious, stop if develops Sedation Rash (monitor carefully for Steven-Johnson syndrome) Abdominal pain or nausea Joint pain Emotional lability

Note: All anticonvulsants can increase suicidal thoughts in pediatric patients (11 AEDs examined). Can see as soon as 1 week. All patients should be followed for hematologic or liver issues

Antidepressants Amitriptyline	Chronic pain: 0.1 mg/kg at bedtime. Increase as tolerated to 0.5–2 mg/kg/d at bedtime Migraine: start 0.1 mg/kg at night. Maximum 1–1.5 mg/kg/d. Should get EEG in patients receiving ≥1 mg/kg/d or if symptomatic	Sedation Arrhythmias Tachycardia Postural hypotension Urinary retention Tremors Constipation Weight gain IOP increased Anxiety Nausea Weakness Paresthesia Blurred vision Hallucinations

(continued on next page)

Table 2
(continued)

Name	Dose	Common side effects
Cymbalta	No data or doses for pediatrics. Use in older, full-sized adolescents only. Start 20 mg at night. Increase as tolerated to 60 mg at night	Somnolence 7%–21% Headache 13%–20% Dizziness 6%–7% Insomnia 8%–16% Fatigue 2%–15% Nausea Constipation Diarrhea Decreased appetite
Muscle Relaxants Baclofen (Lioresal)	2–12 y: 2.5–5 mg at night. Increase as needed. Maximum 80 mg	Sedation Hypotension Fatigue Constipation Nausea Psychiatric disturbance Headache
Cyclobenzaprine (Flexeril)	Children 12 or under: no doses have been established. >12 y: 5–10 mg at night. Increase as needed to 10 mg 3 times a day. Extended release may use 15–30 mg once daily	Tachycardia Hypotension Drowsiness 39% Dizziness 11%

Tizanidine (Zanaflex)	No pediatric doses given Adults 2–4 mg at bedtime. Increase as needed to a maximum of 36 mg/d in 3 doses	Sedation 48% Dizziness 16% Xerostoma 49% Weakness 41% Hypotension 0.8 mg/d 16%–33% Hallucinations Anxiety Depression Constipation Nausea UTI 10% Increased liver enzymes 3%–5%
Methocarbemol (Robaxin)	Children: only use for tetanus Adults: 500 mg at bedtime. Increase as needed to 1.5 mg 3 times a day	Drowsiness Bradycardia Hypotension Rash Metallic taste
Carisoprodol (Soma)	Recommended only for short term use. No dosing for pediatric patients <16 y. 250 mg at night. Increase as needed to a maximum of 350 3 times a day. Potential for drug dependency exists	Sedation 17% Dizziness Headache Withdrawal symptoms

Abbreviations: AED, antiepileptic drug; EEG, electroencephalography; IOP, intraocular pressure; UTI, urinary tract infection.
Data from Lexi-Comp.

Baclofen can be helpful in visceral pain syndromes, because it also affects smooth muscle. Cyclobenzaprine (Flexoril) has the most study results for treatment of fibromyalgia. Tizanidine is a more titratable drug, which is often useful. Carisoprodol (Soma) is metabolized to a tranquilizer and is potentially addictive. For patients with severe anxiety issues this drug may be useful, but the addiction risk must be weighed. Methocarbamol (Robaxin) is the less sedating muscle relaxant, useful for people who need to use daytime doses and not be sedated.

Antidepressants

Antidepressants help with the frequent depression seen with chronic pain as well as strengthening the descending inhibitory pathway to help with pain. There is no ideal antidepressant. Escitalopram (Lexapro) been shown to help with depression in some studies, as have sertraline (Zoloft), paroxetine (Paxil), and fluoxetine (Prozac). Venlafaxine (Effexor) and mirtazapine (Remeron) also have undergone studies suggesting they are helpful in treating pain. Trazedone is useful for helping with sleep, as is mirtazapine and clonazepam. Trazedone is an antidepressant, but is probably a better sedative our first choice is Zoloft.

Topical Agents

Topical agents are attractive because of their limited side effects. Lidoderm patches, which contain lidocaine, can be cut and applied to the affected area. In a full-size patient, 3 patches can be used for 12 hours out of a 24-hour day. Flector patches contain diclofenac, potentially providing less gastrointestinal upset. One patch can be cut and applied every 12 hours. Capsaicin is less helpful in children because of the burning sensation on application. Lidoderm gel or Emla cream can help decrease the burning sensation if applied before the capsaicin.

Mast Cell Stabilizers

Many children with chronic pain tend to show weal and flare easily and have rashes, suggesting easy histamine release. A few have skin pain issues. Cetirizine (Zyrtec) and loratadine (Claritin) are helpful in some children in reducing pain.

HEADACHES

Headaches are common in children. Occasional headaches are seen in up to 20% of children younger than 5 years [7]. Before puberty, tension-type headaches are as common as migraines. Migraine headaches usually become evident in school-aged children. Migraine symptoms are similar to those seen in adults: headaches, often unilateral and/or pulsating, which last 4 to 72 hours and are improved with sleep. Photophobia or phonophobia is common, often with nausea. An aura (lasting less than 60 minutes) is present in about half of children with migraines. The pain is usually increased with physical activity such as stair climbing. Parents who have migraines often recognize the symptoms in their children. Tension headaches are described as a "band-like" tightness in the head. These headaches may be caused by myofascial spasms in the muscles of the head and neck. Both types of headache can exist in the same patient. In some cases, children may develop constant or "daily" headaches.

Migraines may present in primary school–aged children, but more typically present in the preteen or adolescent period. Most "daily" headaches occur in patients with a genetic predisposition to migraines. Patients who have ongoing headaches following concussion (often sports related) or a car accident with a whiplash injury often have an underlying genetic predisposition for migraines. Approximately 5% of the population carries these genes, which are usually inherited as an autosomal dominant. A few families have a hemiplegic migraine pattern whereby migraines involve some degree of hemiparesis. A calcium channel subunit mutation in a gene mapped to chromosome 19 has been implicated [8]. For many patients, nonsteroidal anti-inflammatory drugs (NSAIDs) (ibuprofen, naproxen [Naprosyn], and acetaminophen [Excedrin, Tylenol]) are effective. Triptans are often not as effective as NSAIDs in younger children. However, patients who have 8 or more headaches per month should have a preventive treatment. β-Blockers and calcium channel blockers are frequently used as preventive medications in adult patients. These agents are much less effective in pediatric patients. Preventive medications for the pediatric age group include anticonvulsants, especially topiramate, coenzyme Q10, vitamin B2, and magnesium. There is also evidence that feverfew, butterbur, and α-lipoic acid may help.

If NSAIDs are not adequate for treating headaches, then Excedrin or a caffeine product may be helpful. Nasal dihydroergotamine can be helpful, but the first dose should be under medical supervision with monitoring of blood pressure, and checks for ischemia and possible cardiac symptoms. Prolonged use can lead to fibrotic changes in the heart and pulmonary valves. Usually pediatric patients do not have risk factors for coronary artery disease. Triptans can be effective and should be tried. Midrin (acetaminophen/isometheptene/dichloralphenazone) can also be helpful. Ketorolac (Toradol) injections are useful for many patients. A combination of ondansetron (Zofran) or metoclopramide (Reglan), diphenhydramine (Benadryl), and ketorolac may help especially given when in an emergency room environment. Anticonvulsant infusions, such as levetiracetam (Keppra) or valproic acid, can also be helpful. Tramadol can be effective. Other opioids should be used as a last resort.

Other causes of headaches need to be eliminated in order to diagnose headaches as either migraine or tension-type headaches. These causes include dental braces, sinusitis, visual errors, increase intracranial pressure (including pseudotumor cerebri), epilepsy, drug effects, brain tumors, Chiari malformations, depression, obstructive sleep apnea, and systemic illnesses such as hypertension. Particularly in patients with neurologic changes, other diagnoses should be ruled out. Imaging, including magnetic resonance (MR) imaging, computed tomography scan of the brain, and MR venography/MR angiography, may be helpful. Lumbar puncture may be needed to eliminate diagnosis such as pseudotumor cerebri or infections [9].

Pediatric patients can develop rebound headaches from overtreatment, which can present as a chronic daily headache. No more than 8 days per month should involve treatment with any type of abortive medication. On a given day, a patient may be treated with more than one agent; for example, an NSAID followed by a triptan followed by Reglan and Benadryl. Midrin and triptans should not be combined within 24 hours, nor should Midrin or triptans be combined with dihydroergotamine within 24 hours.

In patients presenting with frequent or daily headaches, it is worthwhile reviewing food and beverage choices. Overuse of caffeine of energy drinks can aggravate headaches. It is important to keep daily caffeine intake consistent. Nitrates, aged cheese, monosodium glutamate, and red wine are also frequent triggers.

In patients who have a constant headache, depression should be ruled out. Severe depression can cause a constant headache and other agents will not work until the depression is corrected. Suicide risk should be assessed in a depressed patient with daily headache because suicide risk is increased in this group.

Many patients who have frequent headaches or daily headaches have a strong muscle component to their pain. Head-forward syndrome, represented by the neck being forward and the ear much more forward than the shoulder, results in muscle spasms of the trapezius, scalene, splenius capitus, and semispidatus. As the patient compensates, tightening occurs in the parascapular muscles, paravertebral muscles, pectoralis muscles, temporalis muscles, and frontalis muscles. Pressure is put on the occipital nerves, auricular nerves, and supraorbital nerves, which can maintain a headache. Occipital, auricular, and supraorbital nerve injections can minimize the nerve irritation, and trigger-point injections into procerus, corregor, frontalis, temporalis, sternocleidomastoid, scalene, splenius capitus, semispinatus, and trapezius muscles can relieve the muscle spasms and help reduce the headaches. Physical therapy with instruction in proper body mechanics and slow stretching exercises can be used to treat the muscle spasm component or to help maintain this improvement. Muscle relaxants such as baclofen, cyclobenzaprine, and tizanidine are helpful in maintaining muscle relaxation. Patients with tight muscles should be evaluated for possible injections to achieve more rapid improvement of their headaches.

COMPLEX REGIONAL PAIN SYNDROME

Complex regional pain syndrome, or CRPS, is increasingly recognized in children. The peak incidence is around puberty. Lower extremity cases are more common than upper extremity cases in CRPS Type 1, which is pain without indications of a specific nerve injury. Girls are more often affected than boys [10]. In many cases specific traumatic incidents can be identified as "causing" the injury, but in some cases there is no specific trauma, merely frequent activities such as sports or dancing with a presumed, but unrecognized injury. CRPS Type 2 occurs with equal frequency among boys and girls. Type 2 CRPS is pain with a partial or complete nerve injury in the affected area. Of note, neonates with Erb palsy from brachial plexus injuries rarely develop pain in the extremities [11].

The diagnosis is based on the history and physical examination. Pain out of proportion to the injury is the major sign. Usually it is not in a dermatomal pattern, but more diffuse, similar to a stocking-glove distribution, spreading a variable length along the affected limb. Usually the foot or hand is involved. The lower extremity is more involved in pediatric cases; in adults upper extremity cases slightly outnumber lower extremity cases. However, the whole limb may be affected. The patient or parents will describe color changes. While bluish purple and pink discoloration is seen, mottling of the extremity when dependent is also frequently seen. Usually there is a temperature difference in the area of severe pain. Allodynia commonly develops and many children present in wheelchairs or on crutches, nonweight bearing. Hair growth and nail growth changes can also be seen from one extremity to another. Swelling of the affected extremity can be significant. Muscle spasms can develop and progress up the body.

Triple-phase bone scans can be helpful for diagnoses. While a normal triple-phase bone scan does not rule out CRPS, it can be helpful in ruling out other orthopedic abnormalities. There is no conclusive test for CRPS. Even sympathetic blocks only indicate if the pain is still sympathetically maintained. Some patients with classic physical findings suggesting CRPS may have no response to the sympathetic blocks, having sympathetically independent or even centralized pain. Other causes of pain should be ruled out before considering a diagnosis of CRPS.

Many medications have been tried for treatment of CRPS. Anticonvulsants, TCAs, NSAIDS, and steroids have all been used. Opioids have also been used, both systemically and neuronally. Recent studies show the benefit of physical therapy in reversing the condition. Aggressive physical therapy programs have been successful in treating children as well as adults [12]. TENS (transcutaneous electrical nerve stimulator) units can be helpful as part of the physical therapy. Use of medications and/or injections may allow the child to participate more in physical therapy, due to decreased pain. Because children rarely tolerate injections without sedation, injections are usually done under heavy sedation or brief general anesthetic. At The Children's Hospital, the authors try one sympathetic injection before placing an indwelling catheter. About 10% of their pediatric patients with CRPS have had complete resolution of their symptoms following one injection combined with physical therapy. Because many injections use fluoroscopy for accurate placement of the injection, use of an indwelling catheter (sciatic nerve or brachial plexus if possible) minimizes radiation risk as well as limiting exposure to anesthetics. Patients with indwelling catheters are kept in the hospital for 5 to 7 days, allowing more aggressive physical therapy with minimal pain. One group has reported good success in a small series of patients using a continuous infusion system supervised at home for up to 96 hours. The authors' referral area includes many remote places where such supervision could be difficult if a problem occurred. For some patients with total limb involvement, a neuraxial catheter is used. There is a higher risk of motor or sensory block, which might affect physical therapy, with a neuraxial catheter. Ropivacaine is frequently used to minimize motor blockade. Use of neuropathic medications, such as amitriptyline and gabapentin, can also decrease pain and help improve function.

Psychological support is critical in treating children with CRPS. The combination of severe pain with often striking physical findings in the affected limb can cause severe anxiety in parents as well as the patient. As in all pediatric patients with chronic pain, anxiety, depression, and environmental stressors are often present.

Although some parents report that they also have CRPS, genetic factors have not been fully studied. If injections, medications, and physical therapy are not successful, then more invasive techniques such as dorsal column stimulators may be helpful. Careful psychological evaluation needs to be done before implanting such a system. In addition, the possible immaturity of the nervous system of the pediatric patient and whether the patient has finished growth should also be weighed when deciding when to recommend this therapy. Although there is moderate evidence supporting the use of dorsal column stimulators in adults, there are no studies in pediatric patients. Sympathectomy should not be recommended or encouraged; this is an irreversible procedure that has not shown long-term success. The initial failure rate has been reported to be 10% [13]. This procedure can lead to sympathalgia, and its long-term physiologic consequences in adolescents are unknown. The procedure helps only the sympathetic portion of the pain. With time the spinal cord can recruit new pathways to carry the pain.

Complementary techniques such as acupuncture can be helpful, but there have been no large controlled studies. Herbal remedies and nutritional supplements may also have anecdotal success, but lack controlled trials.

The potential for recurrence of CRPS is a frequent concern for parents and patients. Estimates have ranged from 30% to 50% [14]. Adults are thought to have a lower risk, which may reflect the fact that fewer get complete resolution of their pain. Even though recurrence may be common, it seems to respond at least as readily to physical therapy and other treatments.

ABDOMINAL PAIN

Abdominal complaints are frequent in childhood, and may be associated with other painful conditions such as headaches. As with other types of chronic pain, organic pathology such as Crohn disease needs to be ruled out. The occurrence of unintentional weight loss, dysuria, anemia, guaic-positive stools, pain causing the child to wake up at night, elevated erythrocyte sedimentation rate, or nonumbilical pain (pain occurring far from the umbilicus) should increase suspicions of a definable cause of pain. Usually various imaging studies such as ultrasonography, endoscopy, colonoscopy, and urinalysis are performed to eliminate definable causes. Abused children may complain about abdominal pain. Testing for celiac disease and *Helicobacter pylori* infections may help identify contributing factors.

The innervation of the abdomen is sparse. Most sensory afferent fibers are C-type nociceptors. Pain tends to be described as dull and poorly localized.

Sensitivity to distension of the intestines fits a bell-shaped curve. Sensitive people may have pain from distension or stretching of the intestinal wall. Their perception can be modified by higher cortical centers. These centers can also affect gastrointestinal function, which has led to the idea of the "brain-gut" axis [15]. Irritable bowel syndrome (IBS) is seen in children as well as adults. IBS is often diagnosed by lack of other findings with a combination of abdominal pain and disordered defecation. Patients may have periods of diarrhea alternating with constipation. There may be evidence of altered transit or other signs of dysfunction. Some children with IBS have significantly more abdominal pain than others.

Abdominal migraines are seen in children who also have migraines. Instead of a severe headache, they have sudden onset of severe abdominal pain and vomiting. The usual treatments for migraines usually help abdominal migraines, and the time course is similar.

Functional abdominal pain or recurrent abdominal pain is a common pediatric pain complaint. Recurrent abdominal pain is defined as monthly episodes of pain for at least 3 consecutive months, separated by pain-free periods, and severe enough to interfere with daily activities. Prevalence estimates have ranged between 9% and 25%, depending on gender and age [16]. Girls tend to have a later age of onset, and a higher incidence as they approach puberty. Children placed in stressful situations also appear to have a higher incidence. Functional abdominal pain is defined as continuous or nearly continuous abdominal pain for 12 weeks with no relationship to eating, menses, or defecation. There is some loss of function in daily activities, no other causes, and no malingering.

Lactose intolerance has been suggested as a cause of both recurrent abdominal pain and functional abdominal pain, but studies have had variable results. A lactose-free diet has helped patients, but placebo effects have not been ruled out. Other carbohydrates such as sorbitol or fructose have also been investigated. Dietary causes are worth discussing because dietary restrictions are a relatively easy form of treatment.

Psychological factors can also affect abdominal pain. Elevated levels of anxiety have been seen in patients with specific as well as nonspecific causes of abdominal pain. An evaluation by a pain psychologist can be very helpful. School attendance needs to be encouraged and monitored.

Neuropathic pain medications may be helpful. Baclofen is a profound muscle relaxant because it can relax smooth muscle. Topiramate also appears to be helpful with visceral pain, but its sedation can be limiting. Dicyclomine (Bentyl) may also be useful. Dietary changes that include fiber are helpful. Constipation needs to be treated because it can increase abdominal pain.

MUSCULOSKELETAL PAIN

Musculoskeletal problems are a frequent cause of pediatric chronic pain. Trauma, overuse, or repetitive strain injuries, normal skeletal growth variants, and growing pains are common causes [17]. As children are encouraged to play aggressively at early ages and are selected for competitive teams that compete outside school team schedules, an increased number of sports injuries and repetitive microtrauma injuries can occur. The increasing occurrence of poor posture, particularly in adolescents, only aggravates the situation. The head-forward syndrome has become increasingly common, putting stress on the muscles of the neck, shoulder, and upper back, spreading to the lower back.

It is important to rule out mild orthopedic abnormalities, including stress fractures. A bone scan may be helpful in addition to the appropriate plain films suggested by physical examination. Usually history and physical examinations are sufficient to guide appropriate evaluation. A complete blood count with differential, inflammatory markers, metabolic profile, and vitamin D-25-OH levels should be checked, particularly to rule out more serious problems. A low vitamin D level (less than 32) can be associated with muscle or nerve pain. Arthropathies should be checked for by laboratory tests. Plain films of the affected limb or joint, as well as possible spine films, should be considered. Mild scoliosis can be associated with significant muscle spasms. Chronic spondylothesis is possible with nerve compression. An MR imaging scan to rule out a tethered cord should be done if there are lower extremity bowel or bladder signs. Patients who are hypermobile are more likely to have spontaneous joint dislocations, and may have ligamentous or tendon strains that are painful.

Fibromyalgia is seen in pediatric populations as well as adults. The diagnostic criteria are nonspecific. Widespread myofascial pain, particularly associated with poor sleep, is suggestive. This diagnosis is one of exclusion. Multiple tender points are seen. However, most of the places examined for tender points will also be tender in head-forward syndrome with paravertebral muscle spasm. The lateral epicondylar point and medial fat pad of the knee will not be as affected by posture. Frequently there is a positive family history; often a parent or close relative will have been diagnosed with fibromyalgia. Girls are more commonly affected. Prevalence has been reported to be as high as 6% [18]. Treatment needs to address the associated sleep disorder as well as encouraging function (school attendance). Physical therapy involving slow stretch exercises, gait correction, core strengthening, and possible TENS unit can be helpful. Cognitive-behavioral therapy has been shown to be very helpful.

Useful medications in adults include muscle relaxants (especially cyclobenzaprine [Flexeril]), amitriptyline, and tramadol. Pregabalin, duloxetine (Cymbalta), and milnacipran (Savella) all have specific indications in adults as a result of placebo-controlled double-blind trials. Pediatric data are lacking. Other anticonvulsants have also been helpful. Opioids have not been shown to be useful. While initially helpful, patients taking chronic opioids had the same level of pain within a year as they had before opiate use. At present, fibromyalgia needs to be approached as a controllable condition, not curable.

Growing pains may be seen in 8% to 11% of children between 6 and 10 years old [19], and again with rapid adolescent growth spurts. The pain is usually bilateral and symmetric in the lower extremities. Episodes are usually of short duration and may wake the child from sleep. Increased physical activity during the day is associated with an increased incidence of night pain. The diagnosis is one of exclusion. There is complete remission of symptoms between attacks, and pain-free intervals of days to months are common. NSAIDs and massage can be helpful, along with reassurance. The presence of a limp, worsening symptoms, joint swelling and/or tenderness, abnormal gait, limited range of motion, severe allodynia, fever, malaise, weight loss, or night sweats should trigger further investigation [20].

Restless leg syndrome, which can be diagnosed with polysomnography, should be checked for. Usually there is a family history of other members with restless leg syndrome [21]. This syndrome usually persists—one does not outgrow it. Drugs like amitriptyline, clonazepam, and ropinirole (Requip) may be helpful.

An MR imaging evaluation may be helpful in patients with low back pain. Those with significant scoliosis should be evaluated by an orthopedist. Patients with mild scoliosis can improve with a muscle relaxant and appropriate physical therapy. Patients with facet arthropathy due to injury may improve with injections, in addition to neuropathic pain medications. Medial branch nerve blocks, as well as facet blocks, have been helpful. In patients with bulging or herniated discs, epidural steroid injections may be helpful. Physical therapy and pain-coping skills should be combined with the injections.

CHRONIC DISEASES
Pediatric patients with chronic problems such as sickle cell disease, epidermolysis bullosa, or severe neurofibromatosis are often referred for pain management. Use of opioids, either for short periods such as sickle cell crises, or on a long-term basis (dressing changes for epidermolysis bullosa patients), combined with neuropathic drugs, are often appropriate. Whenever possible, long-acting opioids should provide the majority of the dose, with short-acting opioids used for short-term functional goals (ie, before physical therapy).

Cancer survivors may have several pain issues; chemotherapeutically induced pain, particularly neuropathies, can be difficult to treat while chemotherapy is ongoing. Topiramate, lamotrigine, and amitriptyline may be better tolerated. Gabapentin and pregabalin can cause edema. Opiates are often necessary, and can be tolerated after successful conclusion of the chemotherapy. α-Lipoic acid and L-carnitine have been indicated in some small studies to help vinca alkaloid–induced neuropathies. Topiramate may also help. However, α-lipoic acid and L-carnitine should not be used during chemotherapy without oncology approval, to avoid interference with chemotherapy effectiveness.

CHRONIC PAIN AND FUNCTION
Chronic pain influences all aspects of a person's functioning. Youths suffering from chronic pain report a global negative impact across all facets of their lives [22]. Youths have specific difficulties frequently found in academic achievement, emotional well-being, and peer and family functioning [23]; they also report significantly lower health-related quality of life than both healthy peers and youths with other chronic health conditions [24]. In addition to general

emotional distress, children with chronic pain have been shown to be at increased risk for psychiatric issues such as anxiety, depression, somatoform disorders, sleep disorders, and substance abuse. As pain becomes more chronic, emotional and psychiatric factors play an increasingly dominant role in the maintenance of pain and functional disability [25].

Unfortunately, pediatric chronic pain predisposes youth for the development of adult chronic pain, which may be even more likely when psychiatric comorbidities are present. Children who were more anxious/depressed at age 10 to 11 years experience high persistent levels of pain over time as well as increasing levels of pain over time [26]. Functional disability associated with chronic pain increases with age in children [27], particularly in the presence of psychological difficulties. Children with pain conditions report more somatic complaints than pain-free individuals [28] and continue to report more somatic complaints once their pain is treated. Not surprisingly, somatoform disorders are more prevalent in chronic pain samples than in the general population [29]. The predisposition for adult chronic pain and the higher probability of diagnosis of a somatoform disorder, which are costly and difficult to treat, are two important reasons to examine and treat psychological correlates of pediatric chronic pain.

Anxiety and depression are the most studied psychological comorbidities of pediatric chronic pain, and have been examined within a variety of pain conditions. Stomach aches, headaches, and musculoskeletal pains are strongly associated with anxiety and depression [30]. Children with recurrent abdominal pain have a significantly higher prevalence of psychopathology, particularly anxiety and depression [31,32]. In fact, children with recurrent abdominal pain have been shown to be 6 times more likely to display internalizing symptoms than healthy controls [30]. A recent study found that two-thirds of a sample of children with fibromyalgia met criteria for a current DSM-IV (*Diagnostic and Statistical Manual of Mental Disorders* Fourth Edition, Text Revised) diagnosis, most often a major depressive episode or anxiety [31]. Similarly, depression and anxiety occur more frequently in adolescents with migraine and tension-type headaches.

DEPRESSION

Depression and pain share many of the same neural pathways and often coexist with no clear directional causality (ie, if depression proceeds pain or pain precedes depression). For example, anxiety and depression have been found to be significant predictors of recurrent headaches, stomach aches, and backaches in youth. Girls with depression are 13 times more likely to report musculoskeletal pain and 4 times more likely to report headaches than girls without depression [33]. One possible explanation for this is that the anhedonia (lack of interest and motivation) and social withdrawal that often accompany depression allow children more time to focus on pain and limit daily distractions from somatic complaints. Depression can disrupt sleep, which often makes pain worse. In addition, depression leaves youngsters with less motivation and energy to participate in treatment plans (eg, physical activity) that may improve their pain and physical functioning.

It is also clear that unremitting pain in children can often lead to the development of depression. High rates of depression have been documented in general pediatric pain samples, as well as within specific pain populations. For example, 22% of a recent sample of juvenile fibromyalgia patients met criteria for a mood disorder (major depression, dysthymia) [31]. Estimates of depression among youth with recurrent abdominal pain are around 40% [34]. Depression is strongly associated with frequent headaches, and one study reported that 13% of adolescents with headaches have "seriously considered" suicide [35]. Depression in the setting of pediatric chronic pain has is associated with more frequent school absence [36]. More globally, within the pediatric chronic pain population depression has been widely shown to correlate with higher levels of functional disability [37] and poorer social and adaptive functioning [38].

ANXIETY

Anxiety and chronic pain also frequently co-occur. Youth with anxiety have nervous systems that are predisposed to being aroused, which lowers the threshold for anxiety and pain. Anxiety activates the sympathetic nervous system, which causes physical symptoms such as increased heart rate. Anxiety also increases activity in the pain perception areas of the brain. Anxiety and fear may also contribute to avoidance in some youth (eg, avoiding physical therapy or exercise because it might hurt), motivating inactivity, and therefore contributing to and maintaining pain. Unfortunately, anxiety also affects the ability to cope with pain and ultimately contributes to greater functional disability.

Anxiety has been shown to correlate with pain complaints in both normal and clinic samples of youth. One pediatric pain clinic found that about 80% of youth meet criteria for an underlying anxiety disorder, regardless of their pain condition. Anxiety is closely related with abdominal pain in youth. The prevalence of anxiety disorders in youngsters with recurrent abdominal pain ranges from 42% to 85% [30,34]. However, anxiety is well documented in other pediatric pain samples. In one study, 57% of children with fibromyalgia met criteria for a current anxiety disorder [31]. Adolescents with chronic headaches also report more anxiety than their healthy peers [35].

PSYCHOLOGICAL TREATMENTS

The American Pain Society recommends a multidisciplinary treatment approach to pediatric pain that typically includes psychological intervention. Specific modalities, such as cognitive-behavioral therapy and acceptance and commitment therapy, may be beneficial for reducing children's experience of pain even when they do not meet diagnostic criteria for a psychiatric disorder. However, because pediatric chronic pain has an emotional component and is often accompanied by clinical levels of depression and/or anxiety, psychological intervention also decreases the pain experience by helping resolve the emotional component that may be contributing to or maintaining the pain. Therapy can reduce psychiatric comorbidities as well as promote improved coping skills and the ability to handle stress, and improve sleep. Psychological treatment can also target change within the family system to improve pain and function. For example, by teaching parents to model appropriate pain behaviors and how they can prevent reinforcement of their children's pain behavior, youth may show less pain-related disability. A recent meta-analysis reported that psychological treatments significantly reduce pain intensity reported by children and adolescents with headache, abdominal pain, and fibromyalgia across various settings. Cognitive-behavioral therapy, relaxation skills training, and biofeedback were the most frequently used and efficacious treatments [39].

There may be times when an outpatient, multidisciplinary treatment approach is not effective in treating pediatric chronic pain. This occurrence is more likely once a child has been diagnosed with a somatoform disorder or pain-associated disability syndrome (PADS), a syndrome of at least 2 months of continuous pain-related dysfunction for which typical pain management strategies have failed. In these circumstances, youth may benefit from participation in a more intensive treatment program that combines medication with daily psychological treatment and complementary and alternative medicine (CAM) approaches to pain. Pain rehabilitation day treatment and inpatient pain rehabilitation programs are becoming more common, and are often affiliated with university-based pediatric pain programs.

COMPLEMENTARY AND ALTERNATIVE THERAPIES FOR PEDIATRIC CHRONIC PAIN

CAM, often defined as interventions that are not generally taught in United States medical schools or provided by medical settings [40], have been increasingly used among pediatric populations in recent years. A recent survey of university-affiliated pediatric pain programs in the United States found that 86% of the programs offered one or more CAM treatments [41]. The most common CAM therapies reported in this study were biofeedback, guided imagery, hypnosis, massage, relaxation therapy, and acupuncture. Art therapy, meditation, therapeutic touch, music therapy, self-help groups, herbal medicine, yoga, and tai-chi were also used. Chiropractic care is often used, particularly for neck pain. Any chiropractic care should be discussed by the patient with a physician, as it can cause permanent damage. Use of megavitamins and herbal medicine should also be discussed with a physician before use.

There is a growing body of research on the use of CAM therapies for pain relief in children. However, much of this research has been plagued by methodological problems and therefore limits conclusions about the safety and efficacy of various CAM approaches. A recent review examined the empirical evidence supporting the use of CAM treatments for pediatric pain conditions [42] using the guidelines for empirically supported therapies that were developed by the American Psychological Association (APA) Division 12 Task Force [43,44]. Few studies that used controlled investigations and methodology meeting the Division 12 guidelines were found. In particular, acupuncture shows promising evidence for pediatric chronic pain, specifically for pediatric migraine. Biofeedback has promising evidence for pediatric migraine and tension headaches. The use of peppermint oil may benefit pain accompanying IBS, and there is evidence that massage therapy reduces pain associated with juvenile rheumatoid arthritis. Finally, hypnosis meets criteria for being an empirically supported treatment for recurrent headaches.

References

[1] Schechter N, Berde C, Yaster M. Pain in infants, children and adolescents, an overview. In : Schechter N, Berde C, Yaster M, editors. Pain in infants, children and adolescents. 2nd edition. Baltimore: Lippincott, Williams and Wilkins; 2003. p. 3–18.

[2] Scharf L, Leichtner A, Rappaport L. Recurrent abdominal pain. In: Schechter N, Berde C, Yaster M, editors. Pain in infants, children and adolescents. 2nd edition. Philadelphia: Lippincott, Williams and Wilkins; 2003. p. 719–31.

[3] Scholz J, Woolf CJ. The neuropathic pain triad: neurons, immune cells, and glia. Nat Neurosci 2007;10:1361–8.

[4] Pocock JM, Kettenmann H. Neurotransmitter receptors on microglia. Trends Neurosci 2007;2:185–93.

[5] Milligan ED, Watkins LR. Pathologic and protective roles of glia in chronic pain. Nat Rev Neurosci 2009;10(1):23–36.

[6] Hutchinson MR, Bland ST, Johnson KW, et al. Opioid-induced glial activation: mechanisms of activation and implications for opioid analgesia, dependence and reward. ScientificWorld Journal 2007;7:98–111.

[7] Winner P. Classification of pediatric headache. Curr Pain Headache Rep 2008;5:357–60.

[8] Ophoff RA, Terwindt GM, Vergouwe MN, et al. Familial hemiplegic migraine and episodic ataxia type-2 are caused by mutations in the Ca^{2+} channel gene CACNLIA4. Cell 1996;87: 543–52.

[9] Hamalainen M, Masek BJ. Diagnosis, classification, and medical management of headache in children and adolescents. In: Schechter N, Berde CB, Yaster M, editors. Pain in infants, children and adolescents. Philadelphia: Lippincott, Williams and Wilkins; 2003. p. 707–18.

[10] Wilder RT. Management of pediatric patients with complex regional pain syndrome. Clin J Pain 2006;22:443–8.

[11] Hocksma AF, Wolf H, Oei SL. Obstetrical brachial plexus injuries: incidence, natural course and shoulder contracture. Clin Rehabil 2000;14:523–6.

[12] Berde CB, Lebel AA, Olsson G. Neuropathic pain in children. In: Schechter N, Berde CB, Yaster M, editors. Pain in infants, children and adolescents. Lippincott, Williams and Wilkins; 2003. p. 620–38.

[13] Bandyk DF, Johnson BI. Surgical sympathectomy for reflex sympathetic dystrophy syndromes. J Vasc Surg 2002;35:269–77.

[14] Lee BH, Scharff L, Sethna NF, et al. Physical therapy and cognitive-behavioral treatment for complex regional pain syndromes. J Pediatr 2002;141:135–40.

[15] Apley J, Naish N. recurrent abdominal pains: a field study of 1,000 schoolchildren. Arch Dis Child 1958;33:165–70.

[16] Ammoury RF, Pfefferkorn Mdel R, Croffie JM. Functional gastrointestinal disorders: past and present. World J Pediatr 2009;5(2):103–12.

[17] de Inocencio J. Musculoskeletal pain in primary pediatric care: analysis of 1000 consecutive general pediatric clinic visits. Pediatrics 1998;102:E63.

[18] Oberklaid F, Amos D, Liu C, et al. "Growing pains": clinical and behavioral correlates in a community sample. J Dev Behav Pediatr 1997;18:102–6.

[19] Buskila D, Press J, Gedalia A, et al. Assessment of nonarticular tenderness and prevalence of fibromyalgia in children. J Rheumatol 1993;20:368–70.

[20] Patel DR, Moore MD, Greydanus DE. Musculoskeletal diagnosis in adolescents. Adolesc Med State Art Rev 2007;18:1–10.

[21] Walters AS, Picchietti DL, Ehrenberg BL, et al. Restless legs syndrome in childhood and adolescence. Pediatr Neurol 1994;11:241–5.

[22] Eccleston C, Jordan A, Crombez G. The impact of chronic pain on adolescents: a review of previously used measures. J Pediatr Psychol 2006;31:684–97.

[23] Hunfeld J, Perquin C, Bertina W, et al. Stability of pain parameters and pain-related quality of life in adolescents with persistent pain: a 3-year follow-up. Clin J Pain 2002;18:99–106.

[24] Gold J, Mahrer N, Yee J, et al. Pain, fatigue, and health-related quality of life in children and adolescents with chronic pain. Clin J Pain 2009;25:407–12.

[25] Gatchel R. Comorbidity of chronic pain and mental health disorders: the biopsychosocial perspective. Am Psychol 2004;59:795–805.

[26] Stanford E, Chambers C, Biesanz J. The frequency, trajectories and predictors of adolescent recurrent pain: a population-based approach. Pain 2007;138:11–21.

[27] Zeltzer L, Tsao J, Bursch B, et al. Introduction to the special issue on pain: from pain to pain-associated disability syndrome. J Pediatr Psychol 2006;31:661–6.

[28] Karwautz A, Wober C, Lang T, et al. Psychosocial factors in children and adolescents with migraine and tension-type headache: a controlled study and review of the literature. Cephalalgia 1999;19:32–43.

[29] Dersh J, Polatin P, Gatchel R. Chronic pain and psychopathology: research findings and theoretical considerations. Psychosom Med 2002;64:773–86.

[30] Dufton L, Dunn M, Compas B. Anxiety and somatic complains in children with recurrent abdominal pain and anxiety disorders. J Pediatr Psychol 2009;34:176–86.

[31] Dorn L, Campo J, Thato S, et al. Psychological comorbidity and stress reactivity in children and adolescents with recurrent abdominal pain and anxiety disorders. J Am Acad Child Adolesc Psychiatry 2003;42:66–75.

[32] Kashikar-Zuck S, Parkins I, Graham T, et al. Anxiety, mood, and behavioral disorders among pediatric patients with juvenile fibromyalgia syndrome. Clin J Pain 2008;24:620–6.

[33] Egger H, Costello E, Erkanli A, et al. Somatic complaints and psychopathology in children and adolescents: stomachaches, musculoskeletal pains, and headaches. J Am Acad Child Adolesc Psychiatry 1998;38:852–60.

[34] Campo J, Bridge J, Ehmann M, et al. Recurrent abdominal pain, anxiety, and depression in primary care. Pediatrics 2004;113:817–24.

[35] Gordon K, Dooley J, Wood E. Self-reported headache frequency and features associated with frequent headaches in Canadian young adolescents. Headache 2004;44:555–61.

[36] Logan D, Simons L, Kaczynski K. School functioning in adolescents with chronic pain: the role of depressive symptoms in school impairment. J Pediatr Psychol 2009;34:882–92.

[37] Claar R, Walker L. Functional assessment of pediatric pain patients: psychometric properties of the functional disability inventory. Pain 2006;121:77–84.

[38] Gauntlett-Gilbert J, Eccleston C. Disability in adolescents with chronic pain: patterns and predictors across different domains of functioning. Pain 2008;131:132–41.

[39] Palermo T. Impact of recurrent and chronic pain on child and family daily functioning: a critical review of the literature. J Dev Behav Pediatr 2009;21:58–69.

[40] Eisenberg D, Davis R, Ettner S. Trends in alternative medicine use in the United States, 1990–1997: results of a follow-up national survey. JAMA 1998;280:1569–75.

[41] Lin Y, Lee A, Kemper K, et al. Use of complementary and alternative medicine in pediatric pain management service: a survey. Pain Med 2005;6:452–8.

[42] Tsao J, Zeltzer L. Complementary and alternative medicine approaches for pediatric pain: a review of the state-of-the-science. Evid Based Complement Alternat Med 2005;2:149–59.

[43] Chambless D, Hollon S. Defining empirically supported therapies. J Consult Clin Psychol 1998;66:7–18.

[44] Palermo T, Eccleston C, Lewandowsky A, et al. Randomized controlled trials of psychological therapies for management of chronic pain in children and adolescents: an updated meta-analytic review. Pain 2010;148:387–97.

Advances in Pediatrics 57 (2010) 163–183

ADVANCES IN PEDIATRICS

Advances in Pediatric Pharmacology, Therapeutics, and Toxicology

Ian M. Paul, MD, MSc[a]

[a]Department of Pediatrics and Public Health Sciences, The Milton S. Hershey Medical Center, Penn State College of Medicine, 500 University Drive, HS83, Hershey, PA 17033, USA

The field of pediatric pharmacology, therapeutics, and toxicology has continued to show marked advancement, and this article highlights many of the tremendous discoveries that have occurred between July 2006 and June 2009. While new therapies and management strategies have been developed, many commonly used drugs and paradigms have been challenged. These aspects include the scrutiny involving over-the-counter (OTC) cough and cold medications and pain relievers, challenges to the routine use of antibiotics for endocarditis and vesicourethral reflux prophylaxis, and controversies over the safety of and monitoring requirements for stimulant medication use for children with attention-deficit/hyperactivity disorder (ADHD).

One of the most important positive developments over the past several years was the reauthorization of the Best Pharmaceuticals for Children Act (BPCA) and the Pediatric Research Equity Act (PREA) in 2007 as part of the Food and Drug Administration Amendments Act of 2007 [1]. BPCA grants pharmaceutical companies an additional 6 months of market exclusivity if pediatric studies have been completed as requested by the Food and Drug Administration (FDA). PREA requires new drugs to be studied in children if they will be used by children and allows FDA to mandate child studies in certain already marketed drugs. Study of drugs used by children is critical, as several recent publications have highlighted the problems of scaling adult doses through weight-based calculations to a pediatric dose [2–4]. Fortunately, pharmaceutical companies continue to study drugs in response to BPCA and PREA as more than 165 drugs have been granted exclusivity [5]. In contrast, the Consortium to Advance the Pediatric Research Infrastructure of the American Academy of Pediatrics (AAP) and others have determined that there is limited capacity to conduct pediatric drug trials in the United States because there is a dearth of adequately trained pediatricians to conduct such trials [6,7]. Nonetheless, scientific advances in pediatric pharmacology, therapeutics, and toxicology have occurred in recent years, which are highlighted in the subsequent sections.

E-mail address: ipaul@psu.edu

0065-3101/10/$ – see front matter
doi:10.1016/j.yapd.2010.08.004

SYMPTOMATIC CARE

As mentioned, there has been significant scrutiny placed on many OTC drugs commonly used by children in recent years. Changes in labeling and manufacturer recommendations have resulted, and more may be forthcoming.

Cough and Cold Medications

Despite evidence-based literature reviews that have determined a lack of proven efficacy [8,9], OTC cough and cold medications are used by 1 in 10 American children each week [10]. For these reasons plus safety concerns, these medications have been reexamined with changes in marketing by manufacturers and recommendations for use in clinical practice (Fig. 1). The first subgroup of these drugs to be affected by federal initiatives was the decongestants. As a result of the Combat Methamphetamine Act [11], pseudoephedrine, the common OTC decongestant, was moved from OTC to being stocked behind the counter because it is a key ingredient in making methamphetamine. Although available without a prescription, the new legislation limited the drug's availability and the amount that can be purchased. The reduced availability did immediately reduce use of pseudoephedrine by children [12]. Several pharmaceutical companies responded to this legislation be replacing pseudoephedrine with phenylephrine in their OTC decongestant preparations, but a commentary by Hendeles and Hatton [13] suggested that phenylephrine is unlikely to provide symptomatic relief at doses recommended by the manufacturers.

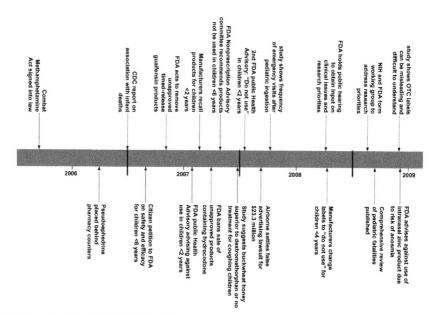

Fig. 1. Selected event timeline involving cough and cold medications between 2006 and June 2009.

Following the changes affecting decongestants, the safety and efficacy of the entire category of OTC cough and cold medications was debated publicly. While studies questioning the efficacy of these medications have been slowly accumulating over the past 20 years, a report published by the Centers for Disease Control and Prevention (CDC) associating infant deaths with cough and cold medications [14] prompted a Citizen Petition to the FDA signed by 14 physicians and an academic pharmacist [15]. In this petition, it was requested that the agency require labels for the medications disclosing the safety risks and lack of proven efficacy of the drugs. It also requested elimination of "infant" or "baby" formulations. The FDA responded in several ways. First, the agency issued a Public Health Advisory in August 2007 urging parents to not use cough and cold medications for children younger than 2 years, not give adult preparations to children, and use caution when giving more than one OTC or prescription medicine along with cough and cold medications [16]. Second, the agency convened the Nonprescription Drugs Advisory Committee in October 2007 to discuss the safety and effectiveness of cough and cold drug product use in children. Just before the committee meeting, the manufacturers of cough and cold medications voluntarily recalled all preparations directed at children younger than 2 years. The committee suggested further action, concluding that it was unacceptable to extrapolate data from adults to children, and that cough and cold products should not be used by children younger than 6 years [17]. After the meeting, the FDA definitively stated that children younger than 2 years should not use cough and cold medications, but delayed judgment for older children [18,19].

The subsequent 12 months further fueled this controversial subject as additional safety and efficacy data were published. Questioning the efficacy of one of the OTC compounds, dextromethorphan, investigators found buckwheat honey to be superior to dextromethorphan or no treatment for the treatment of nocturnal cough and cold symptoms in children aged 2 to 16 years [20]. Another found that a nasal wash with a modified seawater solution was a useful adjunct in aiding resolution of nasal symptoms caused by upper respiratory infections in children aged 6 to 10 years [21].

Safety concerns were also prevalent in the medical literature, with articles published describing the frequency of emergency department visits as a result of ingestions of OTC cough and cold medications [22] as well as a comprehensive examination of pediatric fatalities associated with the drugs over the past 60 years [23]. Of note, both of these studies found that the adverse events were most likely the result of unsupervised ingestions or accidents, and typically involved children younger than 6 years. Improved packaging and labeling has been cited as one potential solution to reducing accidents, which was supported by a publication showing that parents frequently misunderstand the labels on OTC cough and cold medications [24].

The cumulative evidence was debated at a second FDA meeting in October 2008 where clinical and research issues related to OTC cough and cold medications were discussed. Following this meeting, the manufacturers voluntarily agreed to change their labels and marketing, reflecting that the medications should not be used by children younger than 4 years [25]. The labels also were amended to include a statement indicating that antihistamines should not be used for sedative purposes in children.

Changes to therapeutics involving cough and cold medications were not limited to OTC products or the traditional compounds used to treat them. In 2007, the FDA took action to remove unapproved extended-release formulations of guaifenesin as well as unapproved prescription cough suppressants containing hydrocodone [26,27]. Next, the herbal supplement, Airborne, was cited in a 2008 class action lawsuit as making false advertising claims for preventing cold symptoms, resulting in a settlement of more than $23 million [28]. Finally, in 2009 the intranasal zinc product, Zicam, was subject to an FDA advisory after it was associated with long-lasting or permanent anosmia [29].

With this flurry of activity surrounding one group of medications, it is notable that the National Institutes of Health and FDA are actively seeking to increase the evidence base regarding treatments for cough and cold symptoms. In 2009, a working group of experts was developed as part of BPCA to develop research priorities for the treatment of cough and cold symptoms in children.

Analgesics and Antipyretics

The practice of using acetaminophen and ibuprofen together to reduce fever and treat discomfort has been widely employed by parents and health care professionals but with limited evidence to support this strategy. British investigators recently attempted to fill this void in a study that compared acetaminophen (15 mg/kg) given every 6 hours with ibuprofen (10 mg/kg) dosed every 8 hours with a regimen using both drugs [30]. Febrile children 6 months to 6 years old were enrolled and followed for 48 hours. Children in the combined treatment group had less fever over the first 24 hours when compared with the other groups. The combined group also fared better than the acetaminophen-only group, but not the ibuprofen-only group with regard to the rapidity of initial fever reduction and time without fever in the first 4 hours after initial dosing. A second study from the United States compared acetaminophen (15 mg/kg) dosed every 4 hours with acetaminophen followed 3 hours later with ibuprofen (10 mg/kg) [31]. The febrile children aged 6 months to 6 years were followed for 6 hours. Although no difference in temperature between groups was discovered at 0, 3, and 6 hours after the initial acetaminophen, those in the alternating group had lower mean temperatures at hours 4 and 5. Of note, no difference in discomfort was detected between treatment groups in either the British or United States trial.

The topic of analgesia using OTC medications was the primary outcome variable, however, in an emergency department–based study of children presenting with pain from a musculoskeletal injury [32]. Change in pain from baseline was assessed 60 minutes after dosing using a visual analog scale, comparing children receiving acetaminophen (15 mg/kg), ibuprofen (10 mg/kg), or codeine (1 mg/kg). Ibuprofen provided the greatest analgesia 60, 90, and 120 minutes after treatment between the 3 groups. Subgroup analyses demonstrated ibuprofen's superiority in patients with fractures and in those with severe pain.

EAR, NOSE, AND THROAT
Otitis Media and Externa
Acute otitis media continues to be one of the most common pediatric diagnoses, but there is considerable variability in management strategies across the globe, largely because the benefits of antibiotic treatment are marginal. To help clinicians determine which subgroups might benefit most from antibiotic therapy, a meta-analysis was conducted using trials with individual patient data for children ages 6 months to 12 years [33]. The investigators found that the children most likely to benefit from antibiotics were those with otorrhea, and those younger than 2 years with bilateral acute otitis media. This same group of investigators also demonstrated that antibiotics were not helpful in preventing the development of middle ear effusion 1 month after treatment [34].

One of the alternative treatment strategies to an immediate antibiotic course for acute otitis media is a "wait-and-see" prescription. In essence, parents are asked to wait 48 hours to start antibiotics to prevent a treatment course for children whose symptoms would resolve spontaneously without antibiotics. To test this approach versus a standard antibiotic treatment course, investigators randomized children presenting to an emergency department to one of these two approaches [35]. Children in the wait-and-see group were given ibuprofen and otic analgesic drops (antipyrene 54 mg/benzocaine 14 mg/mL). Although the wait-and-see group was much less likely to fill an antibiotic prescription (62% vs 13%), there were no differences in outcomes related to fever, otalgia, or unscheduled office visits.

For chronic otitis media with at least 3 months of continuous otorrhea, a randomized trial compared a 6- to 12-week course of trimethoprim/sulfamethoxazole with placebo [36]. After 6 weeks of treatment, 28% of children in the treatment group had otorrhea compared with 53% of those treated with placebo.

Fluoroquinolones have become an increasingly common treatment for otitis externa, but a randomized trial suggested ofloxacin drops may not be superior to an older, less expensive treatment [37]. Children treated 4 times daily with neomycin sulfate/polymyxin B sulfate/hydrocortisone otic suspension had efficacy comparable with the once-daily ofloxacin treatment in terms of clinical and microbiological cure rates, but the ofloxacin group was more likely to adhere to therapy recommendations.

For all ear complaints, pediatricians often have to overcome the obstacle of cerumen. Not infrequently, cerumen impaction requires treatment, and a new practice guideline on the subject was released by the American Academy of Otolaryngology-Head and Neck Surgery Foundation [38]. The guidelines recommend cerumen removal when impaction causes symptoms or prevents clinical examination. In addition to irrigation and manual removal, cerumenolytics were discussed. The 3 categories described are water-based (eg, acetic acid, Cerumenex [triethanolamine polypeptide oleate condensate], docusate sodium, hydrogen peroxide), oil-based (eg, olive oil, mineral oil), and nonwater-, nonoil-based treatments (eg, Debrox [carbamide peroxide]). Although there is some evidence that these agents may be helpful, there are few data comparing the different treatments.

Rhinitis

In 2008, for the first time in 10 years, the American Academy of Allergy, Asthma, and Immunology published new guidelines for the diagnosis and management of rhinitis in both adults and children [39]. Some key features regarding therapeutics from these extensive guidelines are:

- Intranasal corticosteroids are the most effective medication class for controlling symptoms of allergic rhinitis
- Second-generation antihistamines are generally preferred over first-generation antihistamines for the treatment of allergic rhinitis
- Intranasal antihistamines may be considered for use as first-line treatment for allergic and nonallergic rhinitis
- Oral antileukotriene agents alone, or in combination with antihistamines, have proved to be useful in the treatment of allergic rhinitis
- Intranasal anticholinergics may effectively reduce rhinorrhea, but have no effect on other nasal symptoms.

Sleep Apnea

Because the AAP recommends screening all children for sleep apnea [40], clinicians may be diagnosing sleep apnea at greater frequencies, particularly because sleep apnea has been associated with obesity, itself an increasing problem. For many children, surgical treatment may be necessary, but one recent study showed that a 6-week course of intranasal steroids may reduce the severity of mild obstructive sleep apnea and the magnitude of adenoidal hypertrophy [41]. The treatment effect persisted for 8 weeks after cessation of the study drug, budesonide.

Streptococcal Pharyngitis

Over the past decade, several small studies have suggested that once-daily treatment with amoxicillin is sufficient for the treatment of streptococcal pharyngitis. To more definitively determine the adequacy of this practice, 2 large noninferiority trials were completed with more than 1000 combined participants. The first study found similar outcomes when twice daily treatment with amoxicillin was compared with once-daily amoxicillin at weight-dependent doses [42]. The second study compared twice daily penicillin V with once-daily amoxicillin, and found no difference between treatment outcomes [43]. Both studies had treatment durations of 10 days.

PULMONARY

Asthma

In 2007, the third edition of the national guidelines for the diagnosis and management of asthma were released, with some significant changes to past recommendations [44]. A step-wise approach to treatment was maintained, and several key therapeutic messages emerge for children:

- Consider initiating daily long-term control therapy for (a) children who consistently require short acting β-agonists treatment more than 2 days per week for longer than 4 weeks or (b) children who have 2 exacerbations requiring oral systemic corticosteroids within 6 months
- Inhaled corticosteroids continue as preferred long-term control therapy for all ages
- For children 0 to 4 years old with insufficient control on low-dose inhaled corticosteroids, increasing the dose of inhaled corticosteroids is preferred over the addition of another adjunctive therapy
- For patients at least 5 years old with persistent symptoms on low-dose inhaled corticosteroids, a combination of long-acting β-agonist and inhaled corticosteroids is equally preferred to increasing the dose of inhaled steroids
- For asthma exacerbations, anticholinergics are to be used in emergency care, not hospital care.

In addition to the guideline revisions, several studies focused on the treatment of infants and toddlers with virus-induced wheezing. In one trial, children between the ages of 10 months and 6 years admitted to the hospital were treated with either prednisolone or placebo [45]. There was no significant difference in the duration of hospitalization between groups, although the mean length of hospitalization was relatively brief in both groups (13.9 hours vs 11.0 hours). A second study performed with children aged 1 to 6 years compared a large dose of inhaled fluticasone (750 µg twice daily) with placebo for a duration of up to 10 days initiated at the onset of upper respiratory symptoms [46]. The fluticasone group proved to be superior in terms of reduction in illnesses leading to rescue systemic corticosteroids, but these children had slower linear growth than those given placebo. A third trial comparing inhaled budesonide (1 mg twice daily), montelukast (4 mg daily), and placebo initiated at the onset of respiratory tract illnesses in children 12 to 59 months old with a history of wheezing found no difference in the proportion of episode-free days or oral corticosteroid use, but a modest improvement in symptoms for those treated with budesonide and montelukast [47]. A fourth study compared montelukast with placebo treatment beginning at the onset of respiratory symptoms for a minimum of 7 days and found a modest reduction in acute care use, symptoms, and time missed from school for 2- to 14-year-old children with intermittent asthma. Taken together, there may be some benefit to large doses of corticosteroids or montelukast for illness progression with acute wheezing episodes in known asthmatics, but the decision to initiate this therapy must be balanced against the potential for adverse effects, particularly with repeated courses of corticosteroids.

Bronchiolitis

Like asthma, new guidelines were recently published on the diagnosis and management of bronchiolitis for children younger than 2 years [48]. Key therapeutic messages in the guideline included recommendations against the routine use of bronchodilators, corticosteroids, ribavirin, or antibiotics. It was suggested that a trial of α-adrenergic or β-adrenergic medications may be performed with careful monitoring followed by continued bronchodilator therapy for those with a positive clinical response. These guidelines were supplemented by 2 new publications in the *New England Journal of Medicine*. In the first a multicenter, randomized, controlled trial tested the effects of oral dexamethasone (1 mg/kg) versus placebo in 2- to 12-month-old children with their first episode of wheezing in the emergency department [49]. These children were all diagnosed with bronchiolitis, but there was no difference in rates of hospital admission, respiratory status 4 hours after treatment, or subsequent outcomes regardless of the results of respiratory syncytial virus testing. By contrast, the second study found the combination of nebulized epinephrine (3 mL of epinephrine in a 1:1000 solution per treatment) plus 6 oral doses of dexamethasone (1.0 mg/kg in the emergency department followed by 4 once-daily doses of 0.6 mg/kg at home) to be moderately effective at reducing hospital admissions among infants with bronchiolitis [50].

BEHAVIORAL HEALTH AND PSYCHIATRY
Attention-Deficit/Hyperactivity Disorder
Over the past several years there have been numerous efficacy studies, safety concerns, and published guidelines regarding treatments for ADHD. Regarding efficacy, the setting where effective medication is perhaps most often necessary is in school, and a recent study demonstrated that elementary school-aged children with ADHD taking medications for their condition scored better on standardized math and reading tests than their nonmedicated peers [51].

As for individual medication classes, amphetamine stimulants have long been the first-line treatment choice, but the stimulant transdermal patch represents a relatively new delivery mechanism for the medication. This option offers some attractive differences for clinicians and families because patch size and duration of patch wear can be optimally tailored for the individual child as opposed to fixed-dose oral preparations [52]. Although the patch can cause local skin irritation and has a somewhat slower onset of action than oral preparations, it is generally well tolerated and effective delivery route.

A second class of medications commonly used for ADHD is the α2-adrenergic agonists. A recent review summarized the safety and efficacy of the 2 commonly used drugs from this class, clonidine and guanfacine [53]. In this class, an extended-release formulation of guanfacine was approved, and this preparation was shown to be well tolerated and effective when compared with a placebo [54].

One compound shown not to be superior to placebo for ADHD symptoms was *Hypericum perforatum*, commonly known as St John's wort. In a study involving 54 children, no difference was detected in any ADHD outcome between groups over the 8-week observation period [55]. These results may be disappointing to some families, as complementary and alternative remedies may seem appealing given controversies over stimulant safety now described.

In 2008, the American Heart Association (AHA) issued a scientific statement regarding cardiovascular monitoring of children and adolescents receiving stimulant drugs [56]. In addition to guidance on cardiac history and physical examination measures, among the recommendations in this statement was one to obtain an electrocardiogram (ECG) on all patients being considered for stimulant drug therapy. The investigators acknowledged a lack of data to inform this screen, but nonetheless made the recommendation. The statement further recommended that a cardiologist with pediatric experience review each child's ECG, problematic given the limited workforce capacity to review the volume of ECGs that would result from this recommendation. The routine ECG screening recommendation was also in direct contradiction with policy statements by the AAP and the American Academy of Child Psychiatry, causing a public debate [57,58]. Shortly following the AHA statement's publication, the AAP and AHA issued a joint statement clarifying the recommended screening recommendation [59]. The clarification stated that routine ECG screening is not mandatory, but should be performed if warranted by risk factors presenting during history taking or physical examination. This statement temporarily assuaged fears regarding cardiovascular risk with stimulant medications, but a 2009 publication describing sudden death with use of stimulant medications by children renewed the controversy [60]. In a case-control study, 564 cases of sudden unexplained death in children aged 7 to 19 years were compared with 564 pediatric deaths due to motor vehicle accidents. Whereas 1.8% of children suffering unexplained deaths were taking stimulants, only 0.4% of those in motor vehicle accidents were taking the medications. The FDA promptly responded to the article with a critique of the study, arguing that the study's numerous limitations do not affect the overall risk-benefit profile of stimulant medications used to treat ADHD [61].

Depression and Anxiety

Controversy has also surrounded the use of antidepressants for children and, in particular, the risk of suicidal ideation among children taking selective serotonin reuptake inhibitors (SSRIs). The purported risk appears to have reduced prescriptions of SSRIs for children [62]. A meta-analysis attempted to further examine this issue as well as the efficacy of SSRIs for the treatment of children and adolescents with major depressive disorder, obsessive-compulsive disorder (OCD), and non-OCD anxiety disorders [63]. While there was a small, 0.7% increase in suicidal ideation across treatment indications, no suicides were actually completed in any of the 27 studies involving more than 5000 patients. Further, the SSRIs were at least modestly effective for all treatment indications.

Because many patients do not respond to initial treatment with SSRIs, the question has been raised as to the best next step for treatment. To answer this question for adolescents, a trial compared changing to a second SSRI or changing to venlafaxine, a selective serotonin and noradrenergic reuptake inhibitor [64]. This 4-arm trial tested each of the 2 drugs with and without simultaneous cognitive behavioral therapy (CBT). The results demonstrated that switching to another drug with CBT was superior to medication alone, but the SSRI group had fewer adverse events than the venlafaxine treatment arm. CBT plus sertraline was also found to be superior to each individual treatment for childhood and adolescent anxiety disorders in another study of 488 children between the ages of 7 and 17 years with separation anxiety disorder, generalized anxiety disorder, or social phobia [65].

Pervasive Developmental Disorder and Autism

Although therapeutic breakthroughs in the medical management of children with autism have been limited, the past several years did mark the approval of the first drug that is FDA approved for treatment of autistic behaviors, risperidone [66]. The specific behaviors cited for treatment were irritability and aggression. While exciting, the use of antipsychotics such as risperidone do come with known increased risk of obesity, type 2 diabetes, and orthostatic hypotension [67]. In addition to risperidone, other treatment considerations for clinicians were nicely summarized in a clinical report from the AAP [68]. There, guidance was offered for the various symptoms that are associated with autism as well as references to guide dosing of drugs.

Sleep Difficulty

Sleep disturbances are common in childhood, but there are few proven therapeutic options. Zolpidem is commonly used and has been shown to be effective for adults, but there are limited pediatric data. To help elucidate dosing for children, Blumer and colleagues [69] undertook an open-label dose-escalation study in children with insomnia between ages 2 and 18. The investigators suggested that a dose of 0.25 mg/kg be used in future efficacy trials.

CARDIOVASCULAR DISEASE

Infective Endocarditis

Although the AHA's guideline for use of stimulants initially suggested a more aggressive management strategy, their new guideline for prevention of infective endocarditis invited less aggressive management than previous versions [70]. Whereas previous antibiotic prophylaxis for invasive procedures including dental work in patients with many heart conditions was previously recommended, the new version indicates prophylaxis only for those patients with the highest risk of endocarditis: prosthetic cardiac valve, previous infective endocarditis, unrepaired cyanotic congenital heart disease, congenital heart defect with prosthetic material placed within the prior 6 months, repaired heart defect with residual defects adjacent to prosthetic material, and cardiac transplantation recipients with valvulopathy. Further, administration of antibiotics for patients undergoing gastrointestinal or genitourinary procedures for the sole purpose of preventing endocarditis is no longer recommended.

Obesity and the Metabolic Syndrome

With increasing obesity rates among youth in the United States, the comorbidities of obesity also are on the increase. Using a database from a pharmacy benefits manager, prevalence of prescriptions for antihypertensive, antidiabetic, and dyslipidemic medications were shown to increase by more than 15% among a large population of commercially insured 6- to 18-year-old children between 2004 and 2007 [71]. Regarding which drugs to use for treatment, 2 thorough reviews were recently published to guide management of hypertension and dyslipidemia in children. Flynn and Daniels summarized the currently available data regarding efficacy and safety of antihypertensives for children [72]. These investigators suggest that several classes of agents may be used as first-line treatments including diuretics, β-blocking agents, angiotensin-converting enzyme inhibitors, angiotensin receptor antagonists, and calcium channel blockers. For dyslipidemia, the use of statins was reviewed by Belay and colleagues [73]. Their review acknowledged the lack of long-term data to demonstrate benefit of statin treatment for prevention of cardiovascular disease in children, and the potential for adverse events including elevated liver enzymes, myositis, and rhabdomyolysis. These factors must be balanced with the individual's cardiovascular risk.

UROLOGY AND NEPHROLOGY
Urinary Tract Infections
Because of fears over the long-term consequences of recurrent infections and subsequent renal scarring, clinicians have been treating children with a history of a single urinary tract infection (UTI) and evidence of vesicoureteral reflux with indefinite courses of prophylactic antibiotics. Recently, however, new publications have questioned this practice. The first of these studies examined the time to recurrent UTI as well as resistance patterns of subsequent UTIs in a large primary care practice network [74]. Conflicting with current practice, the study found that antimicrobial prophylaxis was not associated with a decreased risk of subsequent UTIs, but did increase the risk for antibiotic resistant organisms with subsequent infections. A randomized trial in Italy confirmed these results by comparing no prophylaxis following the first febrile UTI with either trimethoprim plus sulfamethoxazole or amoxicillin plus clavulanic acid in children between the ages of 2 months and 7 years [75]. Regardless of the degree of vesicoureteral reflux, no difference was discovered in rate of recurrence of UTI or that of renal scarring [76].

INFECTIOUS DISEASES
Fluoroquinolones
Despite concerns regarding arthrotoxicity, adverse musculoskeletal events, and other side effects, more than 500,000 prescriptions were written for fluoroquinolone use by children in the United States in 2002 [77]. To address this class of antibiotics, an AAP policy statement was published in 2006, which urged caution in using these drugs in children. The main exception where use may be indicated is for multidrug-resistant infections for which no other safe and effective alternative is available, such as drug-resistant strains of *Pseudomonas aeruginosa* and *Escherichia coli*. The caution regarding use of fluoroquinolones in children was supported by

the addition of a "black box" warning to this class of drugs in 2008 because of concerns regarding tendonitis and tendon rupture [78].

Antiviral Therapy for Influenza

The AAP also issued guidance on the use of antiviral medications for children with influenza infections [79]. In this clinical report, oseltamivir and zanamivir were chosen as the first-line treatments of influenza because of resistance to amantadine and rimantadine. Indications for therapy included children at high risk of severe infection or those with moderate to severe infections that might benefit from a shorter duration of illness. Examples of high-risk groups eligible for therapy include children aged 12 to 24 months, those that are immunosuppressed, or those with chronic disease.

Skin and Soft Tissue Infections

In the age of methicillin-resistant *Staphylococcus aureus* (MRSA), choosing the correct antibiotic for community-acquired skin and soft tissue infections requires careful consideration. Two publications offer some guidance on how to approach treatment. The first article analyzed the clinical scenario of skin and soft tissue infections that cannot be drained or cultured in an MRSA-endemic region [80]. Surprisingly for these generally more mild infections, treatment with β-lactam antibiotics was superior to trimethoprim-sulfamethoxazole and equivalent to clindamycin. The investigators hypothesized that these infections may be more likely to be caused by group A streptococcus than lesions that can be drained or cultured.

In contrast to that article, a second report found that for purulent infections that can be drained and cultured, empirical treatment of skin and soft tissue infections with clindamycin or trimethoprim-sulfamethoxazole was superior to cephalexin when the prevalence of community-associated MRSA infections is greater than 10% [81]. When combined, these 2 articles offer some guidance for decision making by the clinician, with ability to drain and culture the lesions being the key clinical feature.

Tinea Capitis and Head Lice

The FDA approved 2 treatments for common pediatric conditions affecting the scalp and hair. For tinea capitis, griseofulvin has been the traditional treatment, but terbinafine oral granules are now an approved alternative for children aged 4 years and up [82]. Similarly, the agency approved benzyl alcohol lotion 5% for the treatment of head lice in children at least 6 months old [83]. For this lotion, 2 10-minute treatments separated by 1 week resulted in a cure rate of greater than 75% 2 weeks after the second application.

GASTROENTEROLOGY

Vomiting

Vomiting is certainly a distressing symptom for children and their parents, and there have been relatively few well-conducted trials evaluating treatment of this symptom when associated with acute gastroenteritis. As an attempt to synthesize the available data, a systematic review and meta-analysis were performed evaluating ondansetron, domperidone, trimethobenzamide, pyrilamine-pentobarbital, metoclopramide, dexamethasone, and promethazine [84]. Although most of the drugs were difficult to evaluate owing to inadequate data or trial design, the investigators found that ondansetron reduced vomiting, need for intravenous fluids, and hospital admission due to acute gastroenteritis. Another drug that has been used by clinicians for nausea and vomiting is trimethobenzamide, a sedating antihistamine that had been marketed under the trade name, Tigan. Citing a lack of evidence of effectiveness, the FDA mandated that companies stop marketing suppositories containing this drug in 2007 [85].

Gastroesophageal Reflux

Another distressing symptom for parents is fussiness during infancy. As treatments for gastroesophageal reflux (GER) have become available, these medications have been frequently prescribed for infants because many "spit up," and it therefore seems logical that this fussiness could be related to GER. Two recent publications question this logic. In the first, infants with persistent regurgitation underwent extended esophageal pH monitoring, and only 8 of 44 pH studies showed abnormal acid reflux [86]. The investigators further reported that discontinuation of the medication did not result in an exacerbation of symptoms.

In the second publication, the use of metoclopramide for infant GER is questioned [87]. In a systematic review of the literature, 12 articles were examined including 5 randomized, blinded clinical trials. Among the 5 randomized trials, 2 showed no benefit from the drug while 2 others reported a significant placebo effect. Based on the current published evidence, the investigators determined that there was insufficient evidence for or against the use of metoclopramide for GER in infants.

Irritable Bowel Syndrome

Irritable bowel syndrome is a common and frustrating cause of abdominal pain for children and adolescents, made more distressing by a lack of therapeutic options. Amitriptyline may be effective, however, as demonstrated by a study of 33 adolescents in which amitriptyline was compared with placebo over a 13-week study period [88]. The medication, dosed according to weight (30–50 kg: 10 mg every bedtime, 50–80 kg: 20 mg every bedtime, >80 kg: 30 mg every bedtime), was associated with improved quality of life, less diarrhea, and reduced abdominal pain when compared with placebo.

NEUROLOGY

Seizures

The number of therapeutic options for chronic seizure management has grown in recent years. To evaluate the efficacy of these newer medications compared with traditional therapies, 2 simultaneous studies were conducted as part of the Standard and New Antiepileptic Drugs (SANAD) trial [89,90]. Participants were at least 4 years old, and could be either children or adults without a history of progressive neurologic disease. One of these studies involved patients with generalized or unclassified epilepsy, and compared valproate with lamotrigine and topiramate [89]. Valproate was superior to topiramate for time to treatment failure and better than lamotrigine for time to 12-month remission, suggesting that it should remain the drug of first choice for these patients. The second study compared carbamazepine with gabapentin, lamotrigine, oxcarbazepine, and topiramate for the treatment of partial epilepsy [90]. Here, the newer drug, lamotrigine, prevailed with the longest time to treatment failure of the group.

For simple febrile seizures, the AAP released an updated clinical practice guideline in 2008 [91]. While the preventive benefits of continuous anticonvulsant therapy was recognized, the use of such a therapeutic strategy was discouraged because of the relatively high prevalence of adverse events associated with antiepileptic therapy and the generally benign nature of febrile seizures. In addition, the use of antipyretics for the prevention of seizures was discouraged, based on data suggesting such an approach is ineffective.

Migraine Headaches

As all clinicians recognize, treatment of migraine headaches often requires preventive therapy as well as medication for acute exacerbations. Important new publications have contributed to our knowledge of treatment options for both domains of migraine therapy. For prevention, topiramate is emerging as a therapeutic option for children and adolescents, supported by a study of adolescents treated with the drug or placebo for 16 weeks [92]. In this trial, a 100-mg daily dose, but not a 50-mg daily dose, was found to be more effective than placebo for reducing rates of migraine headaches.

For acute treatment of migraines, zolmitriptan nasal spray was studied in adolescents with a known diagnosis of migraine, with or without aura [93]. At 1 hour after dosing, relief was seen by 58% of zolmitriptan-treated participants compared with only 43% of those treated with placebo for acute headache, and both pain reduction and sustained relief were better in the active drug arm.

DERMATOLOGY

Hemangiomas

Although most infantile hemangiomas are benign and spontaneously resolve, some interfere with function and/or cause significant disfigurement. In such cases, corticosteroids are often used as treatment, with limited data to support this approach. A new trial compared oral and high-dose pulse corticosteroids for problematic infantile hemangiomas, and found the daily, oral prednisolone treatment to be more effective (2 mg/kg/d for 3 months) [94]. The orally treated group also had higher rates of hypertension and growth retardation, however.

An alternative to corticosteroids, propranolol, was suggested in a letter to the editor of the *New England Journal of Medicine* [95]. This letter, which includes impressive photographs, describes the treatment with 2 mg/kg of propranolol in 11 infants as highly effective, with rapid improvement in these hemangiomas, some of which were inadequately treated with corticosteroids.

RHEUMATOLOGY
Kawasaki Disease
One of the mysteries of Kawasaki disease is that although it is thought to be an immune-mediated vasculitis, corticosteroid therapy has not been definitively shown to benefit children afflicted with this condition. Nonetheless, investigators continue to investigate the role of corticosteroids in the treatment of Kawasaki disease. In addition to intravenous immunoglobulin, a Japanese trial evaluated the addition of daily prednisolone versus placebo, and found that the prednisolone group had fewer coronary artery abnormalities in the first month after diagnosis, shorter duration of initial fever, and more rapid resolution of inflammatory biomarkers [96]. A second study, which differed in corticosteroid treatment (single pulse dose of intravenous methylprednisolone) and study design (placebo controlled with blinded investigators and echocardiogram interpretation), found similar results with regard to initial illness course and biomarker changes, but no difference in coronary artery outcomes, leading these investigators to reject the single-pulse dose of methylprednisolone as a therapy for children with Kawasaki disease [97].

Juvenile Idiopathic Arthritis
New therapeutic options targeting tumor necrosis factor (TNF) are becoming available for children with juvenile idiopathic arthritis (JIA). Adalimumab is a monoclonal anti-TNF antibody that was included in a trial of 4- to 17-year-old children with polyarticular JIA [98]. Adalimumab significantly reduced disease flares for patients taking and not taking concomitant methotrexate, and response rates were sustained over an extended 2 years of open-label treatment. This anti-TNF antibody also was shown to improve JIA-associated and idiopathic uveitis [99].

Two other therapies with different targets were recently studied for children with JIA. Abatacept, which competitively binds to CD80 or CD86 inhibiting T-cell activation, was tested against placebo in a cohort of 6- to 17-year-old children with refractory, polyarticular JIA, and significantly reduced frequency of disease flares [100]. Another trial tested tocilizumab, an anti–interleukin-6 antibody, in children aged 2 to 19 years with refractory, systemic-onset JIA [101]. Following a 6-week open-label course that produced significant improvement in nearly all participants, a double-blind, placebo-controlled 12-week trial demonstrated the treatment's significant benefit for this difficult-to-treat disorder.

EFFECTS OF MATERNAL MEDICATION USE DURING PREGNANCY AND LACTATION
Opioids
Opioid medications are commonly taken by lactating women for pain management. In 2007, the FDA issued a warning regarding codeine use by nursing

mothers following the death of a 13-day-old breastfed infant whose mother was an unknown ultrarapid metabolizer of codeine who was taking the drug for episiotomy pain [102]. Because some codeine is metabolized to morphine, ultrarapid metabolizers may have higher than normal levels of morphine in their blood and breast milk following drug consumption. Following this warning, a case-control study was conducted, which found that among 72 mothers surveyed following treatment with codeine, 17 had infants that were symptomatic. Mothers of symptomatic infants had a significantly higher dose of codeine than those with asymptomatic infants, and there was a 71% concordance between maternal and neonatal central nervous system depression. In addition, 2 infants who exhibited severe nervous system depression both had mothers who were ultrarapid metabolizers. Based on this report, given the lack of routine pharmacogenetic testing of breastfeeding mothers, clinicians should pay close attention to sedation in these mother-baby pairs.

Antidepressants

Antidepressants are commonly taken during pregnancy, with SSRIs serving as the most common treatment option. To evaluate the relationship between first-trimester use of SSRIs and birth defects, investigators at the Slone Epidemiology Center conducted a case-control analysis [103]. While overall use of SSRIs was not associated with birth defects and absolute risks are small, the investigators did find significant associations between sertraline and both omphalocele and septal heart defects as well as between paroxetine and right ventricular outflow tract obstruction defects.

Behavioral symptoms in newborns have also been reported following maternal SSRI use. To study these features among term and preterm infants following maternal SSRI or venlafaxine use during the third trimester, a cohort of exposed neonates was compared with nonexposed newborns [104]. Behavioral symptoms in the first few days after delivery were significantly more common among exposed newborns and included abnormal movements, tone abnormalities, irritability, and insomnia. In general, these symptoms resolved within 5 days of delivery. An additional study found no adverse attentional or activity behaviors among 4-year-old children exposed to SSRIs during the second or third trimester [105].

Antiepileptics

Although most women with epilepsy deliver healthy newborns, the differential treatment effects on cognitive functioning among offspring is an important question. As such, pregnant women with epilepsy taking a single antiepileptic were enrolled in a prospective, observational study seeking to examine neurodevelopmental outcomes [106]. The study with 309 children discovered that at age 3 years, children exposed in utero to valproate had significantly lower IQ scores (mean of 92) than those exposed to lamotrigine (101), phenytoin (99), or carbamazepine (98) after adjustment for relevant confounders.

References

[1] 110th Congress. Food and Drug Administration Amendments Act of 2007. Public Law 110–85. September 27, 2007.

[2] Rodriguez W, Selen A, Avant D, et al. Improving pediatric dosing through pediatric initiatives: what we have learned. Pediatrics 2008;121:530–9.

[3] Johnson TN. The problems in scaling adult drug doses to children. Arch Dis Child 2008;93: 207–11.

[4] Hawcutt DB, Smyth RL. One size does not fit all: getting drug doses right for children. Arch Dis Child 2008;93:190–1.

[5] US Food and Drug Administration. Drugs to which FDA has granted pediatric exclusivity for pediatric studies under section 505A of the Federal Food, Drug, and Cosmetic Act. Available at: http://www.fda.gov/Drugs/DevelopmentApprovalProcess/DevelopmentResources/ucm050005.htm. Accessed July 10, 2009.

[6] Kearns GL, Ritschel WA, Wilson JT, et al. Clinical pharmacology: a discipline called to action for maternal and child health. Clin Pharmacol Ther 2007;81:463–8.

[7] AAP Department of Research. Investigation finds limited capacity to conduct pediatric drug trials. AAP News 2008;29(8):12.

[8] Smith SM, Schroeder K, Fahey T. Over-the-counter medications for acute cough in children and adults in ambulatory settings. Cochrane Database Syst Rev 2008;1:CD001831.

[9] Shields MD, Bush A, Everard ML, et al. BTS guidelines: recommendations for the assessment and management of cough in children. Thorax 2008;63(Suppl 3):iii1–15.

[10] Vernacchio L, Kelly JP, Kaufman DW, et al. Cough and cold medication use by US children, 1999–2006: results from the Slone survey. Pediatrics 2008;122:e323–9.

[11] 109th Congress. USA Patriot Improvement and Reauthorization Act of 2005. Public Law 109–177. March 9, 2006.

[12] Vernacchio L, Kelly JP, Kaufman DW, et al. Pseudoephedrine use among US children, 1999–2006: results from the Slone survey. Pediatrics 2008;122:1299–304.

[13] Hendeles L, Hatton RC. Oral phenylephrine: an ineffective replacement for pseudoephedrine? J Allergy Clin Immunol 2006;118:279–80.

[14] Infant deaths associated with cough and cold medications—two states, 2005. MMWR Morb Mortal Wkly Rep 2007;56:1–4.

[15] Available at: http://www.baltimorehealth.org/press/FDA%20petition%20PDF.pdf. Accessed July 12, 2009.

[16] Available at: http://www.fda.gov/Drugs/DrugSafety/PublicHealthAdvisories/ucm051282.html. Accessed July 13, 2009.

[17] Sharfstein JM, North M, Serwint JR. Over the counter but no longer under the radar—pediatric cough and cold medications. N Engl J Med 2007;357:2321–4.

[18] Kuehn BM. Citing serious risks, FDA recommends no cold and cough medicines for infants. JAMA 2008;299:887–8.

[19] Available at: http://www.fda.gov/Drugs/DrugSafety/PublicHealthAdvisories/ucm051137.html. Accessed July 14, 2009.

[20] Paul IM, Beiler J, McMonagle A, et al. Effect of honey, dextromethorphan, and no treatment on nocturnal cough and sleep quality for coughing children and their parents. Arch Pediatr Adolesc Med 2007;161:1140–6.

[21] Slapak I, Skoupa J, Strnad P, et al. Efficacy of isotonic nasal wash (seawater) in the treatment and prevention of rhinitis in children. Arch Otolaryngol Head Neck Surg 2008;134:67–74.

[22] Schaefer MK, Shehab N, Cohen AL, et al. Adverse events from cough and cold medications in children. Pediatrics 2008;121:783–7.

[23] Dart RC, Paul IM, Bond GR, et al. Pediatric fatalities associated with over the counter (nonprescription) cough and cold medications. Ann Emerg Med 2009;53:411–7.

[24] Lokker N, Sanders L, Perrin EM, et al. Parental misinterpretations of over-the-counter pediatric cough and cold medication labels. Pediatrics 2009;123:1464–71.

[25] Kuehn BM. Debate continues over the safety of cold and cough medicines for children. JAMA 2008;300:2354–6.

[26] Available at: http://www.fda.gov/NewsEvents/Newsroom/PressAnnouncements/2007/ucm108921.htm. Accessed July 11, 2009.

[27] Mitka M. FDA bans sale of unapproved cough suppressants containing hydrocodone. JAMA 2007;298:2251–2.

[28] Available at: http://www.ftc.gov/opa/2008/08/airborne.shtm. Accessed July 9, 2009.

[29] Available at: http://www.fda.gov/Drugs/DrugSafety/PublicHealthAdvisories/ucm166059.htm. Accessed July 10, 2009.

[30] Hay AD, Costelloe C, Redmond NM, et al. Paracetamol plus ibuprofen for the treatment of fever in children (PITCH): randomised controlled trial. BMJ 2008;337:a1302.

[31] Kramer LC, Richards PA, Thompson AM, et al. Alternating antipyretics: antipyretic efficacy of acetaminophen versus acetaminophen alternated with ibuprofen in children. Clin Pediatr (Phila) 2008;47:907–11.

[32] Clark E, Plint AC, Correll R, et al. A randomized, controlled trial of acetaminophen, ibuprofen, and codeine for acute pain relief in children with musculoskeletal trauma. Pediatrics 2007;119:460–7.

[33] Rovers MM, Glasziou P, Appelman CL, et al. Antibiotics for acute otitis media: a meta-analysis with individual patient data. Lancet 2006;368:1429–35.

[34] Koopman L, Hoes AW, Glasziou PP, et al. Antibiotic therapy to prevent the development of asymptomatic middle ear effusion in children with acute otitis media: a meta-analysis of individual patient data. Arch Otolaryngol Head Neck Surg 2008;134:128–32.

[35] Spiro DM, Tay KY, Arnold DH, et al. Wait-and-see prescription for the treatment of acute otitis media: a randomized controlled trial. JAMA 2006;296:1235–41.

[36] van der Veen EL, Rovers MM, Albers FW, et al. Effectiveness of trimethoprim/sulfamethoxazole for children with chronic active otitis media: a randomized, placebo-controlled trial. Pediatrics 2007;119:897–904.

[37] Schwartz RH. Once-daily ofloxacin otic solution versus neomycin sulfate/polymyxin B sulfate/hydrocortisone otic suspension four times a day: a multicenter, randomized, evaluator-blinded trial to compare the efficacy, safety, and pain relief in pediatric patients with otitis externa. Curr Med Res Opin 2006;22:1725–36.

[38] Roland PS, Smith TL, Schwartz SR, et al. Clinical practice guideline: cerumen impaction. Otolaryngol Head Neck Surg 2008;139:S1–21.

[39] Wallace DV, Dykewicz MS, Bernstein DI, et al. The diagnosis and management of rhinitis: an updated practice parameter. J Allergy Clin Immunol 2008;122:S1–84.

[40] Section on Pediatric Pulmonology, Subcommittee on Obstructive Sleep Apnea Syndrome. American Academy of Pediatrics. Clinical practice guideline: diagnosis and management of childhood obstructive sleep apnea syndrome. Pediatrics 2002;109:704–12.

[41] Kheirandish-Gozal L, Gozal D. Intranasal budesonide treatment for children with mild obstructive sleep apnea syndrome. Pediatrics 2008;122:e149–55.

[42] Clegg HW, Ryan AG, Dallas SD, et al. Treatment of streptococcal pharyngitis with once-daily compared with twice-daily amoxicillin: a noninferiority trial. Pediatr Infect Dis J 2006;25:761–7.

[43] Lennon DR, Farrell E, Martin DR, et al. Once-daily amoxicillin versus twice-daily penicillin V in group A beta-haemolytic streptococcal pharyngitis. Arch Dis Child 2008;93:474–8.

[44] National Asthma Education and Prevention Program Expert Panel Report 3. Guidelines for the diagnosis and management of Asthma. U.S. Department of Health and Human Services, National Institute of Health, National Heart Lung and Blood Institute; 2007. Available at: http://www.nhlbi.nih.gov/guidelines/asthma/asthsumm.pdf. Accessed July 10, 2009.

[45] Panickar J, Lakhanpaul M, Lambert PC, et al. Oral prednisolone for preschool children with acute virus-induced wheezing. N Engl J Med 2009;360:329–38.

[46] Ducharme FM, Lemire C, Noya FJ, et al. Preemptive use of high-dose fluticasone for virus-induced wheezing in young children. N Engl J Med 2009;360:339–53.

[47] Bacharier LB, Phillips BR, Zeiger RS, et al. Episodic use of an inhaled corticosteroid or leukotriene receptor antagonist in preschool children with moderate-to-severe intermittent wheezing. J Allergy Clin Immunol 2008;122:1127–35, e8.

[48] American Academy of Pediatrics Subcommittee on Diagnosis and Management of Bronchiolitis. Diagnosis and management of bronchiolitis. Pediatrics 2006;118:1774–93.

[49] Corneli HM, Zorc JJ, Mahajan P, et al. A multicenter, randomized, controlled trial of dexamethasone for bronchiolitis. N Engl J Med 2007;357:331–9.

[50] Plint AC, Johnson DW, Patel H, et al. Epinephrine and dexamethasone in children with bronchiolitis. N Engl J Med 2009;360:2079–89.

[51] Scheffler RM, Brown TT, Fulton BD, et al. Positive association between attention-deficit/hyperactivity disorder medication use and academic achievement during elementary school. Pediatrics 2009;123:1273–9.

[52] Arnold LE, Lindsay RL, Lopez FA, et al. Treating attention-deficit/hyperactivity disorder with a stimulant transdermal patch: the clinical art. Pediatrics 2007;120:1100–6.

[53] Scahill L. Alpha-2 adrenergic agonists in attention deficit hyperactivity disorder. J Pediatr 2009;154:S32–7.

[54] Biederman J, Melmed RD, Patel A, et al. A randomized, double-blind, placebo-controlled study of guanfacine extended release in children and adolescents with attention-deficit/hyperactivity disorder. Pediatrics 2008;121:e73–84.

[55] Weber W, Vander Stoep A, McCarty RL, et al. Hypericum perforatum (St John's wort) for attention-deficit/hyperactivity disorder in children and adolescents: a randomized controlled trial. JAMA 2008;299:2633–41.

[56] Vetter VL, Elia J, Erickson C, et al. Cardiovascular monitoring of children and adolescents with heart disease receiving stimulant drugs: a scientific statement from the American Heart Association Council on Cardiovascular Disease in the Young Congenital Cardiac Defects Committee and the Council on Cardiovascular Nursing. Circulation 2008;117:2407–23.

[57] Perrin JM, Friedman RA, Knilans TK. Cardiovascular monitoring and stimulant drugs for attention-deficit/hyperactivity disorder. Pediatrics 2008;122:451–3.

[58] Hampton T. Group's advice on cardiac testing for children with ADHD draws criticism. JAMA 2008;299:2735.

[59] Available at: http://americanheart.mediaroom.com/index.php?s=43&item=422. Accessed July 19, 2009.

[60] Gould MS, Walsh BT, Munfakh JL, et al. Sudden death and use of stimulant medications in youths. Am J Psychiatry 2009;166(9):992–1001.

[61] Available at: http://www.fda.gov/NewsEvents/Newsroom/PressAnnouncements/ucm 166616.htm. Accessed July 5, 2009.

[62] Kurian BT, Ray WA, Arbogast PG, et al. Effect of regulatory warnings on antidepressant prescribing for children and adolescents. Arch Pediatr Adolesc Med 2007;161:690–6.

[63] Bridge JA, Iyengar S, Salary CB, et al. Clinical response and risk for reported suicidal ideation and suicide attempts in pediatric antidepressant treatment: a meta-analysis of randomized controlled trials. JAMA 2007;297:1683–96.

[64] Brent D, Emslie G, Clarke G, et al. Switching to another SSRI or to venlafaxine with or without cognitive behavioral therapy for adolescents with SSRI-resistant depression: the TORDIA randomized controlled trial. JAMA 2008;299:901–13.

[65] Walkup JT, Albano AM, Piacentini J, et al. Cognitive behavioral therapy, sertraline, or a combination in childhood anxiety. N Engl J Med 2008;359:2753–66.

[66] Available at: http://www.fda.gov/NewsEvents/Newsroom/PressAnnouncements/2006/ucm108759.htm. Accessed July 5, 2009.

[67] McIntyre RS, Jerrell JM. Metabolic and cardiovascular adverse events associated with antipsychotic treatment in children and adolescents. Arch Pediatr Adolesc Med 2008;162:929–35.

[68] Myers SM, Johnson CP. Management of children with autism spectrum disorders. Pediatrics 2007;120:1162–82.

[69] Blumer JL, Reed MD, Steinberg F, et al. Potential pharmacokinetic basis for zolpidem dosing in children with sleep difficulties. Clin Pharmacol Ther 2008;83:551–8.

[70] Wilson W, Taubert KA, Gewitz M, et al. Prevention of infective endocarditis: guidelines from the American Heart Association: a guideline from the American Heart Association Rheumatic Fever, Endocarditis, and Kawasaki Disease Committee, Council on Cardiovascular Disease in the Young, and the Council on Clinical Cardiology, Council on Cardiovascular Surgery and Anesthesia, and the Quality of Care and Outcomes Research Interdisciplinary Working Group. Circulation 2007;116:1736–54.

[71] Liberman JN, Berger JE, Lewis M. Prevalence of antihypertensive, antidiabetic, and dyslipidemic prescription medication use among children and adolescents. Arch Pediatr Adolesc Med 2009;163:357–64.

[72] Flynn JT, Daniels SR. Pharmacologic treatment of hypertension in children and adolescents. J Pediatr 2006;149:746–54.

[73] Belay B, Belamarich PF, Tom-Revzon C. The use of statins in pediatrics: knowledge base, limitations, and future directions. Pediatrics 2007;119:370–80.

[74] Conway PH, Cnaan A, Zaoutis T, et al. Recurrent urinary tract infections in children: risk factors and association with prophylactic antimicrobials. JAMA 2007;298:179–86.

[75] Montini G, Rigon L, Zucchetta P, et al. Prophylaxis after first febrile urinary tract infection in children? A multicenter, randomized, controlled, noninferiority trial. Pediatrics 2008;122:1064–71.

[76] Pennesi M, Travan L, Peratoner L, et al. Is antibiotic prophylaxis in children with vesicoureteral reflux effective in preventing pyelonephritis and renal scars? A randomized, controlled trial. Pediatrics 2008;121:e1489–94.

[77] Committee on Infectious Diseases. The use of systemic fluoroquinolones. Pediatrics 2006;118:1287–92.

[78] Available at: http://www.fda.gov/NewsEvents/Newsroom/PressAnnouncements/2008/ucm116919.htm. Accessed December 30, 2009.

[79] American Academy of Pediatrics Committee on Infectious Diseases. Antiviral therapy and prophylaxis for influenza in children. Pediatrics 2007;119:852–60.

[80] Elliott DJ, Zaoutis TE, Troxel AB, et al. Empiric antimicrobial therapy for pediatric skin and soft-tissue infections in the era of methicillin-resistant Staphylococcus aureus. Pediatrics 2009;123:e959–66.

[81] Hersh AL, Maselli JH, Cabana MD. Changes in prescribing of antiviral medications for influenza associated with new treatment guidelines. Am J Public Health 2009;99(Suppl 2):S362–4.

[82] Available at: http://www.fda.gov/NewsEvents/Newsroom/PressAnnouncements/2007/ucm108996.htm. Accessed December 30, 2009.

[83] Available at: http://www.fda.gov/NewsEvents/Newsroom/PressAnnouncements/ucm149562.htm. Accessed December 30, 2009.

[84] DeCamp LR, Byerley JS, Doshi N, et al. Use of antiemetic agents in acute gastroenteritis: a systematic review and meta-analysis. Arch Pediatr Adolesc Med 2008;162:858–65.

[85] Available at: http://www.fda.gov/NewsEvents/Newsroom/PressAnnouncements/2007/ucm108882.htm. Accessed December 31, 2009.

[86] Khoshoo V, Edell D, Thompson A, et al. Are we overprescribing antireflux medications for infants with regurgitation? Pediatrics 2007;120:946–9.

[87] Hibbs AM, Lorch SA. Metoclopramide for the treatment of gastroesophageal reflux disease in infants: a systematic review. Pediatrics 2006;118:746–52.

[88] Bahar RJ, Collins BS, Steinmetz B, et al. Double-blind placebo-controlled trial of amitriptyline for the treatment of irritable bowel syndrome in adolescents. J Pediatr 2008;152:685–9.

[89] Marson AG, Al-Kharusi AM, Alwaidh M, et al. The SANAD study of effectiveness of valproate, lamotrigine, or topiramate for generalised and unclassifiable epilepsy: an unblinded randomised controlled trial. Lancet 2007;369:1016–26.

[90] Marson AG, Al-Kharusi AM, Alwaidh M, et al. The SANAD study of effectiveness of carbamazepine, gabapentin, lamotrigine, oxcarbazepine, or topiramate for treatment of partial epilepsy: an unblinded randomised controlled trial. Lancet 2007;369:1000–15.

[91] Steering Committee on Quality Improvement and Management, Subcommittee on Febrile Seizures American Academy of Pediatrics. Febrile seizures: clinical practice guideline for the long-term management of the child with simple febrile seizures. Pediatrics 2008;121: 1281–6.

[92] Lewis D, Winner P, Saper J, et al. Randomized, double-blind, placebo-controlled study to evaluate the efficacy and safety of topiramate for migraine prevention in pediatric subjects 12 to 17 years of age. Pediatrics 2009;123:924–34.

[93] Lewis DW, Winner P, Hershey AD, et al. Efficacy of zolmitriptan nasal spray in adolescent migraine. Pediatrics 2007;120:390–6.

[94] Pope E, Krafchik BR, Macarthur C, et al. Oral versus high-dose pulse corticosteroids for problematic infantile hemangiomas: a randomized, controlled trial. Pediatrics 2007;119:e1239–47.

[95] Leaute-Labreze C, Dumas de la Roque E, Hubiche T, et al. Propranolol for severe hemangiomas of infancy. N Engl J Med 2008;358:2649–51.

[96] Inoue Y, Okada Y, Shinohara M, et al. A multicenter prospective randomized trial of corticosteroids in primary therapy for Kawasaki disease: clinical course and coronary artery outcome. J Pediatr 2006;149:336–41.

[97] Newburger JW, Sleeper LA, McCrindle BW, et al. Randomized trial of pulsed corticosteroid therapy for primary treatment of Kawasaki disease. N Engl J Med 2007;356: 663–75.

[98] Lovell DJ, Ruperto N, Goodman S, et al. Adalimumab with or without methotrexate in juvenile rheumatoid arthritis. N Engl J Med 2008;359:810–20.

[99] Vazquez-Cobian LB, Flynn T, Lehman TJ. Adalimumab therapy for childhood uveitis. J Pediatr 2006;149:572–5.

[100] Ruperto N, Lovell DJ, Quartier P, et al. Abatacept in children with juvenile idiopathic arthritis: a randomised, double-blind, placebo-controlled withdrawal trial. Lancet 2008;372:383–91.

[101] Yokota S, Imagawa T, Mori M, et al. Efficacy and safety of tocilizumab in patients with systemic-onset juvenile idiopathic arthritis: a randomised, double-blind, placebo-controlled, withdrawal phase III trial. Lancet 2008;371:998–1006.

[102] Available at: http://www.fda.gov/NewsEvents/Newsroom/PressAnnouncements/2007/ ucm108968.htm. Accessed December 31, 2009.

[103] Louik C, Lin AE, Werler MM, et al. First-trimester use of selective serotonin-reuptake inhibitors and the risk of birth defects. N Engl J Med 2007;356:2675–83.

[104] Ferreira E, Carceller AM, Agogue C, et al. Effects of selective serotonin reuptake inhibitors and venlafaxine during pregnancy in term and preterm neonates. Pediatrics 2007;119: 52–9.

[105] Oberlander TF, Reebye P, Misri S, et al. Externalizing and attentional behaviors in children of depressed mothers treated with a selective serotonin reuptake inhibitor antidepressant during pregnancy. Arch Pediatr Adolesc Med 2007;161:22–9.

[106] Meador KJ, Baker GA, Browning N, et al. Cognitive function at 3 years of age after fetal exposure to antiepileptic drugs. N Engl J Med 2009;360:1597–605.

Advances in Pediatrics 57 (2010) 185–218

ADVANCES IN PEDIATRICS

Therapeutic Use of Immunoglobulins

E. Richard Stiehm, MD[a],*, Jordan S. Orange, MD, PhD[b],
Mark Ballow, MD[c], Heather Lehman, MD[c]

[a]Division of Immunology/Allergy/Rheumatology, Mattel Children's Hospital, UCLA School of Medicine at UCLA, CA, USA
[b]Division of Immunology, Children's Hospital of Philadelphia, University of Pennsylvania School of Medicine, PA, USA
[c]Division of Allergy, Immunology and Pediatric Rheumatology, Women & Children's Hospital of Buffalo, State University of New York at Buffalo School of Medicine and Biomedical Sciences, NY, USA

OVERVIEW

Antibodies have been used for more than a century to prevent and treat illness, neutralize drugs and poisons, and accentuate or depress the immune system. Their specificity and diversity and their relative safety make them potent therapy in antibody deficiencies, certain infections and several autoimmune/inflammatory disorders.

This article discusses 3 principal uses of immunoglobulins: for infectious diseases, for immunodeficiency, and for immunomodulation. These subjects are discussed in that order, because antibody was first used for infections (since the 1890s), next used for immunodeficiency (since the 1950s), and then used for immunomodulation (since the 1970s, after the introduction of intravenous immunoglobulin [IVIG]). The last use, for a great variety of disorders, is now the largest consumer for immunoglobulin products.

This article does not discuss the use of therapeutic monoclonal antibodies, of which 18 are now licensed in the United States, and more are in the pipeline. The therapeutic use of monoclonals for infections and for immunomodulation is in its neonatal period, and, like infants, great expectations have been bestowed upon them.

IMMUNOGLOBULINS FOR PREVENTION AND TREATMENT OF INFECTIOUS DISEASES

Emil von Behring was awarded the first Nobel Prize in Medicine in 1901 for development of equine antiserum for the treatment of diphtheria and tetanus. His citation stated "For his work on serum therapy, especially its application against diphtheria, by which he has opened a new road in the domain of

*Corresponding author. E-mail address: estiehm@mednet.ucla.edu

0065-3101/10/$ – see front matter
doi:10.1016/j.yapd.2010.08.005

medical science and thereby placed in the hands of the physician a victorious weapon against illness and death."

Since then antibodies in multiple forms (animal and human serums, immune globulins and monoclonal antibodies) have been developed, primarily for prevention of infectious diseases, and less commonly for their treatment. These antibodies are presented in Table 1. This section reviews their uses, with an emphasis on their value in the treatment of human infections, as summarized in Table 2.

Antibody works by several mechanisms. It can neutralize viruses and bacterial toxins, lyse bacteria with the aid of complement, prevent the spread of microbes to adjacent cells or along nerve roots, coat bacteria for opsonization by phagocytes, block microbial attachment by saturating microbial receptors, and facilitate lysis of infected cells by binding them to cytotoxic cells with an Fc receptor.

Bacterial Infections

Antibody is particularly valuable in bacterial diseases associated with toxin production because much of the tissue damage results from action of the toxin; these can be neutralized rapidly by antibody before antibiotics kill the bacterium.

Anthrax (Bacillus anthracis)

Anthrax is a rare but serious infection, predominantly of ruminant animals, caused by an aerobic gram-positive rod [1]. Humans are infected through the skin (cutaneous anthrax), by ingestion (gastrointestinal anthrax), or by inhalation of anthrax spores (inhalational anthrax) [1]. The last often results from prolonged exposure to animal hides or carcasses or infected soil, and rarely by deliberate spore exposure in the bioterrorism setting. After inhalation the spores are ingested by alveolar macrophages and transported to regional nodes, where the spores germinate and release potent exotoxins. These toxins damage cell membranes, increase capillary permeability, cause pulmonary damage, and lead to shock and cardiovascular collapse.

A vaccine is available for individuals at high risk for exposure and for the military.

Before the antibiotic era and as early as 1903, anthrax antitoxin (usually equine) was used in therapy [2]. An antitoxin is of value in a bioterrorism attack, both before and after exposure. The US Government is collecting plasma from immunized donors to develop a human high-titer IGIV [3]. A human monoclonal antibody is being tested in animals and humans [4].

Clostridial infections

Diphtheria (Corynebacterium diphtheriae). Many of the adverse effects of diphtheria result from the action of its potent toxin on the heart, central nervous system, and other organs [5]. Thus the prompt use of antitoxin is indicated, in addition to antibiotics [6]. The dose used depends on the localization and severity of infection, ranging from 20,000 units for mild infection of short duration to 120,000 units for severe illness with neck edema. The equine antitoxin

Table 1
Antibody preparations available for passive immunity in the United States

Product	Abbreviation(s)/brand name(s)	Principal use
Standard Human Immune Serum Globulins (HISG, γ-Globulin)		
Immune globulin, intravenous	IVIG, IGIV	Treatment of antibody deficiency, immune thrombocytopenic purpura, Kawasaki disease, other immunoregulatory and inflammatory diseases
Immune globulin, intramuscular	Immunoglobulin, IGIM	Treatment of antibody deficiency; prevention of measles, hepatitis A
Immune globulin, subcutaneous	SCIG	Treatment of antibody deficiency
Special Human Immune Serum Globulins for Intramuscular or Subcutaneous Use		
Hepatitis B immune globulin	HBIG	Prevention of hepatitis B
Varicella-zoster immune globulin	VZIG	Prevention or modification of chickenpox
Rabies immune globulin	RIG	Prevention of rabies
Tetanus immune globulin	TIG	Prevention or treatment of tetanus
Vaccinia immune globulin	VIG	Prevention or treatment of vaccinia, prevention of smallpox
Rho(D) immune globulin	RhoGAM	Prevention of Rh hemolytic disease
Special Human Intravenous Immune Globulins		
Cytomegalovirus immune globulin	CMV-IVIG, CMVIG, CytoGam	Prevention or treatment of cytomegalovirus infection
Hepatitis B immune globulin, intravenous	HepaGam B	Prevention of hepatitis B (including liver transplantation)
Vaccinia immune globulin, intravenous	VIG-IVIG	Prevention or treatment of vaccinia, prevention of smallpox
Rho(D) immune globulin intravenous	WinRho SDF	Treatment of immune thrombocytopenic purpura
Botulinum immune globulin	BIG, Baby BIG	Treatment of newborn botulism
Animal Serums and Globulins		
Tetanus antitoxin (equine)	TAT	Prevention or treatment of tetanus (when TIG unavailable)
Diphtheria antitoxin (equine)	DAT	Treatment of diphtheria
Botulinum antitoxins (equine heptavalent)[a]	HBAT	Treatment of botulism

(continued on next page)

Table 1
(continued)

Product	Abbreviation(s)/brand name(s)	Principal use
Latrodectus mactans antivenin (equine)		Treatment of black widow spider bites
Crotalidae polyvalent antivenin (equine)		Treatment of most snake bites
Crotalidae polyvalent immune Fab (ovine)[a]		Treatment of most snake bites
Micrurus fulvius antivenin (equine)		Treatment of coral snake bites
Digoxin immune Fab fragments (ovine)[a]	Digibind, DigiFab	Treatment of digoxin or digitoxin overdose
Lymphocyte/thymocyte immune globulin (equine)	Equine ATG, Atgam	Immunosuppression
Lymphocyte/thymocyte immune globulin (rabbit)	Rabbit ATG, thymoglobulin	Immunosuppression

[a] Fab fragment.

is given intravenously, so must be preceded by skin testing for hypersensitivity and possible desensitization. The antitoxin is available through the US Centers for Disease Control (CDC).

A smaller dose of antitoxin can be used in asymptomatic, exposed, susceptible individuals. Before the availability of diphtheria vaccine, antitoxins were given to health care workers caring for patients with diphtheria [7].

Tetanus (Clostridium tetani). Equine antitoxin for the treatment of tetanus was initiated by von Behring in the 1890s for toxin neutralization. Extensive studies have been carried out to determine the optimal dose of antitoxin and the possible benefit of intrathecal antitoxin, particularly in tetanus neonatorum, a common problem in developing countries [8]. Since the 1960s a human tetanus immune globulin (TIG) has been available, but in some areas of the world equine antitoxin is still used.

TIG is given to unimmunized or incompletely immunized patients who sustain contaminated or deep puncture wounds [8]. The recommended dose of TIG is 250 IU, along with initiation of active immunization. If TIG is unavailable, human IVIG can also be used; it contains variable titers of tetanus antitoxin but a minimal dose of 200–400 mg/kg is suggested for tetanus prophylaxis [8,9].

Clostridium difficile *gastroenteritis. Clostridium difficile* infection of the gastrointestinal tract is usually associated with antibiotic-associated diarrhea, often with pseudomembranous colitis and sometimes toxic megacolon [10] Toxic strains of *Clostridium difficile* release 2 distinct toxins, both of which have potent cytotoxic and inflammatory properties [11]. Infection generally leads to an antibody response to the toxin, and most individuals older than 2 years have such antibodies. High levels of these antibodies acquired after colonization may result in the asymptomatic carrier state [12].

Table 2
Summary of the efficacy of antibody in the prevention and treatment of infectious diseases

Infection	Prophylaxis	Treatment
Bacterial Infections		
Respiratory infections (streptococcal, Streptococcus pneumoniae, Neisseria meningitidis, Haemophilus influenzae)	Proved (NR)[a]	Proved (NR)
Diphtheria	Unproved (NR)	Proved
Pertussis	Unproved (NR)	Unproved (NR)
Tetanus	Proved	Proved
Other clostridial infections		
Clostridium botulinum	Proved	Proved
Newborn botulism	Unproved	Proved
Clostridium difficile	Unproved	Probable benefit
Staphylococcal infections		
Toxic shock syndrome	Unproved (NR)	Probable benefit
Antibiotic resistance	Unproved	Possible benefit (NR)
Staphylococcus epidermidis in newborns	Unproved	Possible benefit
Toxic shock	Unproved (NR)	Probable benefit
Newborn sepsis	Possible benefit (NR)	Probable benefit
Shock, intensive care, and trauma	Unproved	Possible benefit (NR)
Pseudomonas infections		
Cystic fibrosis	Unproved (NR)	Unproved (NR)
Burns	Unproved (NR)	Unproved (NR)
Viral Diseases		
Hepatitis A	Proved	No benefit
Hepatitis B	Proved	No benefit
Hepatitis C	Unproved (NR)	No benefit
HIV infection	Unproved (NR)	Unproved (NR)
RSV infection	Proved	Unproved (NR)
Herpesvirus infections		
CMV	Proved	Possible benefit
EBV	Unproved (NR)	Unproved (NR)
HSV	Unproved (NR)	Unproved (NR)
VZV	Proved	Unproved (NR)
Parvovirus	Possible benefit	Proved (NR)
Enterovirus infections		
In newborns	Unproved	Possible benefit
Encephalomyelitis	Possible benefit	Probable benefit (NR)[a]
Poliovirus	Proved (NR)	Unproved (NR)
Ebola	Unproved	Unproved
Rabies	Proved	No benefit
Measles	Proved	No benefit
Rubella	Unproved (NR)	No benefit
Mumps	Unproved (NR)	No benefit
Tick-borne encephalitis	Possible benefit	No benefit
Vaccinia	Proved	Proved
Variola	Proved	Unproved

Abbreviations: CMV, cytomegalovirus; EBV, Epstein-Barr virus; HIV, human immunodeficiency virus; HSV, herpes simplex virus; NR, not recommended; RSV, respiratory syncytial virus; VZV, varicella-zoster virus.
[a] Recommended for immunodeficient patients.
Modified from Stiehm ER, Keller MA. Passive immunization. In: Feigen RD, Cherry JD, Demmler-Harrison GJ, et al, editors. Textbook of pediatric infectious diseases. 6th edition. Philadelphia: Saunders/Elsevier; 2009. p. 3447-79.

Some patients with symptomatic infection, many of whom are immunodeficient or immunosuppressed, develop antibiotic-resistant diarrhea; many have low or absent IgG antibodies to toxin A. Such patients may respond to IVIG given 300 to 500 mg/kg every 1 to 3 weeks [13]. Such therapy increases antitoxin levels, controls the diarrhea, and prevents relapses [14,15]. Controlled trials have not been performed.

Botulism (Clostridium botulinum). Botulism is a severe paralytic poisoning resulting for the ingestion or absorption of neurotoxin or spores of *Clostridium botulinum.* Several variants are recognized: food poisoning from ingestion of contaminated canned food, wound botulism from a contaminated soft-tissue infection, inhalational botulism among individuals working with the toxin or in a bioterrorist event, infantile botulism (see next section), and adult-type infant botulism in adults with preexisting gastrointestinal disease [16–18]. In the last 2 types, ingested spores multiply in the gastrointestinal tract to elaborate toxin; the absorbed toxin results in a paralytic disorder.

A few cases of botulism have been associated with use of botulism toxin for cosmetic use [19,20].

An heptavalent fab fragment equine antitoxin (HBAT) to types A, B, C, D, E, F and G is available in the United States through the CDC [21,22]. Sensitivity testing must be conducted before their use. Antitoxin to all 3 types is given unless the toxin type is known. Additional doses may be needed in severe wound botulism. Antitoxin can also by used prophylactically in individuals known to have ingested contaminated food. It is not used for infantile botulism.

Infantile botulism (Clostridium botulinum). This severe paralytic disorder of infants results from the ingestion of *Clostridium botulinum* spores in baby formulae or food, resulting in slow onset of constipation, abdominal bloating, poor feeding, and respiratory paralysis [22]. Such infants must be hospitalized for prolonged periods for tube feeding and respiratory support, often for as long as 6 to 9 months. Human IV botulism immune globulin is available for treatment of infantile botulism [23]. Despite its high cost ($50,000 per vial) it is cost-effective because of the shortened hospital stay needed.

Gas gangrene (Clostridium perfringens). There is no antitoxin for gas gangrene.

Bacterial respiratory infections
Respiratory infections with Streptoccocci, *Streptococcus pneumonia, Haemophilus influenzae,* and *Neisseria meningitides* are reduced in immunodeficient patients receiving immunoglobulin therapy. These patients include young infants with poor antibody responses to polysaccharide antigens, patients infected with the human immunodeficiency virus (HIV), and patients with primary antibody immunodeficiencies. Before antibiotics, immune serum or animal serum was used as therapy for severe bacterial infection [24,25].

Other studies suggest that a large dose of IVIG decreases the frequency of otitis in patients with recurrent otitis and normal immunity [26].

Thus regular use of IVIG in antibody-deficient patients in doses of 400 to 600 mg/kg every 3 to 4 weeks or an equivalent amount given subcutaneously decreases the frequency and severity of otitis and other respiratory tract infections [27,28].

Streptococcal infection

Circulating antibody may play a role in the prevention and treatment of invasive group A streptococcal infection [29]. Newborns with transplacental antibody and patients on IVIG rarely develop streptococcal illnesses. Equine antitoxin was used with some success in the treatment of erysipelas and scarlet fever in the 1920s and 1930s [30]. A preventive vaccine against the streptococcal M protein has been contemplated but is not yet unavailable.

Treatment with IVIG, in addition to antibiotics, is probably beneficial [25,31]. Streptococcal pyrogenic exotoxins types A, B, and C and mitogenic factor elaborated by certain strains of streptococci may be responsible for these complications. These exotoxins are potent superantigens that activate certain T lymphocytes directly, leading to synthesis and/or release of multiple cytokines with resultant shock, fever, and organ failure.

IVIG contains neutralizing antibodies to these antigens of varying titers from batch to batch [32]. Despite this variability IVIG is recommended, in addition to antibiotics, in the management of these infections, not only to neutralize pyrogenic toxins but to dampen cytokine storm and release [33]. Controlled trials are unavailable but case reports and large series compared with historical controls are encouraging [34]. Large doses of IVIG are recommended (eg, 1–2 g/kg over several days).

Staphylococcal infections

Staphylococcal infections are ubiquitous and of varying severity, ranging from superficial skin infections to deep-seated cellulitis, osteomyelitis, and overwhelming shock [35,36]. These severe infections occur when the organism is resistant to antibiotics or is a strain associated with toxin production.

One well-recognized syndrome is toxic shock associated with tampon use in menstruating women [36]. This syndrome results from release of the toxic shock syndrome toxin-1, a potent superantigen that initiates the release of multiple cytokines and a clinical picture of rapidly progressive fever, shock, and organ failure. Most authorities recommend a high dose of IVIG to neutralize the toxin and dampen cytokine storm [35,37].

A second situation in which IVIG may be of value is in neonatal staphylococcal infection, usually coagulase-negative *Staphylococcus epidermidis*. This is the most common cause of sepsis in premature infants and is aggravated in part by the use of catheters and central lines [38,39].

One controlled study indicated that IVIG was of value in decreasing the incidence of this infection [40]. Other studies were not confirmatory, possibly because of differences in titer for the protective antibodies [39].

Immunoglobulin is also used in the treatment of antibiotic-resistant staphylococcal infection. Older studies from Waisbren [41] and current studies from

Russia suggest clinical benefit [42]. Animal studies support such a combined approach [43].

Infection in high-risk newborns

Newborns, particularly premature newborns with birth weight less than 2000 g are potential candidates for immunoglobulin therapy in view of the frequency and severity of infections. All newborns have low levels of IgM and IgA, and, if premature, a deficiency of transplacental maternal IgG, the deficiency of which is proportional to the degree of immaturity [44]. Premature infants also have defects in antibody synthesis, complement levels, opsonic activity, neutrophil mobilization and killing, and cellular immune responses [44].

Accordingly several studies sought to determine the value of IGIV in the prevention or early treatment of infection in premature infants. These studies differ in terms of entry criteria, immunoglobulin dose and duration, and end points (eg, type and severity of infection, survival). Meta-analyses of prospective, randomized, placebo-controlled prevention studies suggest a slight reduction (3%) in the frequency of sepsis but no difference in mortality, length of nursery stay, or other complications of prematurity [45–47].

By contrast meta-analysis of 6 controlled studies for the treatment of proven sepsis, involving 262 premature infants, showed that IGIV therapy reduced mortality from 20% to 11%, a significant difference [48]. There was a suggestive benefit for infants with suspected sepsis also. Infants with neutropenia may particularly benefit.

Because a common cause of neonatal sepsis is *Staphylococcus epidermidis*, a hyperimmune staphylococcal IVIG may be of particular benefit in the prevention of neonatal sepsis. Two recent studies of IGIV from either immunized donors (Altastaph) [49] or selected donors with high titers to a fibrinogen-binding protein (Veronate) [50] did not show a significantly decreased incidence of infection. Studies of monoclonal antibodies to staphylococcal antigens are in progress.

Thus the 1990 National Institutes of Health consensus statement that IGIV should not be given routinely to infants of low birth weight but that it may be of value in selected premature newborns with proven or suspected infection remains valid [51].

Shock, intensive care, and trauma

Patients undergoing severe stress associated with trauma, extensive surgery, or intensive care have profound exposure to and susceptibility to infection, usually as a result of enteric gram-negative infections [52,53]. Monoclonal antibodies, IgM-enriched IGIV, and regular IGIV have been studied in these situations with inconclusive results [5]. Laupland and colleagues [54] reviewed 14 randomized trials of IGIV and found suggestive benefit in terms of length of stay in the intensive care unit (ICU) and mortality. Similar studies in pediatric patients in the ICU have not been performed.

Despite the lack of controlled trials, IGIV is often used in critically ill patients, particularly neutropenic patients, because of possible benefit and rare side effects.

Viral Diseases

Although many viral diseases are prevented by immunoglobulin, just a few are amenable to antibody therapy, as presented in Table 2. This section focuses on some viral diseases in which antibodies can be used in therapy.

Vaccinia and smallpox (variola)

Although smallpox (variola) has been eradicated from the world since 1977, immunization with live vaccinia virus (cowpox virus) is still used by the military and by certain laboratory personnel working with vaccinia [5]. Further, smallpox is a potential bioterrorism weapon so a supply of vaccinia immune globulin (VIG) is being stockpiled by the US Government for complications of smallpox vaccine and for a response to biological warfare.

Kempe [55] used immune globulin from vaccinated individuals (VIG) to prevent the spread in a 1953 outbreak of smallpox in Madras, India. He also showed that VIG could be used to treat the not infrequent complications of smallpox vaccine including vaccinia eczematum, generalized vaccinia, autoinoculation, and prevention of spread to high-risk individuals exposed to a recently vaccinated individual.

VIG, both for IV and intramuscular (IM) use, is prepared from vaccinated donors and is commercially available. The usual dose is 100 mg/kg [56].

Parvovirus B19

Parvovirus is a DNA virus that causes fifth disease (slapped cheek syndrome, a common exanthem of childhood that usually provides lifelong immunity to subsequent exposure [57]). Parvovirus infects erythroid progenitors (its receptor is the common red cell P antigen) to cause red cell aplasia in patients with congenital or acquired immunodeficiencies including HIV, immunosuppressed organ transplant recipients, and patients with sickle cell disease [57–59].

IGIV contains neutralizing antibody to parvovirus such that prolonged high-dose therapy can eradicate the infection. Parvovirus infection during pregnancy can also cause fetal hydrops [60]. Arthritis and chronic fatigue syndrome are uncommon manifestations of chronic parvovirus infections [60,61].

The IVIG dose needed to eradicate parvovirus in not established but is large (1–2 g/kg) and should be repeated until the virus is eradicated as indicated by serum polymerase chain reaction analysis [62,63].

Cytomegalovirus

Antibodies to cytomegalovirus (CMV) either in the form of hyperimmune IV CMV immune globulin (CMVIG-Cytogam) or regular IGIV have been used for more than a decade to prevent CMV infection in recipients of bone marrow and solid organ transplant [64]. CMVIG is prepared from donors with high anti-CMV titers but regular IGIV also contains CMV antibodies at lower titers. Testing of donor and recipient for CMV infection, the use of CMV antibody-negative blood donors, and the use of antiviral drugs have greatly reduced the indications for CMV antibody [65]. CMVIG is still used in heart and heart-lung transplants (along with antivirals) if either the donor or the recipient is

CMV-seropositive [66]. CMVIG is also of suggestive benefit in severe CMV pneumonitis along with antiviral treatment [67].

CMVIG may also be of value for in utero CMV infection; infusions of CMVIG were given intraperitoneally at 28 and 29 weeks to a CMV-infected fetus, with possible benefit [68]. Nigro and colleagues [69] gave 31 pregnant women with primary CMV infection CMVIG during pregnancy; some women received additional CMVIG into the amniotic sac or umbilical cord. Only one woman gave birth to an infant with CMV infection compared with CMV infection in 7 of 14 infants of control women who did not receive antibody therapy. These data are encouraging but are not from well-controlled studies.

Thus the use of CMVIG in recipients of organ transplant, severe CMV infections, or in utero CMV infections is unproved but of suggestive therapeutic benefit.

Herpes simplex
Transplacental maternal antibody has a proven preventive effect in herpes simplex virus (HSV) infection in the newborn period: mothers with a reactivated herpex infection (ie, preexisting infection) during delivery are 10-fold less likely to transmit HSV to their newborn infants during vaginal delivery than are mothers with primary HSV infection acquired during late pregnancy [70].

Masci and colleagues [71] used IVIG to prevent recurrent genital HSV infection with suggestive benefit. The value of HSV monoclonal antibody or IVIG is being evaluated for treatment of disseminated neonatal disease.

Epstein-Barr virus infection
Epstein-Barr virus (EBV) antibodies are present in variable titers in IVIG, particularly in CMVIG, because donors with high titers of CMV often have high titers of EBV. A few patients with posttransplant EBV-induced lymphoproliferative syndrome or hepatitis have been treated successfully with a combination of IGIV or CMVIG, antiviral therapy and interferon-α [72–74]. Similar results have been achieved in EBV infection in X-linked lymphoproliferative syndrome: such patients have a hereditary predisposition to overwhelming EBV infection [75].

Varicella-zoster infection
Varicella-zoster immune globulin (VZIG), available since 1978, is prepared from plasma with high titers to VZ virus [76]. The commercial product Vari-ZIG is used for the prevention or modification of susceptible high-risk immunodeficient or immunosuppressed children exposed to chickenpox or shingles. It is also used in susceptible women during late pregnancy, newborn infants whose mother develops chickenpox perinatally, and exposed premature infants of less than 28 weeks' gestation. It is not of benefit in established chickenpox or zoster infection [77].

Enteroviral infections
Encephalomyelitis. Before poliovirus vaccine was introduced, immunoglobulin was used in the prevention of poliomyelitis [78]. Immunodeficient individuals are

susceptible to chronic enteroviral encephalitis, usually echovirus or coxsackievirus or less commonly, attenuated poliovirus vaccine strains [79–82]. Regular doses of IGIV given to antibody-deficient patients have markedly reduced the frequency of enterovirus encephalitis in these patients. Attenuated poliovirus has been replaced in many countries by inactivated (Salk) vaccine.

High-dose IVIG (sufficient to increase the serum IgG levels to 1000 mg/mL) has been used successfully in immunodeficient patients with enteroviral encephalomyelitis [80–83]. Some patients have been given intrathecal infusions [80,81]. Not all IVIG-treated patients are cured: some may have viral strains for which the IVIG has no neutralizing antibody. For these instances typing of the cerebrospinal fluid and treatment with selective IVIG units with antibodies to the infecting serotype may be necessary. Antiviral therapy with pleconoril has also been used [83].

Neonatal enteroviral infection. Severe and sometimes fatal disseminated enterovirus infection can develop in neonates [84–86]. High-dose IVIG has been used in such infants with suggested benefit in decreasing the severity of the illness [84]. Maternal plasma may also be used in the likelihood that the mother has antibody to the organism involved [85].

IVIG has also been used to prevent spread to unaffected infants in a nursery [86]. Unless the titer in the IVIG is known, large doses are recommended.

Hepatitis B immune globulin in recipients of liver transplant

An increasingly important use of hyperimmune hepatitis B immune globulin (HBIG) is to prevent hepatitis B recurrence in hepatitis B-seropositive recipients of liver transplant, many of whom are transplanted because of complications of hepatitis B [87,88]. Hepatitis B reoccurs in half of the patients in 3 years [89].

Such recurrences can be reduced significantly by giving large doses of HBIG for a prolonged period beginning at the time of transplantation and continuing indefinitely after transplantation [89]. Antiviral agents such as lamivudine are also given simultaneously. The dose of HBIG after transplantation is varied so as to maintain a continuous serum anti-HbS titer. Hepatitis B vaccine can also be given to induce active immunity.

The 2 types of HBIG available include the 16% IGIM used for prophylaxis in newborns of hepatic B-positive mothers and for unimmunized exposed susceptibles and a 5% HBIG for IV use in liver transplantation. The use of the latter adds a considerable cost to liver transplantation. The University of California at Los Angeles Medical Center spends $500,000 per year on HBIG, nearly all for the liver transplant program.

A hyperimmune hepatitis C immune globulin for hepatitis C liver transplantation is also under study. Monoclonal antibodies to hepatitis B and C are under development.

Regional viral infections

West Nile fever. West Nile fever, caused by the West Nile virus, is common in many tropical regions where *Culex* mosquitoes are endemic. It has spread to

Europe and the United States, and can also be transmitted by infected blood and organ transplantation. Several case reports and animal studies suggest that IVIG prepared from seropositive donors modifies the severity and mortality [90,91].

Ebola. Ebola virus, a filivirus, causes severe and often fatal hemorrhagic fever in tropical Africa. There is no effective antiviral agent. Goat hyperimmune serum protected guinea pigs from experimental infection if given within 72 hours of exposure. This product was used for emergency prophylaxis in 4 patients exposed by a laboratory accident. Only one developed mild infection [92].

Equine serum has protected monkeys against low-dose virus challenge but not high-dose virus challenge [93]. Blood from convalescing patients has also been used with promising results [94]. Other animal antisera have been developed, as have monoclonal antibodies.

Tick-borne encephalitis. Tick-borne encephalitis caused by a flavivirus is endemic in central Europe. A vaccine is available as is a hyperimmune immune globulin. A combination has been also used [95,96].

Argentine hemorrhagic fever. Argentine hemorrhagic fever caused by the Junin virus has a high mortality from vascular or neurologic complications. Maiztegui and colleagues [97] found that immune plasma given before the ninth day of illness reduced mortality to 1% among 91 patients given immune plasma compared with 16.5% mortality among 97 patient given normal plasma.

Severe acute respiratory distress syndrome. Convalescent plasma and IVIG have been used in the treatment of severe acute respiratory distress syndrome caused by a corona virus. Studies were inconclusive [98].

Summary of Antibody Use in Infectious Diseases

Antibody is a time-honored way to prevent viral infection after exposure, and has a crucial role in the treatment of bacterial diseases associated with toxin production. It is also of value in prevention of certain viral infections as well as in the treatment of parvovius, enterovirus infection, and certain regional viral infections.

IMMUNOGLOBULINS IN PRIMARY IMMUNODEFICIENCIES

Polyclonal immunoglobulin, now used in scores of diverse disorders [99–101], was first used in the prevention of infectious diseases. In 1952, Ogden Bruton [102] reported a child with agammaglobulinemia and initiated the first use of repeat injections of immunoglobulin as replacement therapy. In his report γ-globulin fractionated from human plasma was administered subcutaneously to an 8-year-old boy who had no known γ-globulin in a serum protein electorophoresis. This child had multiple infections, including 19 episodes of septicemia, which were ameliorated by chronic treatment with the immunoglobulin. This experience represented the dawn of immunoglobulin therapy for primary immunodeficiency and defined its use in a disease for which no therapeutic alterative was available.

Since then, the study of primary immunodeficiency has expanded markedly. There are now more than 140 distinct diagnoses, most of which have defects of humoral immunity [103]. Approximately 1 in 2000 people are living with a primary immunodeficiency in the United States, of whom greater than 50% have an antibody deficiency potentially requiring immunoglobulin replacement therapy [104]. Other primary immunodeficiency registries confirm that greater than 50% have an antibody deficiency [105–108]. Treatment with immunoglobulin remains the best therapeutic option for most of these patients.

Primary Antibody Deficiencies

Characteristics of antibody immunodeficiencies appropriate for replacement therapy are presented in Table 3. The clearest indications for immunoglobulin therapy are those associated with an absence of B cells (category I). These patients are unable to make antibodies or immunoglobulin I. Examples include agammaglobulinemia and certain types of severe combined immunodeficiency. Several gene defects may be responsible for these illnesses [109], but all need immunoglobulin replacement therapy.

The next category (II) of patients needing immunoglobulin are those who have B cells but cannot make IgG and generate specific IgG antibodies. Because IgG represents the major defense of humoral immunity against infection, these patients also require immunoglobulin replacement therapy. This diagnostic category includes the hyper IgM syndrome (HIGM) and common variable immunodeficiency (CVID). HIGM is caused by several specific gene mutations [110], but most CVID cases have no identifiable genetic lesions [111].

Diagnosis can be made by either identifying a specific gene mutation, or by defining the quantitative and qualitative deficit of IgG [112]. As in patients in category I, continuous and uninterrupted replacement therapy with immunoglobulin is warranted. If the diagnosis is confirmed molecularly, immunoglobulin therapy must be continued. In a few cases, it may be clinically appropriate to stop immunoglobulin therapy once during a lifetime to determine if the defect is fixed [1]. This strategy should not be repeated if the single trial indicates a persistent deficit. If a trial off immunoglobulin therapy is considered, this should be performed in late spring or summer, when respiratory infections are less prevalent.

A third diagnostic category (III) of antibody deficiencies is those associated with qualitative defects in humoral immunity [113]. These patients have B cells and produce normal quantities of IgG but the quality of IgG is diminished. These individuals are unable to respond appropriately to specific antigenic challenges such as vaccinations or infections. This category includes those with specific antibody deficiency with normal immunoglobulins [113] and certain patients with NEMO (NF-kappa;-B essential modulator) deficiency [114,115]. Diagnosis is made after documentation of an ineffective vaccination

Table 3
Conceptual classification of the primary antibody immunodeficiencies

Category	B cells	IgG quantity	IgG quality (antigen-specific antibody)	Diagnostic examples	Immunoglobulin replacement therapy	Cessation of therapy for reevaluation
I	Absent	Absent	Absent	Agammaglobulinemia Severe combined deficiency disease	Absolute indication, provide immediately	Inappropriate
II	Present	Low	Low	Hyper IgM CVID NEMO deficiency (subset)	Absolute indication, provide after firm diagnosis	Inappropriate
III	Present	Normal	Low	Specific antibody deficiency NEMO deficiency (subset) Subclass deficiency with specific antibody defect	Provide if diagnosis is firm	Single trial appropriate only if diagnosis is not related to a specific genetic defect
IV	Present	Low	Normal	Transient hypogammaglobulinemia of infancy	Provide when clinically indicated	Reassess if indicated with a single trail
V	Present	Normal, but IgG subclass deficient	Normal	Primary hypogammaglobulinemia IgG1, IgG2, or IgG3 subclass deficiency	Provide when clinically indicated	Reassess if indicated with a single trail
VI	Present	Normal	Normal	Recurrent infection	As adjunct therapy only where indicated	As appropriate

response, a failed humoral response to an infection, or a specific molecular/ genetic diagnosis linked to this category [112].

A fourth category (IV) includes patients with lower than expected levels of IgG but who are able to mount effective antibody responses. This category forms a subset of individuals referred to as having "isolated hypogammaglobulinemia" when only the IgG level is low. Although hypogammaglobulinemia can be a component of many immunologic defects, in isolated hypogammaglobulinemia antibody quality is adequate, with normal responses to vaccination or infection.

Because the normal age-specific ranges of IgG define the lower limit at the 2.5th percentile, one of 40 individuals has low levels of IgG. The question becomes, when there is no deficit of antibody quality, is isolated hypogamma-globulinemia clinically a problem? It is also important to discern when hypo-gammaglobulinemia represents a primary versus a secondary problem with increased loss of IgG. Examples of the latter include draining chylothorax [116] or intestinal lymphangiectasia [117]. In these individuals, the hypogam-maglobulinemia is less likely to cause a problem because antibody synthesis is intact and often accelerated.

In patients with primary hypogammaglobulinemia, the level of IgG that is associated with a definitive risk for infection is not defined, especially when antibody quality is intact [112]. Some insurance companies recommend replace-ment therapy for patients who have an IgG level less than 400 mg/dL and a history of recurrent infection. Although that situation may be reasonable, questions still exist about how to manage the patient recognized as having primary hypogammaglobulinemia with low IgG levels (ie, <150) but no history of infection.

Diagnostic examples include transient hypogammaglobulinemia of infancy (THI) [118–120] or otherwise unexplained primary hypogammaglobulinemia [121]. The former diagnosis is established in retrospect, as the IgG level normalizes with age. Thus, in select cases of THI immunoglobulin replacement may be considered as a temporizing measure. However, primary hypogamma-globulinemia remains a difficult diagnostic and therapeutic dilemma.

Other patients (a fifth diagnostic category [V]) have a deficiency of one of the 3 major IgG subclasses, IgG1, IgG2, or IgG3. IgG4 deficiency is common and should not be considered an abnormality [99]. Although a deficiency of one of the major IgG subclasses indicates some immunologic deviation, most of these patients have a normal total IgG level, intact responses to specific antigens, and are not candidates for immunoglobulin replacement therapy. Those with impaired antibody specificity do not fall in to this category, but into the third category. However, even without impairment in antibody quality, immuno-globulin replacement in some patients in a deficiency subclass does reduce the incidence of infections [122,123]. Nevertheless, most insurers in the United States have additional criteria for justifying therapy in patients with IgG in defi-ciency subclasses.

A final diagnostic category is patients with recurrent infection who do not have hypogammaglobulinemia subclass deficiency or deficits of antibody quality.

Thus, they have infectious susceptibility without evidence of identifiable immune abnormality. The infectious burden in these individuals can be high and most certainly has an explanation, so nonhumoral diagnoses should be aggressively sought. There are also patients an explanation of whose infectious susceptibility presently evades clinical science. immunoglobulin replacement therapy has been considered in these individuals under certain circumstances.

Immunoglobulin Preparations for Antibody Immunodeficiencies

Although Bruton [102] gave immunoglobulin to his patient by the subcutaneous (SC) route, subsequent patients until 1970 received immunoglobulin by weekly IM injections [124]. This strategy was necessary because the immunoglobulin preparations were not purified to the degree required for IV administration. In the early 1970s, immunoglobulin preparations with low quantities of immunoglobulin aggregates were developed for IV administration. IVIG and IGIV have numerous advantages, including achieving high peak and trough IgG levels and convenient monthly dosing regimens. Although limited studies have compared IVIG with IMIG, the IV route has become the preferred route of immunoglobulin administration worldwide [125].

Seven IVIG preparations are currently approved by the US Food and Drug Administration (FDA) for replacement therapy in primary immunodeficiency (Table 4). Each has been studied in a licensing trial in patients with primary immunodeficiency and found to be safe and effective. The primary end point in most of these clinical trials has been the prevention of serious bacterial infection compared with the expected frequency of such infections before diagnosis [126]. The rate of infection can be surprisingly high, as shown by Bruton's [102] first patient mentioned earlier. The early diagnosis and treatment of primary immunodeficiency with immunoglobulin products has reduced morbidity and mortality and considerable savings of health care expenditures [127,128].

All IVIG products are purified from human plasma pools under strict manufacturing guidelines. Although each manufacturer has its own process there are more similarities than differences in the various methods. All processes remove non-IgG impurities and IgG aggregates and add stabilizers to prevent in vitro aggregate formation. Despite these efforts, adverse reactions during IVIG administration are not uncommon [129]. All immunoglobulin manufacturers have robust measures to screen donors and to inactivate blood-borne pathogens; the safety of immunoglobulin preparations in the last decade has been superb [130].

There are subtle differences among different IVIG products from different companies; several companies have more than one product on the market [131]. This situation can lead to confusion about which IVIG to administer to which patient.

In general, most IVIG products are tolerated by most patients. The characteristics of the individual IVIG preparations, as outlined in Table 2, may help in selecting the best product for each patient. They differ as to concentration, stabilizers, sugar content, IgA content, sodium content, and osmality. The

Table 4
IVIG products for replacement therapy in primary immunodeficiency available in the United States in 2010

Product	Form	Stabilizer/Sugar	IgA (µg/ml)	Osm (mOsm/kg or L)	Sodium (mg/ml)	Storage	Manufacturer
Carimune	Lyophilized	Sucrose	Trace	768 (12%)	<2.4	RT (24 m)	CSL
Flebogamma	5% liquid	Sorbitol	<50	240–370	?	RT (24 m)	Grifols
Gammagard liquid	10% liquid	Glycine	37	240–300	None added	RT (6 m) 4° (36 m)	Baxter
Gammagard SD	Lyophilized	Glucose	<2.2	1250 (10%)	8.5	RT (24 m)	Baxter
Gammunex	10% liquid	Glycine	46	258	Trace	RT (9 m) 4° (36 m)	Talecris
Octagam	5% liquid	Maltose	<200	310–380	<0.7	RT (24 m)	Octapharma
Privigen	10% liquid	Proline	<25	240–440	Trace	RT (24 m)	CSL

Abbreviation: RT, room temperature.

volume of individual vials, storage requirements, need to reconstitute a lyophilized product before use, local availability, and price are also variable. Many patients may tolerate one product more effectively than another. Thus, when a patient tolerates a particular immunoglobulin product it is advisable to continue with that product whenever possible [99].

Three other preparations of immunoglobulin are approved by the US FDA (Table 5). One is approved for IM administration and two for SC administration. Few patients receive their immunoglobulin by the IM route.

Subcutaneous Immunoglobulin

The SC administration of immunoglobulin resurfaced in 1980 in the United States [132]. Subcutaneous immunoglobulin (SCIG) is usually given in the abdominal wall or thigh with a thin bored needle and an infusion pump, delivered over several hours. Although its initial use in the United States was limited, the SC route gained popularity in Europe; extensive clinical experience indicated that it was equivalent to IVIG therapy [133,134]. A crossover trial with IVIG and a US FDA licensing trial showed that SCIG was equivalent to IVIG in preventing infection in primary immunodeficiency [135,136].

SCIG has advantages and disadvantages compared with IVIG therapy (many related to patient preferences) and these have been reviewed extensively [137–139]. One advantage of SCIG over IVIG is the markedly decreased incidence of systemic reactions [134,135]. Another is eliminating the need for IV access or indwelling IV access devices. The most serious disadvantage is the need for more frequent administration (at least weekly) to administer sufficient immunoglobulin [140]. Another disadvantage is less frequent physician encounters because most SCIG infusions are given at home by caretakers or home infusion companies.

Dose and Administration of IVIG and SCIG

The dose and frequency of immunoglobulin therapy is a complex topic and draws on both evidence- and experience-based sources. These recommendations are presented in a several reviews and consensus statements [99,112,138,139,141]. The recommendations include starting doses of 400 to 600 mg/kg/mo. After several months this dose can be altered depending on the trough level and the clinical response. Patients vary as to their requirement to maintain reasonable resistance to infection [141,142].

Table 5
Other immunoglobulin products for replacement therapy in primary immunodeficiency available in the United States in 2010

Product	Approved route	Form	Stabilizer/ Sugar	IgA (µg/ml)	Sodium (mg/ml)	Storage	Manufacturer
Gammastan	IM	~16% liquid	Glycine	?	3.0	4°	Talecris
Vivaglobin	SC	16% liquid	Glycine	1700	<3.2	4°	CSL
Hizentra	SC	20% liquid	Proline	<50	Trace	RT	CSL

SCIG is typically used after the patient has been on IVIG for several months. The weekly SCIG dose is usually one-fourth of the previous monthly IVIG dose. Some immunoglobulin-naive patients are started on immunoglobulin therapy with SCIG so the number of initial doses may need to be increased.

The amount of SCIG given at a single site for an adult is usually 20 mL of the 16% solution (ie, 3.2 g). More than one site can be used simultaneously to deliver the target dose. This procedure has been facilitated by the availability of special tubing, needle sets, catheters, and pumps. Infusion site reactions are not uncommon but are rarely severe [136].

IVIG is usually administered monthly and SCIG is usually administered weekly, but other schedules are often used. These schedules include shorter or longer intervals between infusions of IVIG to achieve a satisfactory clinical response. SCIG can be given biweekly, or divided into more frequent injections, even small daily doses. The latter is generally self-administered at home, well tolerated, and preferred by some patients because of the small daily dose needed [143,144].

Trough levels of immunoglobulin achieved must be considered. Several studies have correlated resistance to infection with specific IgG trough levels. Targeting a specific trough level may be feasible for patients with agammaglobulinemia who have a profound deficiency of IgG [126] but more difficult for other antibody deficiencies [145–147]. In agammaglobulinemia, a trough level of 500 mg/dL is a minimally acceptable level and 800 mg/dL a more desirable trough level [99,126]. These recommendations may not be appropriate in other disorders in which baseline IgG levels and antibody titers are variable; in these cases the clinical response must be considered.

Summary of Immunoglobulin Use in Primary Immunodeficiency

Polyclonal immunoglobulin is essential therapy for the primary antibody immunodeficiency diseases. The different disorders in which immunoglobulin therapy are used are reviewed. Several immunoglobulin products are available for their treatment; they have similar therapeutic properties but there are individual differences among the available products. immunoglobulin can be given either intravenously (IVIG) or subcutaneously (SCIG). Dosage, frequency of infusions, achieved trough levels, and advantages and disadvantages of IVIG and SCIG are discussed.

IVIG IN AUTOIMMUNE AND INFLAMMATORY DISEASES

The early 1980s witnessed an increase in the use of IVIG as an immunomodulator for inflammatory and autoimmune disorders. More than 70% of the IVIG prescribed is for patients with autoimmune and inflammatory diseases, despite the fact that IVIG is approved for just a handful of indications (Box 1). In the late 1990s, this situation led to an IVIG shortage, compromising those patients who depend on IgG replacement therapy to correct their underlying antibody deficiency.

In 2006, the American Academy of Allergy, Asthma and Immunology's Committee on Primary Immunodeficiency evaluated the use of IVIG for multiple disorders. The strength of the evidence for a beneficial effect and the basis for this recommendation were classified (Box 2). This section reviews the use of IVIG for the autoimmune and inflammatory conditions in this report (Box 3), in the context of a review of the mechanisms of action of IVIG in these conditions.

The multiple effects of IVIG on the innate and adaptive immune system are illustrated in Fig. 1.

Historical Note: IVIG in Immune Thrombocytopenic Purpura

The first use of IVIG for an autoimmune process was in children with immune thrombocytopenic purpura (ITP). Imbach and colleagues [148] observed that antibody-deficient patients receiving IVIG who also had ITP had a marked increase in platelet count after IVIG infusions. Subsequently, these investigators examined the therapeutic effects of IVIG in children with a primary diagnosis of ITP; they used high-dose IVIG (400 mg/kg) for 4 consecutive days. The investigators reported a dramatic increase in platelet count within hours of the administration of IVIG. In some patients, the increase in platelet count was sustained; in others, repeat IVIG treatments were necessary.

Fc Receptor Blockade

Box 3 presents the indications for IVIG in autoimmune cytopenias as well its likely benefit. Several hypotheses have been proposed to explain the rapid increase in platelet count (or other antibody-coated cells) after IVIG administration. The most accepted hypothesis is that high-dose IVIG induces an Fc receptor blockade of reticuloendothelial cells in the liver and spleen, preventing them from removing antibody-sensitized cells.

Box 1: FDA-approved indications for IVIG

- Primary immunodeficiency
- Idiopathic thrombocytopenic purpura
- Kawasaki disease
- B-cell chronic lymphocytic leukemia
- Pediatric HIV
- Bone marrow transplantation
    Graft-versus-host disease (GVHD)
    Interstitial pneumonia
    Infections
- Chronic inflammatory demyelinating polyneuropathy

Box 2: Levels of evidence-based medical decisions

- Categorization of evidence and basis of recommendation

  Ia. From meta-analysis of randomized controlled studies

  Ib. From at least one randomized controlled study

  IIa. From at least one controlled trial without randomization

  IIb. From at least one other type of quasiexperimental study

  III. From nonexperimental descriptive studies, such as comparative, correlation, or case-control studies

  IV. From expert committee reports or opinions or clinical experience of respected authorities or both

- Strength of recommendation

  A. Based on category I evidence

  B. Based on category II evidence or extrapolated from category I evidence

  C. Based on category III evidence or extrapolated from category I or II evidence

  D. Based on category IV evidence or extrapolated from category I, II, or III evidence

---

Debre and colleagues [149] provided evidence for this hypothesis when they infused Fcγ fragments in children with ITP, and showed an increase in platelet count after the infusion. The Fc receptor blockade theory may account for the rapid increase in platelet count after the IVIG infusion, but not for the long-term benefits of IVIG. Thus additional mechanisms have been sought.

Fc Receptor Modulation

One such mechanism, supported by animal studies, is that IVIG stimulates inhibitory FcγRIIB receptors found on a variety of cell types including B cells that in turn inhibit antibody and immune function [150]. Samuelsson and colleagues [151] showed in a mouse model of ITP that IVIG suppresses or inhibits antiplatelet antibody production through this FcγRIIB receptor.

Subsequently Ravetch and colleagues [152,153] identified distinct motifs in the IVIG that have a propensity to engage and activate the FcγRIIB inhibitor receptor that inhibits antibody synthesis. These distinct properties were attributed to the carbohydrate moiety in the IVIG molecule, representing about 5% of the total IgG molecule. More than 30 different covalently attached carbohydrate glycans in the IgG molecule have been identified. Glycosylation of the IgG is essential for binding to all Fcγ receptors. The important glycan moiety in the IgG molecule is attached to the asparagine (Asn^{297}) in the second domain of the constant region of the IgG molecule.

Using a K/BxN serum-induced arthritis model in mice, Kaneko [152] showed that IgG at 1 g/kg inhibited the inflammatory arthritic process.

Box 3: Strength of the evidence for the effectiveness of IVIG in autoimmune/inflammatory diseases

Autoimmune cytopenias

- Definitely beneficial:
  Idiopathic thrombocytopenic purpura (Ia-A)
- Might provide benefit
  Autoimmune neutropenia (III-D)
  Autoimmune hemolytic anemia (III-D)
  Fetomaternal alloimmune thrombocytopenia (III-D)
  Neonatal isoimmune hemolytic anemia (III-D)
  Posttransfusion purpura (III-D)

Inflammatory neuropathies

- Definitely beneficial:
  Guillain-Barré syndrome (Ia-A)
  Chronic inflammatory demyelinating polyneuropathy (Ia-A)
  Multifocal motor neuropathy (Ia-A)
- Probably beneficial:
  Myasthenia gravis (Ib-IIa-B)
  Lambert-Eaton myasthenic syndrome (Ib-A)
  IgM antimyelin-associated glycoprotein paraprotein-associated peripheral neuropathy (Ib-A)
  Stiff man syndrome (Ib-A)
- Might provide benefit:
  Relapsing-remitting multiple sclerosis (Ia-A)
  Intractable childhood seizures (Ia-A)
  Rasmussen syndrome (IIB-B)
  Acute disseminated encephalomyelitis (III-C)
  Lumbosacral or brachial plexitis (III-C)
  Human T-lymphotropic virus-1–associated myelopathy (III-C)
  Postinfectious cerebellar ataxia (III-D)
  Acute idiopathic dysautonomia (III-D)
- Unlikely to be beneficial:
  Demyelinating neuropathy associated with monoclonal IgM (Ib-A)
  Amyotrophic lateral sclerosis (III-C)
  POEMS syndrome (III-C)
  Paraneoplastic neuropathies (III-C)

Rheumatologic and organ-specific autoimmune diseases
- Definitely beneficial:
  Graves ophthalmopathy (Ib-A)
- Probably beneficial:
  Autoimmune uveitis (IIA-B)
- Might provide benefit:
  Severe rheumatoid arthritis (IIb-B)
  Autoimmune diabetes mellitus (IIb-B)
  Vasculitides and antineutrophil antibody syndromes (III-D)
  Systemic lupus erythematosus (III-D)
- Unlikely to be beneficial:
  Antiphospholipid antibody syndrome (III-D)

IVIG in other inflammatory disorders
- Definitely beneficial:
- Probably beneficial:
  Toxic epidermal necrolysis/ Stevens-Johnson syndrome (IIa-B)
- Might provide benefit:
  Steroid-dependent asthma (Ib-A)

  Prevention of acute humoral rejection in renal transplants (Ib-A)

  Treatment of acute humoral rejection in renal transplants (III-C)

  Pediatric autoimmune neuropsychiatric disorder associated with streptococcus (PANDAS) (IIb-B)

  Delayed pressure urticaria (IIb-B)

  Chronic urticaria (III-C)

  Acute myocarditis (III-C)

  Autoimmune blistering diseases (III-C)

  Autoimmune liver disease (III-D)

  Prevention of pregnancy loss in a subset of women (repeat second-trimester loss) with spontaneous recurrent abortions (Ia-A)
- Unlikely to be beneficial:
  Nonsteroid-dependent asthma (Ib-A)

  Prevention of chronic GVHD after bone marrow transplantation (Ib-A)

  Chronic fatigue syndrome (Ib-A)

  Atopic dermatitis (IIa-B)

  Autism (III-C)

Adapted from Orange JS, Hossny EM, Weiler CR, et al. Use of intravenous immunoglobulin in human disease: a review of evidence by members of the Primary Immunodeficiency Committee of the American Academy of Allergy, Asthma and Immunology. J Allergy Clin Immunol 2006;117:S525–53.

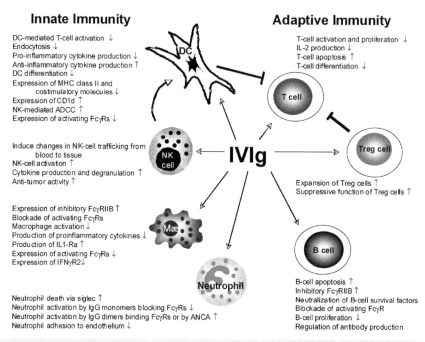

Innate Immunity

DC-mediated T-cell activation ↓
Endocytosis ↓
Pro-inflammatory cytokine production ↓
Anti-inflammatory cytokine production ↑
DC differentiation ↓
Expression of MHC class II and
    costimulatory molecules ↓
Expression of CD1d ↑
NK-mediated ADCC ↑
Expression of activating FcγRs ↓

Induce changes in NK-cell trafficking from
    blood to tissue
NK-cell activation ↑
Cytokine production and degranulation ↑
Anti-tumor activity ↑

Expression of inhibitory FcγRIIB ↑
Blockade of activating FcγRs
Macrophage activation ↓
Production of proinflammatory cytokines ↓
Production of IL1-Ra ↑
Expression of activating FcγRs ↓
Expression of IFNγR2↓

Neutrophil death via siglec ↑
Neutrophil activation by IgG monomers blocking FcγRs ↓
Neutrophil activation by IgG dimers binding FcγRs or by ANCA ↑
Neutrophil adhesion to endothelium ↓

Adaptive Immunity

T-cell activation and proliferation ↓
IL-2 production ↓
T-cell apoptosis ↑
T-cell differentiation ↓

Expansion of Treg cells ↑
Suppressive function of Treg cells ↑

B-cell apoptosis ↑
Inhibitory FcγRIIB ↑
Neutralization of B-cell survival factors
Blockade of activating FcγR
B-cell proliferation ↓
Regulation of antibody production

Fig. 1. Multiple effects of IVIG on the innate and adaptive immune system. (*Adapted from* Tha-In T, Bayry J, Metselaar HJ, et al. Modulation of the cellular immune system by intravenous immunoglobulin. Trends Immunol 2008;29:613; with permission.)

Deglycosylated or neuraminidase-treated IVIGs were unable to inhibit this inflammation. Kaneko then showed that IVIG enriched for the sialylated glycan moiety had comparable inhibitory effects on the inflammatory process at one-tenth of the dosage used with intact IVIG. This investigator showed that this inhibitory activity resided in the IgG Fc fragment, and was dependent on FcγRIIB expression on effector macrophages.

Anthony and colleagues [154] have engineered a recombinant/sialylated human IgG1 Fc protein that had the same immune modulating activity as native IVIG. These investigators showed that the action of sialylated Fc in the rheumatoid arthritis mouse model is mediated through the interaction of sialylated Fc with the SIGN-R1 receptor on macrophages [154]. The investigators propose that the interaction between sialylated Fc and SIGN-R1 produces an antiinflammatory state that upregulates inhibitory FcγRIIB receptors on effector cells, making these cells more resistant to triggering by immune complexes. They suggest that DC-SIGN, the human homolog of SIGN-R1, has a comparable role for the antiinflammatory effects of IgG Fc fragments.

Acceleration of IgG Catabolism

Another mechanism proposed by Yu and Lennon [155] suggested that the administration of high-dose IVIG augments the catabolism of endogenous serum IgG.

IgG catabolism occurs through a process by which the IgG molecule binds to a specialized Fc receptor found on endothelial cells (eg, FcRn), which protects the IgG molecule from normal catabolism and its removal from the plasma. This process accounts for the long serum IgG half-life (21 days). High-dose IVIG saturates the FcRn receptor, resulting in the accelerated catabolism of auto-antibodies [156–157]. Hansen and Balthasar [157] have supporting data in a rat model of immune thrombocytopenia using monoclonal antibodies.

Presence of Antiidiotypic Antibodies

The uses of IVIG in several autoimmune inflammatory neuropathies are presented in Box 3. The FDA has recently approved the use of IVIG in chronic inflammatory demyelinating polyneuropathy. This table also shows the evidence-based efficacy of IVIG in rheumatic disorders. Aside from the mechanisms involving the FcγRIIB inhibitory receptor and the accelerated catabolism of autoimmune antibodies through the FcRn receptor, it has also been proposed that the administration of IVIG can regulate autoreactive B cells by restoring the idiotypic-antiidiotypic network.

Other autoimmune diseases may be associated with a deficiency of these antiidiotypic antibodies, which are believed to regulate the production and activity of these autoantibodies (Box 4). Kazatchkine and colleagues [158] showed that $F(ab')_2$ fragments prepared from IVIG could bind to several auto-antibodies (eg, antifactor VIII, antithyroglobulin, anti-DNA, antiintrinsic factor, neutrophil cytoplasmic antigens), and thus lead to increased catabolism of these autoimmune antibodies and prevent them from inducing tissue injury [159]. These investigators postulated that IVIG may work, at least in part, in certain autoimmune diseases by neutralizing the functional activity of various autoantibodies or inhibiting their binding to their respective autoantigens [160].

Inhibition of Complement Activation

Another mechanism by which IVIG may benefit autoimmune disease is by preventing the uptake of complement on target tissues. Berger and colleagues [161] showed that high concentrations of IgG inhibit the uptake of C3 on antibody-sensitized erythrocytes. Thus, any inflammatory or autoimmune process that involves a C3b-or C4b-dependent process could be modulated by IVIG therapy. This situation is best exemplified in patients with dermatomyositis

---

Box 4: Diseases that may be associated with deficiencies of antiidiotypic antibodies

- Myasthenia gravis
- Autoimmune neuropathies
- Guillain-Barré syndrome
- Antifactor VIII autoimmune disease
- Autoimmune thyroiditis
- Systemic lupus erythematosus

in whom the disease is mediated by activation of C3 and deposition of the membrane attack complex on the endomysial capillaries [162]. Treatment with IVIG inhibits complement-induced inflammation by decreasing complement deposition on the endomysial capillaries of muscle tissues [163,164]. This mechanism of IVIG is relevant not only in dermatomyositis but also in Guillain-Barré syndrome and myasthenia gravis [165,166].

Fas Ligand Inhibition

As shown in Box 3, IVIG is used in many other inflammatory diseases. However, the evidence-based data for several of these diseases are not so strong as some of the autoimmune disorders discussed earlier. Nevertheless, one inflammatory disease in which IVIG may be beneficial is toxic epidermal necrolysis or Stevens-Johnson syndrome. Patients with toxic epidermal necrolysis have high levels of serum-soluble Fas ligand that bind to Fas receptors on keratinocytes to induce apoptosis (cell death). Viard and colleagues [167] showed that the anti-Fas antibodies in IVIG block the interaction of Fas ligand with Fas receptors on the keratinocytes, preventing destruction of the epithelium.

Inhibition of Neutrophil Adhesion

IVIG contains antibodies to several cell-surface molecules [168] including antibodies to a 10-peptide sequence containing the (Arg-Gly-Asp) motif that is expressed on cell surfaces and matrix proteins that are part of the integrin adhesion system. IVIG inhibits the adhesion of B cells to fibronectin and inhibits platelet aggregation [169]. Turhan and colleagues [170] and Chang and colleagues [171] investigated the effect of IVIG on a mouse model of sickle cell acute vasoocclusive crisis, in which the adhesion of sickled red blood cells to leukocytes causes the vasoocclusive disease. In this model, high-dose IVIG given after the onset of a crisis resulted in improved blood flow and prolonged survival. These investigators showed that IVIG reverses acute vasoocclusive crisis in sickle cell mice by inhibiting neutrophil adhesion to the capillary endothelial cells.

Summary of IVIG Use in Inflammatory/Autoimmune Disorders

The various mechanisms of the antiinflammatory and immunomodulatory properties of IVIG are reviewed. The first use of IVIG was in the treatment of immune thrombocytopenia, presumably because of Fc receptor blockade. Other mechanisms are reviewed as well as the evidence for the value of IVIG in multiple disorders. IVIG may have yet undiscovered immunomodulating properties on both the innate and adaptive immune systems. Future advances will include a better understanding of its mechanisms of action and modification of the IgG molecule to enhance its immunomodulating properties.

References

[1] Lucey D. Anthrax. In: Mandel G, Bennett JE, Donin R, editors. Principles and practice of infectious diseases. 6th edition. Philadelphia: Elsevier/Churchill Livingston; 2005. p. 3618–24, 2485–91.

[2] Gold H, Chester PA. Studies on anthrax: clinical report of ten human cases. J Lab Clin Med 1935;21:134–52.

[3] Cidrap. HHS to buy 20,000 courses of anthrax antitoxin. Available at: cidrap.umn.edu/cidrap/content/bt/anthrax/news/jun2006anthrax.html. Accessed June 20, 2006.

[4] Migone T, Subramanian M, Zhong J, et al. Raxibacumab or the treatment of inhalational anthrax. N Engl J Med 2009;361:135–44.

[5] Stiehm ER, Keller MA. Passive immunization. In: Feigen RD, Cherry JD, Demmler-Harrison GJ, et al, editors. Textbook of pediatric infectious diseases. 6th edition. Philadelphia: Saunders/Elsevier; 2009. p. 3447–79.

[6] American Academy of Pediatrics. Diphtheria. In: Pickering LK, Baker CJ, Kimberlin DW, et al, editors. Red Book: 2009 Report of the Committee on infectious diseases. 28th edition. Elk Grove Village (IL): American Academy of Pediatrics; 2009. p. 280–3.

[7] Faber HK, McIntosh R. History of the American Pediatric Society 1887–1965. New York: McGraw-Hill; 1966. p. 35–6.

[8] American Academy of Pediatrics. Tetanus. In: Pickering LK, Baker CJ, Kimberlin DW, et al, editors. Red Book: 2009 Report of the Committee on infectious diseases. 28th edition. Elk Grove Village (IL): American Academy of Pediatrics; 2009. p. 655–60.

[9] Lee DC, Lederman HM. Anti-tetanus toxoid antibodies in intravenous gamma globulin: an alternative to tetanus immune globulin. J Infect Dis 1992;166:642–5.

[10] Wilcox MH. Treatment of Clostridium difficile infection. J Antimicrob Chemother 1998;41-(Suppl C):41–6.

[11] Cleary R. Clostridium difficile-associated diarrhea and colitis: clinical manifestations, diagnosis, and treatment. Dis Colon Rectum 1998;41:1435–49.

[12] Kyne L, Warny M, Qamar A, et al. Asymptomatic carriage of Clostridium difficile and serum levels of IgG antibody against toxin. N Engl J Med 2000;342:390–7.

[13] McPherson S, Rees CJ, Ellis R, et al. Intravenous immunoglobulin for the treatment of severe, refractory, and recurrent Clostridium difficile diarrhea. Dis Colon Rectum 2006;49:640–5.

[14] Leung D, Kelly YM, Boguniewicz CP, et al. Treatment with intravenously administered gamma globulin of chronic relapsing colitis induced by Clostridium difficile toxin. J Pediatr 1991;118:633–7.

[15] Salcedo J, Keates S, Pothoulakis C, et al. Intravenous immunoglobulin therapy for severe Clostridium difficile colitis. Gastroenterology 1997;41:366–70.

[16] Arnon SS, Schechter R, Inglesby TV, et al. Botulinum toxin as a biological weapon: medical and public health management. JAMA 2001;285:1059–71.

[17] Berg BO. Syndrome of infant botulism. Pediatrics 1977;59:321–2.

[18] Centers for Disease Control. Botulism in the United States, 1899–1977. Handbook for epidemiologists, clinicians and laboratory workers. Atlanta (GA): Centers for Disease Control; 1979.

[19] Chertow DS, Tan ET, Maslanka SE, et al. Botulism in 4 adults following cosmetic injections with an unlicensed, highly concentrated botulinum preparation. JAMA 2006;2476–9.

[20] Souayah N, Karim H, Kamin SS, et al. Severe botulism after focal injection of botulinum toxin. Neurology 2006;67:1855–6.

[21] Centers for Disease Control and Prevention (CDC). Investigational heptavalent botulinum antitoxin (HBAT) to replace licensed botulinum antitoxin AB and investigational botulinum antitoxin E. MMWR Morb Mortal Wkly Report 2010;59(10):299.

[22] American Academy of Pediatrics. Botulism and infant botulism. In: Pickering LK, Baker CJ, Kimberlin DW, et al, editors. Red Book: 2009 Report of the Committee on infectious diseases. 28th edition. Elk Grove Village (IL): American Academy of Pediatrics; 2009. p. 259–62.

[23] Arnon SS, Schechter R, Maslanka SE, et al. Human botulism immune globulin for the treatment of infant botulism. N Engl J Med 2006;345:462–71.

[24] Alexander HE. Treatment of Haemophilus influenzae infection and of meningococcic and pneumococcic meningitis. Am J Dis Child 1943;66:172–87.

[25] Casadevall A, Scharff MD. Return to the past: the case for antibody-based therapies in infectious diseases. Clin Infect Dis 1995;21:150–61.

[26] Simoes EAF, Groothuis JR, Tristram DA, et al. Respiratory syncytial virus-enriched globulin for the prevention of acute otitis media in high risk children. J Pediatr 1996;129:214–9.

[27] Mofenson LM, Moye J Jr, Bethel J, et al. Prophylactic intravenous immunoglobulin in HIV-infected children with CD4$^+$ counts of 0.20 $\times$ 10^9/L or more: effect on viral, opportunistic, and bacterial infections. JAMA 1992;268:483–8.

[28] National Institute of Child Health and Human Development (NICHHD) Intravenous Immunoglobulin Study Group. Intravenous immune globulin for the prevention of bacterial infections in children with symptomatic human immunodeficiency virus infection. N Engl J Med 1991;325:73–80.

[29] Casadevall A. Passive antibody therapies: progress and continuing challenges. Clin Immunol 1999;93:5–15.

[30] Lucchesi PF, Bowman JE. Antitoxin versus no antitoxin in scarlet fever. JAMA 1930;103:1049–51.

[31] Perez CM, Kubak BM, Cryer HG, et al. Adjunctive treatment of streptococcal toxic shock syndrome using intravenous immunoglobulin: case report and review. Am J Med 1997;102:111–3.

[32] Schrage B, Duan G, Yang LP, et al. Different preparations of intravenous immunoglobulin vary in their efficacy to neutralize streptococcal superantigens: implications for treatment of streptococcal toxic shock syndrome. Clin Infect Dis 2006;43:743–6.

[33] Lamothe F, D'Amico P, Ghosen P, et al. Clinical usefulness of intravenous human immunoglobulins in invasive group A streptococcal infections: case report and review. Clin Infect Dis 1995;21:1469–70.

[34] Kaul R, McGeer A, Norrby-Tegllund A, et al. Intravenous immunoglobulin for streptococcal toxic shock syndrome—a comparative observational study. Clin Infect Dis 1999;28:800–7.

[35] American Academy of Pediatrics. Staphylococcal infections. In: Pickering LK, Baker CJ, Kimberlin DW, et al, editors. Red Book: 2009 Report of the Committee on infectious diseases. 28th edition. Elk Grove Village (IL): American Academy of Pediatrics; 2009. p. 601–15.

[36] Melish ME, Murata S, Fukunaga C, et al. Vaginal tampon model for toxic shock syndrome. Rev Infect Dis 1989;11(Suppl 1):219–28, 238–46.

[37] Suen J, Chesney PJ, Davis JP. Toxic shock syndrome. In: Feigen RD, Cherry JD, Demmler-Harrison GJ, et al, editors. Textbook of pediatric infectious diseases. 6th edition. Philadelphia: Saunders/Elsevier; 2009. p. 862–84.

[38] Fischer GW, Cieslak TJ, Wilson SR, et al. Opsonic antibodies to *Staphylococcus epidermidis*: in vitro and in vivo studies using human intravenous immune globulin. J Infect Dis 1994;169:324–9.

[39] Jenson HB, Pollock BH. The role of intravenous immunoglobulin for the prevention and treatment of neonatal sepsis. Semin Perinatol 1998;22:50–63.

[40] Baker CJ, Melish ME, Hall RT. Intravenous immune globulin for the prevention of nosocomial infection in low-birth-weight neonates. N Engl J Med 1992;327:213–9.

[41] Waisbren BA. The treatment of bacterial infections with the combination of antibiotics and gamma globulin. Antibiot Chemother 1957;7:322–32.

[42] Kelly J. Immunotherapy against antibiotic-resistant bacteria: the Russian experience with an antistaphyloccocal hyperimmune plasma and immunoglobulin. Microbes Infect 2000;2:1383–92.

[43] Fisher MW. Synergism between human gamma globulin and chloramphenicol in the treatment of experimental bacterial infections. Antibiot Chemother 1956;7:315–21.

[44] Lewis DB, Tu W. The physiologic immunodeficiency of immaturity. In: Stiehm ER, Ochs HD, Winkelstein JW, editors. Immunologic disorders in infants and children. 5th edition. Philadelphia: Elsevier/Saunders; 2004. p. 687–760.

[45] Jenson HB, Pollock BH. Meta-analyses of the effectiveness of intravenous immune globulin for prevention and treatment of neonatal sepsis. Pediatrics 1997;99:E2.

[46] Lacy JB, Ohlsson A. Administration of intravenous immunoglobulins for prophylaxis or treatment of infection in preterm infants: meta-analysis. Arch Dis Child 1995;72: F151–5.

[47] Ohlsson A, Lacy JB. Intravenous immunoglobulin for preventing infection in preterm and/ or low birth-weight infants (Cochrane Review). The Cochrane Library. Oxford. Issue 1. 2001.

[48] Ohlsson A, Lacy JB. Intravenous immunoglobulin for suspected or subsequently proven infection in neonates. Cochrane Database Syst Rev 2004;1: CD001239.

[49] Benjamin DK, Schelonka R, White R, et al. A blinded, randomized, multicenter study of an intravenous Staphylococcus aureus immune globulin. J Perinatol 2006;26:290–5.

[50] Bloom B, Schelonka R, Kueser T, et al. Multicenter study to assess safety and efficacy of INH-A21, a donor-selected human staphylococcal immunoglobulin, for prevention of nosocomial infections in very low birth weight infants. Pediatr Infect Dis J 2005;24:858–66.

[51] NIH Consensus Development Conference: diseases, doses, recommendations for intravenous immunoglobulin. HLB Newsletter. Natl Inst Heart Lung Blood Dis 1990;6:73–8.

[52] Glinz PW, Nydegger UE, Ricklin T, et al. Polyvalent immunoglobulins for prophylaxis of bacterial infections in patients following multiple trauma. Intensive Care Med 1985;11: 288–94.

[53] Sandberg ET, Kline MW, Shearer WT. The secondary immunodeficiencies. In: Stiehm ER, editor. Immunologic disorders in infants and children. 4th edition. Philadelphia: WB Saunders; 1996. p. 553–601.

[54] Laupland KB, Kirkpatrick AW, Delaney A. Polyclonal intravenous immunoglobulin for the treatment of severe sepsis and septic shock in critically ill adults: a systematic review and meta-analysis. Crit Care Med 2007;35:2686–92.

[55] Kempe CH. Studies on smallpox and complications of smallpox vaccination. Pediatrics 1960;26:176–89.

[56] American Academy of Pediatrics. Smallpox (variola). In: Pickering LK, Baker CJ, Kimberlin DW, et al, editors. Red Book: 2009 Report of the Committee on infectious diseases. 28th edition. Elk Grove Village (IL): American Academy of Pediatrics; 2009. p. 596–8.

[57] Brown KE. Parvovirus B19. In: Mandell GL, Bennett JE, Doling R, editors. Mandell, Douglas and Bennett's principles and practice of infectious diseases. 5th edition. Philadelphia: Churchill Livingstone; 2000. p. 1685–93.

[58] Inoue S, Kinra NK, Mukkamala SR, et al. Parvovirus B19 infection: aplastic crisis, erythema infectiosum and idiopathic thrombocytopenic purpura. Pediatr Infect Dis J 1991;10: 251–3.

[59] Young NS. Parvovirus infection and its treatment. Clin Exp Immunol 1996;104(Suppl 1): 26–30.

[60] American Academy of Pediatrics. Parvovirus B19. In: Pickering LK, Baker CJ, Kimberlin DW, et al, editors. Red Book: 2009 Report of the Committee on infectious diseases. 28th edition. Elk Grove Village (IL): American Academy of Pediatrics; 2009. p. 491–4.

[61] McGhee SA, Kaska B, Liebhaber M, et al. Persistent parvovirus-associated chronic fatigue treated with high dose intravenous immunoglobulin. Pediatr Infect Dis J 2005;24:272–4.

[62] Frickhofen NJ, Abkowitz L, Safford M, et al. Persistent B19 parvovirus infection in patients infected with human immunodeficiency virus type 1 (HIV-1): a treatable cause of anemia with AIDS. Ann Intern Med 1990;113:926–33.

[63] Koduri PR, Kumapley RJ, Valladares J, et al. Chronic pure red cell aplasia caused by parvovirus B19 in AIDS: use of intravenous immunoglobulin: a report of eight patients. Am J Hematol 1999;61:16–20.

[64] Bulinski P, Toledo-Pereyra LH, Dalal S, et al. Cytomegalovirus infection in kidney transplantation: prophylaxis and management. Transplant Proc 1996;28:3310–1.

[65] Jassal SV, Roscoe JM, Zaltzman JS, et al. Clinical practice guidelines: prevention of cytomegalovirus disease after renal transplantation. J Am Soc Nephrol 1998;9: 1697–708.

[66] Bonaros NE, Kocher A, Dunkler D, et al. Comparison of combined prophylaxis of cytomegalovirus hyperimmune globulin plus ganciclovir versus cytomegalovirus hyperimmune globulin alone in high-risk heart transplant recipients. Transplantation 2004;77:890–7.

[67] Paar DP, Pollard RB. Immunotherapy of CMV infections. Adv Exp Med Biol 1996;394: 145–51.

[68] Negishi H, Yamada H, Hirayama E, et al. Intraperitoneal administration of cytomegalovirus hyperimmunoglobulin to the cytomegalovirus-infected fetus. J Perinatol 1998;18:466–9.

[69] Nigro G, Adler SP, La Torre R, et al. Passive immunization during pregnancy for congenital cytomegalovirus infection. N Engl J Med 2005;353:1350–62.

[70] American Academy of Pediatrics. Herpes simplex. In: Pickering LK, Baker CJ, Kimberlin DW, et al, editors. Red Book: 2009 Report of the Committee on infectious diseases. 28th edition. Elk Grove Village (IL): American Academy of Pediatrics; 2009. p. 363–73.

[71] Masci S, De Simone C, Famularo G, et al. Intravenous immunoglobulins suppress the recurrences of genital herpes simplex virus: a clinical and immunological study. Immunopharmacol Immunotoxicol 1995;17:33–47.

[72] Delone PJ, Corkill J, Jordan M, et al. Successful treatment of Epstein-Barr virus infection with ganciclovir and cytomegalovirus hyperimmune globulin following kidney transplantation. Transplant Proc 1995;27(Suppl 1):58–9.

[73] Oettle H, Wilborn F, Schmidt CA, et al. Treatment with ganciclovir and Ig for acute Epstein-Barr virus infection after allogeneic bone marrow transplantation. Blood 1993;82: 2257–62.

[74] Taguchi Y, Purtilo DT, Okano M. The effect of intravenous immunoglobulin and interferon-alpha on Epstein-Barr virus-induced lymphoproliferative disorder in a liver transplant recipient. Transplantation 1994;57:1813–5.

[75] Filipovich AH, Gross T, Jyonouchi H, et al. Immune-mediated hematologic and oncologic disorders, including Epstein-Barr virus infection. In: Stiehm ER, editor. Immunologic disorders in infants and children. 4th edition. Philadelphia: WB Saunders; 1996. p. 855–88.

[76] Brunell PA, Gershon AA. Passive immunization against varicella zoster infections. J Infect Dis 1973;127:415–23.

[77] American Academy of Pediatrics. Varicella-zoster infections. In: Pickering LK, Baker CJ, Kimberlin DW, et al, editors. Red Book: 2009 Report of the Committee on infectious diseases. 28th edition. Elk Grove Village (IL): American Academy of Pediatrics; 2009. p. 714–27.

[78] Bodian D. Experimental studies on passive immunization against poliomyelitis: I. Protection with human gamma globulin against intramuscular inoculation and combined passive and active immunization. Am J Hyg 1951;54:132–43.

[79] McKinney RE, Katz SL, Wilfert CM. Chronic enteroviral meningoencephalitis in agammaglobulinemic patients. Rev Infect Dis 1987;9:334–56.

[80] Dwyer JM, Erlendsson K. Intraventricular gamma-globulin for the management of enterovirus encephalitis. Pediatr Infect Dis J 1988;7:S30–3.

[81] Kondoh HK, Kobayashi Y, Sugio K, et al. Successful treatment of echovirus meningoencephalitis in sex-linked agammaglobulinaemia by intrathecal and intravenous injection of high titer gammaglobulin. Eur J Pediatr 1987;146:610–2.

[82] Misbah SA, Spickett GP, Ryba CJ, et al. Chronic enteroviral meningoencephalitis, in agammaglobulinemia: case report and literature review. J Clin Immunol 1992;12: 266–70.

[83] Desmond RA, Accortt NA, Talley L, et al. Enteroviral meningitis: natural history and outcome of pleconaril therapy. Antimicrob Agents Chemother 2006;50:2409–14.

[84] Abzug MJ, Keyserling HL, Lee ML, et al. Neonatal enterovirus infection: virology, serology, and effects of intravenous immune globulin. Clin Infect Dis 1995;20:1201–6.

[85] Rentz AC, Libbey JE, Fujinami RS, et al. Investigation of treatment failure in neonatal echovirus 7 infection. Pediatr Infect Dis 2006;25:259–62.

[86] Nagington J, Gandy G, Walker J, et al. Use of normal immunoglobulin in an echovirus 11 outbreak in a special-care baby unit. Lancet 1983;ii:443–6.

[87] Terrault NA, Zhou S, Combs C, et al. Prophylaxis in liver transplant recipients using a fixed dosing schedule of hepatitis B immunoglobulin. Hepatology 1996;24:1327–33.

[88] Grazi GL, Mazziotti A, Sama C, et al. Liver transplantation in HBsAg-positive HBV-DNA-negative cirrhotics: immunoprophylaxis and long term outcome. Liver Transpl Surg 1996;2:418–25.

[89] Samuel D, Bismuth A, Serres C, et al. HBV-infection in liver transplantation in HBsAg positive patients: experience with long-term immunoprophylaxis. Transplant Proc 1991;23:1492–4.

[90] Makhoul B, Braun E, Herskovitz M, et al. Hyperimmune gammaglobulin for the treatment of West Nile virus encephalitis. Isr Med Assoc J 2009;11:151–3.

[91] Ben-Nathan D, Gershoni-Yahalom O, Samina I, et al. Using high titer West Nile intravenous immunoglobulin from selected Israeli donors for treatment of West Nile virus infection. Available at: http://www.biomedcentral.com/1471-2334/9/18.

[92] Kudoyarova-Zubavichene NM, Sergeyev NN, Chepurnov AA, et al. Preparation and use of hyperimmune serum for prophylaxis and therapy of Ebola virus infections. J Infect Dis 1999;179(Suppl 1):218–23.

[93] Jahrling PB, Geisbert TW, Geisbert JB, et al. Evaluation of immune globulin and recombinant interferon-α2b for treatment of experimental Ebola virus infections. J Infect Dis 1999;179(Suppl):224–34.

[94] Mupapa K, Massamba M, Kibadi K, et al. Treatment of Ebola hemorrhagic fever with blood transfusions from convalescent patients. J Infect Dis 1999;179(Suppl 1):S18–23.

[95] Dumpis U, Crook D, Oksi J. Tick-borne encephalitis. Clin Infect Dis 1999;28:882–90.

[96] Von Hedenström M, Heberle U, Theobald K. Vaccination against tick-borne encephalitis (TBE): influence of simultaneous application of TBE immunoglobulin on seroconversion and rate of adverse events. Vaccine 1995;13:759–62.

[97] Maiztegui JI, Fernandez NJ, De Damilano AJ. Efficacy of immune plasma in treatment of Argentine haemorrhagic fever and association between treatment and a late neurological syndrome. Lancet 1979;ii:1216–7.

[98] Stockman LJ, Bellamy R, Garner P. SARS: systematic review of treatment effects. PLoS Med 2006;3:e343 10.1371/journal pmed0030343.

[99] Orange JS, Hossny EM, Weiler CR, et al. Use of intravenous immunoglobulin in human disease: a review of evidence by members of the Primary Immunodeficiency Committee of the American Academy of Allergy, Asthma and Immunology. J Allergy Clin Immunol 2006;117:S525–53.

[100] Constantine MM, Thomas W, Whitman L, et al. Intravenous immunoglobulin utilization in the Canadian Atlantic provinces: a report of the Atlantic Collaborative Intravenous Immune Globulin Utilization Working Group. Transfusion 2007;47:2072–80.

[101] Provan D, Chapel HM, Sewell WA, et al. Prescribing intravenous immunoglobulin: summary of Department of Health guidelines. BMJ 2008;337:a1831.

[102] Bruton OC. Agammaglobulinemia. Pediatrics 1952;9:722–8.

[103] Geha RS, Notarangelo LD, Casanova JL, et al. Primary immunodeficiency diseases: an update from the International Union of Immunological Societies Primary Immunodeficiency Diseases Classification Committee. J Allergy Clin Immunol 2007;120:776–94.

[104] Boyle JM, Buckley RH. Population prevalence of diagnosed primary immunodeficiency diseases in the United States. J Clin Immunol 2007;27:497–502.

[105] Leiva LE, Zelazco M, Oleastro M, et al. Primary immunodeficiency diseases in Latin America: the second report of the LAGID registry. J Clin Immunol 2007;27:101–8.

[106] Kirkpatrick P, Riminton S. Primary immunodeficiency diseases in Australia and New Zealand. J Clin Immunol 2007;27:517–24.

[107] Luzi G, Businco L, Aiuti F. Primary immunodeficiency syndromes in Italy: a report of the national register in children and adults. J Clin Immunol 1983;3:316–20.

[108] Stray-Pedersen A, Abrahamsen TG, Froland SS. Primary immunodeficiency diseases in Norway. J Clin Immunol 2000;20:477–85.

[109] Conley ME, Dobbs AK, Farmer DM, et al. Primary B cell immunodeficiencies: comparisons and contrasts. Annu Rev Immunol 2009;27:199–227.

[110] Notarangelo LD, Lanzi G, Peron S, et al. Defects of class-switch recombination. J Allergy Clin Immunol 2006;117:855–64.

[111] Yong PF, Tarzi M, Chua I, et al. Common variable immunodeficiency: an update on etiology and management. Immunol Allergy Clin North Am 2008;28:367–86.

[112] Bonilla FA, Bernstein IL, Khan DA, et al. Practice parameter for the diagnosis and management of primary immunodeficiency. Ann Allergy Asthma Immunol 2005;94:S1–63.

[113] Wolpert J, Knutsen A. Natural history of selective antibody deficiency to bacterial polysaccharide antigens in children. Pediatr Asthma Allergy Immunol 1998;12:183–91.

[114] Hanson EP, Monaco-Shawver L, Solt LA, et al. Hypomorphic nuclear factor-kappaB essential modulator mutation database and reconstitution system identifies phenotypic and immunologic diversity. J Allergy Clin Immunol 2008;122:1169–77.

[115] Orange JS, Levy O, Brodeur SR, et al. Human nuclear factor kappa B essential modulator mutation can result in immunodeficiency without ectodermal dysplasia. J Allergy Clin Immunol 2004;114:650–6.

[116] Orange JS, Geha RS, Bonilla FA. Acute chylothorax in children: selective retention of memory T cells and natural killer cells. J Pediatr 2003;143:243–9.

[117] Strober W, Wochner RD, Carbone PP, et al. Intestinal lymphangiectasia: a protein-losing enteropathy with hypogammaglobulinemia, lymphocytopenia and impaired homograft rejection. J Clin Invest 1967;46:1643–56.

[118] Dalal I, Reid B, Nisbet-Brown E, et al. The outcome of patients with hypogammaglobulinemia in infancy and early childhood. J Pediatr 1998;133:144–6.

[119] Dorsey MJ, Orange JS. Impaired specific antibody response and increased B-cell population in transient hypogammaglobulinemia of infancy. Ann Allergy Asthma Immunol 2006;97:590–5.

[120] Whelan MA, Hwan WH, Beausoleil J, et al. Infants presenting with recurrent infections and low immunoglobulins: characteristics and analysis of normalization. J Clin Immunol 2006;26:7–11.

[121] Yong PF, Chee R, Grimbacher B. Hypogammaglobulinaemia. Immunol Allergy Clin North Am 2008;28:691–713.

[122] Barlan IB, Geha RS, Schneider LC. Therapy for patients with recurrent infections and low serum IgG3 levels. J Allergy Clin Immunol 1993;92:353–5.

[123] Abdou NI, Greenwell CA, Mehta R, et al. Efficacy of intravenous gammaglobulin for immunoglobulin G subclass and/or antibody deficiency in adults. Int Arch Allergy Immunol 2009;149:267–74.

[124] Janeway CA, Rosen FS. The gamma globulins. IV. Therapeutic uses of gamma globulin. N Engl J Med 1966;275:826–31.

[125] Cunningham-Rundles C, Siegal FP, Smithwick EM, et al. Efficacy of intravenous immunoglobulin in primary humoral immunodeficiency disease. Ann Intern Med 1984;101:435–9.

[126] Quartier P, Debre M, De Blic J, et al. Early and prolonged intravenous immunoglobulin replacement therapy in childhood agammaglobulinemia: a retrospective survey of 31 patients. J Pediatr 1999;134:589–96.

[127] Pickett D, Modell V, Leighton I, et al. Impact of a physician education and patient awareness campaign on the diagnosis and management of primary immunodeficiencies. Immunol Res 2008;40:93–4.

[128] Simoens S. Pharmacoeconomics of immunoglobulins in primary immunodeficiency. Expert Rev Pharmacoecon Outcomes Res 2009;9:375–86.

[129] Carbone J. Adverse reactions and pathogen safety of intravenous immunoglobulin. Curr Drug Saf 2007;2:9–18.

[130] Quinti I, Pierdominici M, Marziali M, et al. European surveillance of immunoglobulin safety–results of initial survey of 1243 patients with primary immunodeficiencies in 16 countries. Clin Immunol 2002;104:231–6.

[131] Gelfand EW. Differences between IGIV products: impact on clinical outcome. Int Immunopharmacol 2006;6:592–9.

[132] Berger M, Cupps TR, Fauci AS. Immunoglobulin replacement therapy by slow subcutaneous infusion. Ann Intern Med 1980;93:55–6.

[133] Gardulf A, Andersen V, Bjorkander J, et al. Subcutaneous immunoglobulin replacement in patients with primary antibody deficiencies: safety and costs. Lancet 1995;345:365–9.

[134] Gardulf A, Hammarstrom L, Smith CI. Home treatment of hypogammaglobulinaemia with subcutaneous gammaglobulin by rapid infusion. Lancet 1991;338:162–6.

[135] Chapel HM, Spickett GP, Ericson D, et al. The comparison of the efficacy and safety of intravenous versus subcutaneous immunoglobulin replacement therapy. J Clin Immunol 2000;20:94–100.

[136] Ochs HD, Gupta S, Kiessling P, et al. Safety and efficacy of self-administered subcutaneous immunoglobulin in patients with primary immunodeficiency diseases. J Clin Immunol 2006;26:265–73.

[137] Berger M. Subcutaneous immunoglobulin replacement in primary immunodeficiencies. Clin Immunol 2004;112:1–7.

[138] Berger M. Subcutaneous administration of IgG. Immunol Allergy Clin North Am 2008;28: 779–802.

[139] Moore ML, Quinn JM. Subcutaneous immunoglobulin replacement therapy for primary antibody deficiency: advancements into the 21st century. Ann Allergy Asthma Immunol 2008;101:114–21.

[140] Bonilla FA. Pharmacokinetics of immunoglobulin administered via intravenous of subcutaneous routes. Immunol Allergy Clin North Am 2008;28:803–19.

[141] Schiff RI. Individualizing the dose of intravenous immune serum globulin for therapy of patients with primary humoral immunodeficiency. Vox Sang 1985;49(Suppl 1):15–24.

[142] Bonagura VR, Marchlewski R, Cox A, et al. Biologic IgG level in primary immunodeficiency disease: the IgG level that protects against recurrent infection. J Allergy Clin Immunol 2008;122:210–2.

[143] Gardulf A, Nicolay U. Replacement IgG therapy and self-therapy at home improve the health-related quality of life in patients with primary antibody deficiencies. Curr Opin Allergy Clin Immunol 2006;6:434–42.

[144] Fasth A, Nystrom J. Quality of life and health-care resource utilization among children with primary immunodeficiency receiving home treatment with subcutaneous human immunoglobulin. J Clin Immunol 2008;28:370–8.

[145] Eijkhout HW, van Der Meer JW, Kallenberg CG, et al. The effect of two different dosages of intravenous immunoglobulin on the incidence of recurrent infections in patients with primary hypogammaglobulinemia. A randomized, double-blind, multicenter crossover trial. Ann Intern Med 2001;135:165–74.

[146] Roifman CM, Schroeder H, Berger M, et al. Comparison of the efficacy of IGIV-C, 10% (caprylate/chromatography) and IGIV-SD, 10% as replacement therapy in primary immune deficiency. A randomized double-blind trial. Int Immunopharmacol 2003;3:1325–33.

[147] Busse PJ, Razvi S, Cunningham-Rundles C. Efficacy of intravenous immunoglobulin in the prevention of pneumonia in patients with common variable immunodeficiency. J Allergy Clin Immunol 2002;109:1001–4.

[148] Imbach P, Barandun S, d'Apuzzo V, et al. High dose intravenous gammaglobulin for idiopathic thrombocytopenic purpura in childhood. Lancet 1981;i:1228–31.

[149] Debre M, Bonnet MC, Fridman WH, et al. Infusion of Fc gamma fragments for treatment of children with acute immune thrombocytopenic purpura. Lancet 1993;342:945–9.

[150] Nimmerjahn F, Ravetch J. Fcg receptor as regulators of immune responses. Nat Rev Immunol 2008;8:34–47.

[151] Samuelsson A, Towers TL, Ravetch JV. Anti-inflammatory activity of IVIG mediated through the inhibitory Fc receptor. Science 2001;291:484–6.

[152] Kaneko Y, Nimmerjahn F, Ravetch J. Anti-inflammatory activity of immunoglobulin G resulting from Fc sialylation. Science 2006;313:670–3.

[153] Anthony R, Nimmerjahn F, Ashline D, et al. Recapitulation of IVIG anti-inflammatory activity with a recombinant IgG Fc. Science 2008;320:373–6.

[154] Anthony RM, Wermeling F, Karlsson MC, et al. Identification of a receptor required for the anti-inflammatory activity of IVIG. Proc Natl Acad Sci U S A 2009;10:19571–8.

[155] Yu Z, Lennon VA. Mechanism of intravenous immune globulin therapy in antibody-mediated autoimmune diseases. N Engl J Med 1999;340:227–8.

[156] Bleeker W, Teeling J, Hack C. Accelerated autoantibody clearance by intravenous immunoglobulin therapy: studies in experimental models to determine the magnitude and time course of the effect. Blood 2001;98:3136–42.

[157] Hansen RJ, Balthasar JP. Effects of intravenous immunoglobulin on platelet count and anti-platelet antibody disposition in a rat model of immune thrombycytopenia. Blood 2002;100:2087–93.

[158] Kazatchkine M, Dietrich G, Ronda N, et al. V region-mediated selection of autoreactive repertoires by intravenous immunoglobulin (IVIG). Immunol Rev 1994;139:79–107.

[159] Nydegger U, Sultan Y, Kazatchkine M. The concept of anti-idiotypic regulation of selected autoimmune diseases by intravenous immunoglobulin. Clin Immunol Immunopathol 1989;53:S72–82.

[160] Sultan Y, Kazatchkine MD, Maisonneuve P, et al. Anti-idiotypic suppression of autoantibodies to factor VIII (antihaemophilic factor) by high-dose intravenous gammaglobulin. Lancet 1984;ii:765–8.

[161] Berger M, Rosenkranz P, Brown CY. Intravenous and standard immune serum globulin preparations interfere with uptake of 125I-C3 onto sensitized erythrocytes and inhibit hemolytic complement activity. Clin Immunol Immunopathol 1985;34:227–36.

[162] Basta M. Modulation of complement-mediated immune damage by intravenous immune globulin. Clin Exp Immunol 1996;104:21–5.

[163] Dalakas MC. Intravenous immune globulin for dermatomyositis. N Engl J Med 1994;330:1392–3.

[164] Dalakas MC. Controlled studies with high-dose intravenous immunoglobulin in the treatment of dermatomyositis, inclusion body myositis, and polymyositis. Neurology 1998;51:S37–45.

[165] Basta M, Illa I, Dalaskas M. Increased in vitro uptake of the complement C3b in the serum of patients with Guillain-Barré syndrome, myasthenia gravis and dermatomyositis. J Neuroimmunol 1996;71:227–9.

[166] Dalakas MC. Intravenous immune globulin therapy for neurologic diseases. Ann Intern Med 1997;126:721–30.

[167] Viard I, Wehrli P, Bullanim R, et al. Inhibition of toxic epidermal necrolysis by blockade of CD95 with human intravenous immunoglobulin. Science 1998;282:490–3.

[168] Negi V, Elluru S, Siberil S, et al. Intravenous immunoglobulin: an update on the clinical use and mechanisms of action. J Clin Immunol 2007;27:233–45.

[169] Vassilev T, Kazatchkine M, Van Huyen J, et al. Inhibition of cell adhesion by antibodies to Arg-Gly-Asp (RGD) in normal immunoglobulin for therapeutic use. Blood 1999;93:3624–31.

[170] Turhan A, Jenab P, Bruhns P, et al. Intravenous immune globulin prevents venular vaso-occlusion in sickle cell mice by inhibiting leukocyte adhesion and the interactions between sickle erythrocytes and adherent leukocytes. Blood 2004;103:2397–400.

[171] Chang J, Shi PA, Chiang EY, et al. Intravenous immunoglobulins reverse acute vaso-occlusive crises in sickle cell mice through rapid inhibition of neutrophil adhesion. Blood 2008;111:915–23.

Advances in Pediatrics 57 (2010) 219–245

ADVANCES IN PEDIATRICS

Pediatric Outpatient Parenteral Antimicrobial Therapy: An Update

Nizar F. Maraqa, MD[a], Mobeen H. Rathore, MD[a,b,*]

[a]Pediatric Infectious Diseases and Immunology, University of Florida-Jacksonville, 653-1 West 8th Street, LRC-3, Pediatrics, L-13, Jacksonville, FL 32209, USA
[b]Wolfson Children's Hospital, 800 Prudential Drive, Jacksonville, FL 32207, USA

Many terms have been used to describe the delivery of antimicrobials (antiviral, antifungal, or antibacterial agents) to patients in the outpatient setting through the parenteral (ie, intravenous, intramuscular, or subcutaneous) route, including *outpatient intravenous antimicrobial therapy* (*OPIVAT*), *community-based parenteral anti-infective therapy* (*CoPAT*), *hospital at home*, *home intravenous antimicrobial therapy* (*HIAT*), and *outpatient parenteral antimicrobial therapy* (*OPAT*) [1–6]. The latter term, OPAT, is the most widely used in the United States. It broadly refers to the parenteral administration of at least two doses of an antimicrobial to a patient on two different days without an intervening hospitalization [1].

OPAT arose from the recognition that some infectious diseases will require management with parenteral therapy, although the patient may not require hospitalization [7]. In 1974, Rucker and Harrison [8] used antibiotics intravenously for the management of pulmonary infections in children with cystic fibrosis in the outpatient setting. Subsequently, in 1978 Antoniskis and colleagues [9] described the first use of self-administered intravenous antibiotics in adult outpatients. Since then, many of the standard techniques of infusion therapy that were previously performed exclusively in the hospital setting have been introduced into the outpatient arena. An estimated 1 in 1000 Americans use OPAT annually and more than 250,000 OPAT courses are administered in the United States every year. The use of OPAT has been increasing at an estimated rate of 10% per annum in the past decade [1,3,10].

OPAT is considered safe, therapeutically effective, and economical [1,6,7,11]. It offers increased comfort and convenience in appropriately selected patients and provides one approach for cost containment, because hospitalization generally represents the most costly aspect of patient care [6,12–16]. OPAT has become a popular alternative that replaces or shortens hospital admissions. Many investigators, from various countries, reported the cost of

*Corresponding author. 653-1 West 8th Street, LRC-3, Pediatrics, L-13, Jacksonville, FL 32209. *E-mail address*: mobeen.rathore@jax.ufl.edu

0065-3101/10/$ – see front matter
doi:10.1016/j.yapd.2010.09.002

OPAT to be 12% to 25% of similar inpatient treatment [2,6,15,16]. The benefits of OPAT, however, should be measured in terms of not only clinical outcomes and cost but also patient preferences and health-related quality of life. OPAT has been shown to improve physical, social, and emotional quality of life parameters [17–20], especially for children, in whom the undesirable psychosocial impact of hospitalization for treatment of serious infections was minimized by OPAT without compromising outcome [21].

OPAT is continually evolving in parallel with the advances in pharmaceuticals, technologic improvements in vascular access devices and infusion methods, and the provision of specialist services [1,17].

Provision of OPAT, despite the multiple benefits mentioned, is not without financial, legal, ethical, and clinical administrative challenges [1,22]. To date, truly evidence-based studies of OPAT are lacking. OPAT administration guidelines usually reflect the collective experiences of members of the infectious disease community and other involved health care disciplines [1,3]. Standards of care are comparable to those expected in the hospital, even though OPAT delivery is unique and usually different from the controlled hospital setting. Although the special needs of children receiving OPAT and the particular importance of safety of neonates, infants, and young children receiving OPAT are realized, even less literature specific to OPAT use is available in this vulnerable group of patients [1,22].

This article reviews the current state of OPAT use in pediatrics. The scope of the discussion will not address in detail the related topics of duration of therapy or management strategies of various infections nor will it include infusion therapies other than antimicrobials that may be administered outside the hospital.

OPAT MODELS

Traditional models of OPAT delivery are the infusion center model, the visiting nurse model, and the self-administration model. Another proposed model is the nursing home model, which is less applicable to children receiving OPAT. The choice of OPAT model is usually dictated by the local needs and available resources. Various publications have delineated the advantages and disadvantages of each of these models [10,22,23].

The Infusion Center Model

The site of OPAT delivery functions as a day-hospital facility extending hospital-level care into the outpatient setting. It requires that the patient be able to come to the infusion site, which is difficult for immobile patients or those receiving multiple antimicrobial infusions per day. Locations that have been used for this model include the physician office, where there is more control over quality of staff and equipment (although cost savings may be significant compared with the hospital, reimbursement issues remain a constant challenge) [23,24], and the hospital-based infusion center, where the pharmacy (owned by the hospital or an independent affiliate) provides the medications and equipment while hospital nurses deliver it to the patients. A variation of this model has been the use of a hospital emergency room for OPAT administration. Patients are usually scheduled during emergency room slow times and kept in observation beds away from acute emergency beds while receiving their antimicrobials.

The Visiting Nurse Model

In this model, the nurse travels to the patient's home, making it a convenient model for immobile patients or families unable to travel. These visits allow the nurse to assess the suitability of the home environment for OPAT and allows the provision of additional services during the same visit (eg, physical therapy, occupational therapy, social services). Among its limitations are the prohibitive cost that may be incurred and the concerns for patient privacy. In certain settings, concern for the safety of the visiting nurse may preclude using this delivery model [22].

The Home Self-Administration Model

The home-based OPAT delivery model with patient or caregiver self-administration of drugs is the most commonly used approach in the United States [12]. There have been multiple reports of successful self-administration of total parenteral nutrition and various other medications by patients or their caregivers at home [25,26]. This model requires that the patient or caregiver (and usually another backup household member) receive adequate training in the techniques of OPAT administration and care for the particular vascular access device being used. This model allows the patient or caregiver to become an integral member of the health care team and to assume a great deal of the responsibility for the therapy to ensure an adequate outcome [27].

Although the hospital or an infusion facility is usually still needed for the initial medical supervision, establishing vascular access, first antimicrobial dose administration, pharmacy services coordination, and patient training, this model results in significant overall financial savings through eliminating personnel and overhead costs at home and allowing for a quicker return to daily activities (eg, work or school) [22]. This model has been shown to be a safe and feasible strategy in appropriately selected patients under the supervision of a specialist OPAT team [17].

Potential concerns for the home self-administration model of OPAT may arise from the absence of medical supervision during the actual infusion and the possibility of anaphylactoid reactions occurring subsequent to the first dosing or mechanical failure of infusion devices [28]. Immediate and ready access to communication with the OPAT team and a mode of transportation are absolutely necessary to reduce the risks of life-threatening complications [29,30]. Intermittent visits to a clinic or an infusion center allow for regular assessment of clinical status, drug and supply distribution, maintenance of vascular access device, and patient compliance with the program.

A home infusion agency model combines the self-administration and visiting nurse delivery models. Initial patient assessment and training typically occurs in the hospital and, after discharge, the home infusion agency provides the anti-microbials and expert infusion nurse backup and support.

OPAT TEAM

Successful delivery of OPAT is usually the result of coordinated effort and excellent communication between the various members of an OPAT program. The core individuals in an OPAT team are the physician, nurse, and pharmacist. Other members may include a social worker, a microbiologist or laboratory technician, an interventional radiologist, and a third-party payer representative. Members of a pediatric OPAT program should be proficient and skilled in the unique requirements of caring for neonates, infants, and children [1,22,30].

Physicians

The physician plays the role of director for many OPAT programs. Regardless of the model of delivery used, the prescribing physician is ultimately responsible for the patient's care and outcome [22]. The participating physician should preferably be knowledgeable about infectious diseases and OPAT [1]. Curricula of infectious diseases educational programs incorporate training in the outpatient use of parenteral antimicrobials, which should help minimize therapeutic failures, adverse events, or vascular access and infusion device complications. A physician can also acquire OPAT certification offered by the American Academy of Home Care Physicians (AAHCP) [1,31]. Physician responsibilities include establishing a diagnosis, prescribing treatment, determining the appropriate site of care, monitoring the patient during therapy, and assuring the overall quality of care [1].

Despite the rapid expansion of the OPAT industry, physician involvement has not kept pace with this growth, partly because of low reimbursement offered for OPAT program management and direct patient care in the home setting [22].

Nurses

A nurse's responsibility varies with the OPAT model and site of care. The nurse usually plays a lead role in recommending the type of vascular access device appropriate for the patient, and usually inserts and maintains the vascular access device. This procedure can be more challenging in pediatric OPAT and may require specialized expertise. A few recent technological advancements have facilitated catheter insertion in patients with difficult vascular access. At many institutions, a team of pediatric nurses specialized in placing vascular access devices use infrared vein-contrast enhancement technology (eg, VeinViewer, Luminetx Technologies, Memphis, Tennessee) and portable ultrasound and fluoroscopy guidance for successful placement of catheters in these patients [30].

OPAT nurses also evaluate the safety of the home environment, educate the patient or caregiver, prevent and manage infusion-related complications, obtain and interpret laboratory results, monitor patient compliance, and assist the patient with waste management. Nurses usually function as a liaison between the patient and the OPAT team and help coordinate various aspects of their care.

Nursing standards in all care settings, including outpatient or home, have been established and published by the Infusion Nurse Society [1,32]. OPAT nurses can acquire accreditation offered by the Infusion Nurses Certification Corporation (INCC) [33].

Pharmacists

The American Society of Health-System Pharmacist (ASHP) has established guidelines for the OPAT pharmacist [34,35]. Responsibilities of the pharmacist include assisting in the choice of drug and appropriate dosage; reviewing the history of allergies or intolerance; monitoring for potential drug-drug interactions; compounding, storage and dispensing of the medication; advising on drug stability and infusion device programming; monitoring laboratory results; and educating the patient regarding potential adverse events [22,34].

Patient and Caregivers

Allowing the patient or caregiver to play an integral part and participate actively in planning their OPAT course is essential for its success. Patients and caregivers usually feel empowered by assuming some degree of responsibility for the outcome of their own care. Before participating in OPAT, patients and caregivers should be trained in aseptic technique and educated about potential venous access and infusion device and medication complications [27].

OPAT programs should have written policies and procedures that outline the responsibilities of the team members and addresses all issues from the selection of the patient for OPAT until their discharge from the program [1].

OPAT team members should be trained on bloodborne pathogen exposure, which seems to occur less than in the hospital setting [36]. All communications among OPAT team members must comply, at all times, with the Health Insurance Portability and Accountability Act (HIPAA) regulations (available at http://www.hhs.gov/ocr/privacy/).

PATIENT SELECTION

OPAT delivery increases the convenience and comfort for patients, caregivers, and family members [20], Treatment at home may be particularly psychologically advantageous in children [12]. Responsible provision of OPAT demands selective patient enrollment, detailed training for patient or caregiver, regular outpatient follow-up, and continuous support [1,17–19,37–39].

Usually, an experienced physician should determine that a patient needs parenteral therapy before consideration of OPAT. However, not every patient is a suitable candidate for OPAT [27]. Patient selection depends on several interrelated parameters. Physical factors (ie, the type, severity, and etiology of the infection), choice of available antimicrobials, presence of concomitant or underlying conditions, type of monitoring and follow-up frequency required, and the ability and motivation of the patient or caregiver are most important when determining whether a patient is a suitable candidate for OPAT [22].

Economic aspects should also be addressed and taken into account when deciding to use OPAT. Although some health insurance plans cover 100% of OPAT costs, patients must be informed of any anticipated out-of-pocket costs they may incur. Additionally, the patient or family's willingness to participate in OPAT delivery and the financial resources available to support all other aspects of OPAT care should be evaluated. Nevertheless, the patients' overall well-being must always take precedence over any financial considerations [1,22].

OPAT delivery in the home requires individuals in the household to be physically and emotionally ready household to support the care of the patient and perform the responsibilities of an OPAT provider. Adequate utilities, running water, a functioning refrigerator, and a phone, and ready access to transportation must be assessed before or at the initial therapy.

In pediatric practice, adolescents being considered for OPAT may present with issues related to high-risk behavior (eg, drug and alcohol abuse) that may not be frequently encountered in younger children. The prescribing physician must weigh the risks of abusing OPAT against its potential benefits in each individual case and consider continuing delivery of care in the hospital for the duration of treatment or until circumstances change [1,39].

To initiate OPAT directly and without any prior hospitalization should be avoided, especially in children. It should only be undertaken when minimal risk is present of sudden or life-threatening changes in health (eg, a patient with cystic fibrosis who is experienced with OPAT receiving an antimicrobial for pulmonary exacerbation). Hospitalization allows monitoring of the early course of the illness, performance of any required procedures or interventions, observation of the patient's tolerance of the antimicrobials, and stabilization of the medical condition before consideration for OPAT.

After a patient and caregiver are selected for OPAT, they must be educated regarding the infection being treated, the antimicrobial agent being infused, the procedure for medication administration, vascular access care, care of the catheter infusion site, and the potential adverse effects and complications. Teaching usually begins in the hospital as OPAT is being arranged. The hospital nurse can begin teaching the actual OPAT drug administration, which also allows for monitoring the patient's response and tolerance of the first dose of the antimicrobial being used [1]. Teaching plans should be individualized for each patient or caregiver, home setting, infection being treated, drug infused, vascular access device being used, and other factors [22]. Preprinted educational materials may also be very helpful. Telemedicine technology and interactive audiovisual devices may be appropriate and helpful in certain settings [40,41].

Continuous accessibility of the OPAT participant to the team members is required. Patients should be clear about how to proceed in case of an emergency and who to call for support in less urgent instances. All communication must preserve the patient's confidentiality.

THE INFECTIONS AMENABLE TO OPAT

Infections that can be effectively managed with oral therapy should not involve the use of OPAT [7]. A paucity of published randomized controlled studies, especially in children, support the use of OPAT as an alternative to the traditional management of some infections in the hospital setting. Nevertheless, overwhelming cumulative evidence and experience in support of this practice now exists, partly because of the availability of safer, more effective infusion devices and improved antimicrobial agents with favorable properties for outpatient administration [1,22,29,42–50].

Osteoarticular infections have been the predominant type of infection for which OPAT delivery is used in children. Various programs have reported their experience with OPAT for childhood osteomyelitis [42,51–56]. Therapy may vary depending on the extent of the infection, the bones and organisms involved, and the patient's age and immune status. Overall, however, uncomplicated acute hematogenous osteomyelitis responds very well to 1 to 2 weeks of intravenous therapy followed by another 2 to 4 weeks of oral antimicrobials.

Staphylococcus aureus remains the most common cause of osteomyelitis in children; however, an increase has occurred in the number of infections caused by community-acquired methicillin-resistant *S aureus* (CA-MRSA), which seems to be more severe and have a potentially worse outcome than methicillin susceptible *S aureus* [57]. Serum bactericidal titers, which have been shown to correlate with efficacy of OPAT when they exceed one to eight in treatment of childhood osteomyelitis, are not clinically practical and not used routinely in the management of childhood osteomyelitis [22,42,51–54].

Osteoarticular infections caused by unusual organisms or as a result of spread from a contiguous site of infection are less commonly seen in children. The use of multiple antimicrobials in an OPAT regimen and for longer therapy duration is not uncommon in these circumstances. Additionally, surgical intervention might be required for the management of osteoarticular infections before or after the initiation of OPAT [51,56].

Infections of skin and soft tissues have also been successfully managed with OPAT when antibiotic therapy is deemed necessary [1,58–60]. These infections have increasingly been caused by CA-MRSA in recent years [61,62]. Patients are stabilized in the hospital, where they may require a drainage procedure, before they are discharged home on OPAT. Patients must be switched to oral antibiotic therapy as soon as the clinical condition allows.

Children with complicated lower respiratory tract infection can be treated with OPAT, especially those with cystic fibrosis, whose OPAT courses lead to fewer hospitalizations, which reduces cross-contamination with resistant organisms and cost [63–67]. Children with complicated pneumonia, especially after video-assisted thoracoscopic surgery for empyema, can usually be discharged on OPAT after clinical stabilization in the hospital to complete their recovery at home [68,69].

In the older child or adult with infective endocarditis, OPAT may be a consideration once the patient is clinically stable and the risk for complications is low.

Patients with endocarditis who have infected prosthetic valves, persistently positive blood cultures, *S aureus* origin, large vegetations, conduction abnormality, or poorly controlled heart failure are usually poor candidates for outpatient management [1,22,70–73].

Genitourinary infections are usually amenable to treatment with oral antimicrobial agents. However, when the infecting organism is resistant to oral agents or the infection is complicated in nature, parenteral therapy may be required and can be delivered using OPAT after the patient is clinically stable [68,74,75].

Meningitis and other serious invasive infections may lead to potentially life-threatening complications during the course of the illness, especially in younger children. Nevertheless, these infections may be amenable for outpatient therapy during the patient's convalescence [21,76–79]. Most experts advocate adherence to strict criteria for selecting children who are clinically improving, whose disease is caused by susceptible pathogens, and who have highly motivated and capable caregivers [80]. These children may require daily physician or skilled pediatric nurse assessment while receiving their OPAT course. Educating the parents about the potential complications and acquiring their informed consent is especially important in this setting. If caregivers are unable or unwilling to assume this increased responsibility for outpatient care, patients should be treated in the hospital setting where they can be monitored closely [79].

SELECTION OF ANTIMICROBIALS FOR OPAT

Selecting antimicrobials for an OPAT regimen should be based on clinical and microbiological evidence that they are effective for the infections being treated while being safe. Cost and dosing convenience should only be considered once those essential determinants are fulfilled [7]. Since the advent of OPAT, the antimicrobial agents used have changed to reflect the changing types of infections and infecting organisms. For example, a decline has occurred in the use of cefazolin, a first-generation cephalosporin, for treatment of musculoskeletal infections, and an increase has been seen in the use of clindamycin, which reflects the changes in the susceptibility of the causative *S aureus*.

Pharmacokinetic and pharmacodynamic properties of antimicrobial agents should be considered when designing an OPAT regimen [7]. Agents with prolonged half-lives, allowing once-daily administration, have generally been preferred for OPAT. This dosing schedule facilitates compliance and is associated with less infectious and/or mechanical catheter complications, minimal disruption of daily activities, and reduced cost of ancillary items [12,22]. Understanding the pharmacokinetics of antimicrobials enables the clinician to achieve serum concentrations that are associated with a desired pharmacologic effect and avoid those associated with failure or toxicity [7]. Many antimicrobials do not distribute well into all body tissues and fluids. This consideration may be a critical when selecting a regimen for treatment of a deep-seated infection (eg, endocarditis, osteomyelitis). Drug elimination and clearance properties may also play a role in selecting the most appropriate agent for patients on

OPAT. Dosage reduction or changes in dosing frequency may be required for antimicrobials cleared by the liver (eg, macrolides, trimethoprim-sulfamethoxazole) or the kidneys (eg, aminoglycosides) in patients with impaired functions of the respective organs [7]. Additionally, the stability of the drug after its mixing in solution should be appropriate for the OPAT delivery model used [81].

Antimicrobials used for OPAT should be well tolerated, minimally veno-irritative and have minimal side effects. Cephalosporins (particularly ceftriaxone) and vancomycin (a glycopeptide) are the most commonly prescribed antimicrobials in OPAT series because of their advantageous spectrum of action, cost, tolerability, and pharmacokinetic profile [17]. In recent years, antifungal (including amphotericin B and fluconazole) and antiviral (including acyclovir and ganciclovir) agents have been safely administered to outpatients with appropriate monitoring for side effects [10].

Some antimicrobials (eg, penicillins, some cephalosporins, macrolides, clindamycin, carbapenems) have a time-dependant killing mechanism, for which the important determinant of efficacy is the length of time that the drug serum levels remain above the minimum inhibitory concentration (MIC) or minimum bactericidal concentration (MBC) for the causative organism. These agents have a short post-antibiotic effect (PAE), allowing the organism to quickly recover and start reproducing again after a decrease in the drug level below the MIC. Administration of these drugs should be either at frequent intermittent dosing or, ideally, through continuous intravenous infusion. Conversely, antimicrobials with concentration-dependant killing and prolonged PAE (eg, aminoglycosides, metronidazole, quinolones) exert the highest rate and extent of bacterial killing at the highest drug concentration, allowing these drugs to be administered at longer intervals using higher doses. A third group of drugs (eg, vancomycin, azithromycin, tetracycline) exert their bactericidal effect at the MIC level but continue to effectively inhibit the bacteria after the drug levels fall below the MIC for a considerable portion of the dosing interval. This mechanism of action allows less frequent administration at the appropriate doses.

The stability of the drugs used for OPAT could affect the choice of agent and the infusion delivery method used [81]. Drugs that are stable for fewer than 12 hours in solution are best infused intermittently and may pose a problem for some portable infusion devices. Ampicillin and imipenem solutions have poor stability at room temperature, requiring intermittent shorter infusions, whereas ceftriaxone and nafcillin solutions are stable for longer periods, allowing preparation of more than one day's dosage and placement in an infusion device reservoir [22,81]. Prolonged exposure of a prepared drug solution may lead to the accumulation of toxic degradation products, which may increase the risk of adverse events [82]. Most drugs used may be refrigerated for 3 to 10 days or even frozen to be rewarmed before infusion. OPAT drugs are usually reconstituted by the OPAT pharmacy; however, simplified systems (eg, ADD-vantage, Hospira Inc, Lake Forest, IL, USA or the Mini-Bag Plus, Baxter Inc, Deerfield, IL, USA) may allow patients or caregivers to perform drug reconstitution at home after appropriate training [22]. Infusion bags or reservoirs should be inspected for signs of drug degradation, precipitation, crystal formation, or change in color [81].

General and local tolerability of an antimicrobial is important when it is being administered away from the closely supervised hospital setting [12]. Anaphylaxis is a rare but potentially fatal condition that usually occurs after the administration of the first dose of an antimicrobial. Therefore, it is accepted practice that the first dose should be administered in a medical facility with immediate availability of resuscitation equipment and personnel needed to manage this condition.

Delayed anaphylactoid reactions may occur as late as 2 to 3 weeks after the start of OPAT. They usually represent a slow angioedema developing progressively with dosing over several days. These reactions, which occur at a rate of 0.5% [28], are usually easier to manage through discontinuing the offending drug and administering antihistamines. Patients and caregivers should be educated regarding the signs and symptoms of these reactions, and special kits with antianaphylactic agents may be kept in the home while the patient is receiving OPAT [1].

Infusion-related reactions also may occur with antimicrobials used for OPAT. The "red-man" syndrome occurring with the use of vancomycin is probably the most famous infusion reaction among OPAT users. It is primarily managed through slowing the rate of infusion and is rarely a reason to discontinue the drug's use, because it seems to occur less with subsequent doses of vancomycin [83].

Monitoring of patients receiving OPAT should be a close and continuous process. It should be more frequent as the duration of therapy increases along with the chance of some drug toxicities. OPAT registries for adult patients have reported that 3% to 10% of OPAT courses may be stopped because of adverse effects of antimicrobials [1]. Data from pediatric OPAT patients suggest a higher rate of discontinuation than in adults. Reports estimate that 24% to 32% of OPAT courses in children may be stopped because of adverse effects to antimicrobials [29,55].

MONITORING OF PATIENTS ON OPAT

The type and frequency of clinical and laboratory monitoring of patients undergoing OPAT should be individualized according to factors related to the patient, the infection treated, the drugs used, and the type of vascular access and infusion device.

The physician usually determines the frequency of clinical monitoring at the start of OPAT. Most children using OPAT are evaluated at least weekly, but they may be seen more frequently if they have certain infections. Nurses and pharmacist assessments are usually separate from face-to-face physician encounters. A physician should continue to evaluate patients after OPAT is stopped to be sure of the clinical response and the lack of late occurring adverse events [1].

Some adverse effects of antimicrobials used for OPAT may be identified with laboratory testing before they manifest clinically in the patient [29,55,84]. Clinical practice standards require periodic, at least weekly, laboratory monitoring for children undergoing OPAT [1,22]. This monitoring is usually performed with as little inconvenience to the child as possible by an OPAT nurse through the vascular access catheter. Tests usually include a complete blood cell (CBC) count to detect potential bone marrow suppressive effects of drugs (eg, beta-lactams, vancomycin). Hepatic function is tested when using agents with hepatotoxic potential (eg, oxacillin, nafcillin, fluconazole, caspofungin). Serum creatinine is followed when using potentially nephrotoxic agents (eg, aminoglycosides, vancomycin, amphotericin-B).

For infants and children scheduled to undergo prolonged therapy (ie, 4–6 weeks) with aminoglycosides, OPAT guidelines suggest considering audiometric screening. Additionally, some experts advocate screening for vestibular dysfunction [1].

Although toxicity may not always be related to drug serum levels, determining these levels may be necessary to avoid drug toxicities or ensure therapeutic efficacy. A controversial issue has been the value of vancomycin serum concentration determination. Most experts still recommend that vancomycin peak and trough serum levels should be determined in children until further studies are available given its potential for adverse effects and to assure effective therapeutic levels [1,85–89].

Laboratory monitoring is also used to follow the response of the infection to therapy. Weekly erythrocyte sedimentation rate, C-reactive protein, or other inflammatory markers may allow for early detection of failed therapy or the occurrence of an unexpected complication of the infection being treated.

OPAT VASCULAR ACCESS DEVICES

Safe and reliable venous access devices that can remain in place for extended periods without incident have made it easier to provide intravenous infusion therapy in the outpatient setting [90,91]. Biocompatible plastic catheters consisting of polyurethane and polytetrafluoroethylene (Teflon) are less likely to allow formation of a thrombus or adherence of microorganisms to them [81,92]. They are now available in various lengths and internal lumen sizes. Some multiple-lumen catheters allow simultaneous administration of medications that cannot be premixed [10,27,93]. Most of these catheters are radio-opaque (or contain a radio-opaque stripe within them), which allows radiographic visualization to ensure proper placement. These advances in vascular access devices have contributed to the safe and successful delivery of various medications in the outpatient setting [94,95].

Often, the OPAT team's preference and local experience and custom determine which device is used in a given situation. The short peripheral intravenous catheter, commonly known as the *intravenous cannula*, is flexible and less likely to rupture a vein or cause infiltration. However, it is only suitable for very short-term OPAT use. Midline catheters are longer but may be associated with higher incidence of phlebitis. Central venous tunneled catheters (eg, Hickman, BARD Access Systems, Inc, Salt Lake City, UT, USA) and subcutaneous venous ports are most difficult and costly to insert but may be used for many months to administer not only antimicrobials but also chemotherapy and parenteral nutrition, or even to perform hemodialysis. Peripherally inserted central catheters (PICC) have emerged as the most convenient means to prolonged vascular access for delivery of OPAT and for blood sampling while having very few complications [1,22,42,43,96,97].

Peripheral Short Catheters (Intravenous Cannula)

Originally made of stainless steel needles, these catheters are now made of biocompatible materials (eg, polyvinyl chloride, polyurethane, silicone, polytetrafluoroethylene). Despite this development, they provide limited access and questionable reliability. An intravenous cannula has a tendency to clot, infiltrate, or cause phlebitis within a few days after insertion. National nursing standards recommend daily assessment and regular flushing with saline (and maybe heparin) solution, and advocate changing the catheter every few days [32]. However, most providers do not necessarily replace a functioning cannula for at least 2 weeks in adult patients. In children, cannulas are often retained for longer periods as long as they are functional. Peripheral short catheters may still have a role in select settings but are rarely used when an OPAT course is expected to last more than 10 days [98].

Midline Catheters

Introduced in 1989, these catheters are a compromise between short peripheral lines and longer central catheters. A midline catheter advances 7.5 to 20 cm from its insertion point as opposed to the 2- to 3-cm insertion length of a peripheral intravenous cannula. It is typically placed in the forearm and advanced beyond the antecubital fossa into the axillary vein. This placement creates less risk for infiltration and phlebitis than a cannula but is not suitable for infusing hyperosmolar solutions (eg, parenteral nutrition solutions with osmolarity approaching 1200 mOsm/l) or chemotherapy agents that require adequate dilution on infusion into the circulation.

Midline catheters are best used for short to intermediate-length OPAT courses of 1 to 4 weeks. They can be placed in the home setting and do not require radiographic confirmation of placement [22,27]. They are less expensive than central catheters [81,94].

Central Venous Catheters

A central venous catheter (CVC; eg, Broviac or Hickman, BARD Access Systems, Inc, Salt Lake City, UT, USA) is typically inserted in the subclavian vein; the internal jugular and femoral veins are used less commonly. A drug infused through a CVC may be infused in larger volumes and at higher concentrations as it becomes adequately diluted into a large vein . The CVC may be tunneled under the skin for about 10 cm to create a barrier to infection and an easier access to its exit site. A Dacron cuff surrounds the catheter in the subcutaneous tunnel a few centimeters from the entrance site. The cuff stimulates growth of fibrous tissue, which serves as a barrier to microorganisms and a natural anchor [81]. Properly maintained CVCs may be used for years for drug infusions and blood sampling.

CVC insertion usually requires a surgical procedure and may be costly. Potential complications may occur during insertion of a CVC, such as bleeding, nerve injury, and pneumothorax (eg, for subclavian CVC). However, the risk of phlebitis is considerably low [22,29,96].

Ports

Generally, a port catheter is concealed beneath the patient's skin, making it almost impervious to the outside environment. It is usually inserted by a surgeon in the operating room while the patient is under general anesthesia. A port typically has a solid cast chamber embedded in a subcutaneous pocket, allowing attachment of the venous-dwelling catheter and introduction of the flushing device. A multilayered leak-proof septum, typically made of silicone material, creates a barrier between the circulation and the outside environment. The port is accessed with a specially curved needle without causing damage. Ports may be easily accessed a few thousand times without incident. The permanent nature of ports makes their use uncommon for OPAT, unless the patient has one already in place [1,22,81].

PICCs

Use of PICCs for OPAT has surpassed that of other types of vascular access devices in the United States [1,94]. These devices are central lines that are inserted peripherally into the desired vein and passed into the central venous circulation. The basilic vein is usually easier (larger and less tortuous) to use than the cephalic vein for PICC insertion into the mid-distal superior vena cava [81,94]. The axillary vein is more commonly used in neonates, in whom it has a lesser chance of accidental dislodgement.

PICCs are safe, easy to insert and remove at the bedside, cost-effective, and less invasive than other types of central vascular access devices [27,99–101]. PICCs provide direct access to the central venous circulation, allowing infusion of a wide variety of medications (eg, highly concentrated drug solution) [22,27]. They may have single, double, or triple lumens, increasing their versatility. Special PICCs are now available that are designed for maximum injection rates (ie, power injection) to allow infusion of contrast media for contrast-enhanced CT (CECT) scans and MRI (eg, PowerPICC, BARD Access Systems, Inc, Salt Lake City, UT, USA) [102].

PICCs also preserve the peripheral vascular system and eliminate the need for multiple painful peripheral intravenous site rotations. These catheters are routinely used for blood sampling as an alternative to venipuncture [103].

PICCs come in various lengths and sizes; most are equipped with a guide wire or a breakaway needle that leaves only a small piece of plastic at the site of insertion. This device is typically left unsutured and covered with sterile dressing. The length of catheter insertion should be recorded and checked again once the catheter is removed. A radiograph is usually required to confirm proper placement after PICC insertion. A qualified OPAT nurse changes the PICC dressing at least weekly and assures its proper functioning. PICC insertion in newborns and premature infants requires special skills. Insertion with the assistance of real-time sonography has been shown to reduce the attempts needed for successful placement. Fig. 1 depicts various steps during PICC placement using the modified sledinger technique in a child at our institution [81,95,104].

Mechanical complications, mainly catheter dislodgement, dislocation, leakage, or occlusion, are more likely to occur with PICCs than other types of central catheters [22,28,29,60,96]. However, infectious complications seem to be less likely with PICCs than with CVCs [1,22,29]. The incidence of overall PICC complications in pediatric patients ranges from 29% to 41%, whereas 69% to 82% of these patients complete the OPAT course with a single PICC [1,22,29,96,97,101,105]. PICC complications increase with increasing catheter dwell time, and require close follow-up and immediate management by the OPAT team [1,22,29,96,101,105]. Early detection and intervention provides the best opportunity to save the catheter and prevent further complications. The patient or caregiver is usually a great resource for early identification of potential PICC complications [27]. Each PICC manufacturer has product-specific guidelines for use and maintenance of the catheter; however, clear general instructions should be provided to the patient or caregiver, especially regarding the infusion technique and maintaining a dry and sterile environment.

Although a PICC may cost more than a peripheral intravenous cannula, overall they are cost-effective because they require less overall nursing care and fewer intravenous line restarts [22,106–109].

Care and Maintenance of Catheters

Various professional groups have attempted to establish criteria for care of patients undergoing OPAT [110,111]. In 2004, the Practice Guidelines Committee of the Infectious Diseases Society of America (IDSA) updated the 1997 guidelines for OPAT [1,3]. The Infusion Nurses Society (INS) developed standards of practice for administering intravenous medications and maintenance of vascular access sites [10,32]. Additionally, the Centers for Disease Control and Prevention (CDC) issued guidelines for prevention of catheter-related infections in various settings [110]. Nevertheless, no accepted universal guidelines are available for catheter care in OPAT, especially in children. OPAT users tend to extrapolate from available knowledge and guidelines for catheter care in the hospital setting and adapt those to the unique circumstances that present themselves in the outpatient setting [22,111].

Exit-site infection, tunnel infection, and catheter-related bloodstream infection can all occur in patients receiving OPAT. Most catheter-related infections are caused by skin flora that invades the cutaneous tract during catheter insertion or during the course of therapy. Outpatients are thought to be at lower risk of contracting catheter-related infections than hospitalized patients, especially

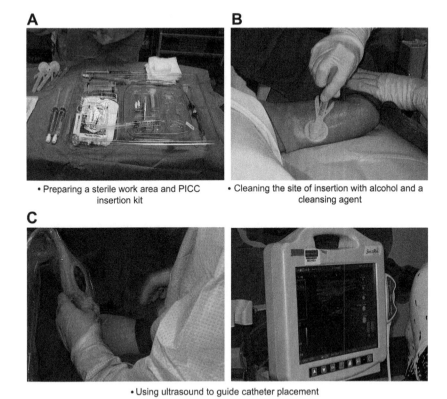

A
• Preparing a sterile work area and PICC insertion kit

B
• Cleaning the site of insertion with alcohol and a cleansing agent

C
• Using ultrasound to guide catheter placement

Fig. 1. (A) Cleaning the site of insertion with alcohol and a cleansing agent. (B) Cleaning the site of insertion with alcohol and a cleansing agent. (C) Using ultrasound to guide catheter placement. (D) Injecting local anesthetic. (E) Insertion of an intravenous cannula into the vein. (F) Threading a guide wire into the cannulated vein. (G) The cannula is removed leaving the guide wire in place (not advanced beyond the shoulder). (H) Insertion of an introducer sheath into the vein over the guide wire. (I) In neonates, a small skin incision next to the guide wire may be required before insertion of the introducer sheath. (J) The guide wire is ready to be removed so as to advance the catheter through the introducer sheath. (K) Preparation of the catheter for insertion; cutting to the desired length. (L) Inserting the PICC into the vein through the intoducer sheath. (M) The introducer sheath is pulled back and removed after PICC is inserted. (N) Catheter tip position is confirmed with ultrasound. (O) Cleaning the site of catheter placement. (P) Securing the catheter with an anchoring device at the entrance site to skin. (Q) Applying sterile transparent dressing; flushing with Normal Saline solution. (R) Inspecting the extremity after PICC is secured and dressing is applied. PICC is ready for use.

infections caused by resistant bacteria [1,22,111]. Noninfectious complications can also be encountered during OPAT, including thrombosis and emboliza-tion, catheter migration, catheter occlusion, leakage, breakage, or dislodge-ment. Preventing and managing each of these complications is critical for the success of OPAT. A detailed description of each is beyond the scope of this discussion.

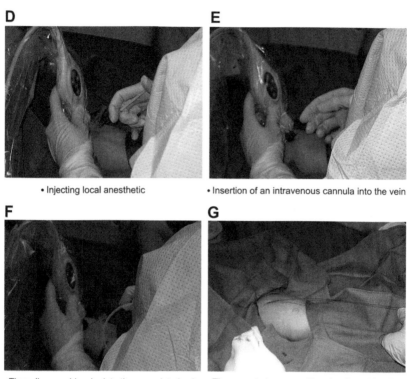

D

• Injecting local anesthetic

E

• Insertion of an intravenous cannula into the vein

F

•Threading a guide wire into the cannulated vein

G

• The cannula is removed leaving the guide wire
in place (not advanced beyond the shoulder)

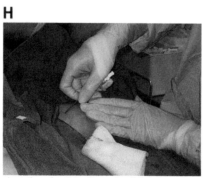

H

• Insertion of an introducer sheath into the vein
over the guide wire

Fig. 1 (continued)

Studies are needed that address infection control issues in the outpatient settings
and provide data to help formulate guidelines for infection control and care of
outpatient vascular access devices. The CDC's guidelines for Standard Precautions [112] and Occupational Safety and Health Administration (OSHA) bloodborne pathogen standards [113,114] should be adhered to when handling

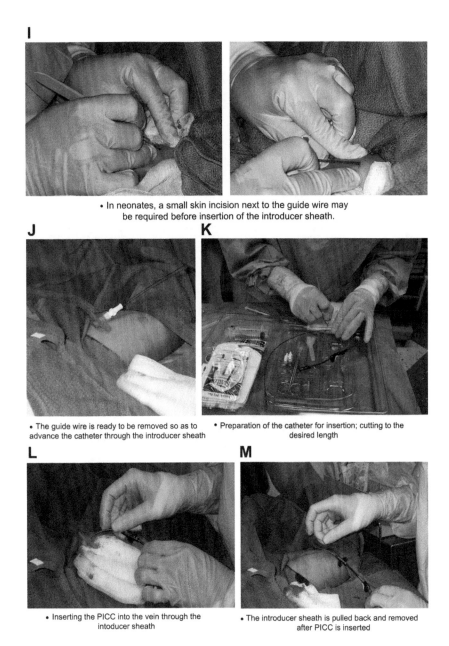

• In neonates, a small skin incision next to the guide wire may
be required before insertion of the introducer sheath.

• The guide wire is ready to be removed so as to
advance the catheter through the introducer sheath

• Preparation of the catheter for insertion; cutting to the
desired length

• Inserting the PICC into the vein through the
intoducer sheath

• The introducer sheath is pulled back and removed
after PICC is inserted

Fig. 1 (continued)

outpatients with vascular access devices to protect the patient and health care worker [111].

Most providers agree that exit-site cleansing and sterile dressing changes are necessary for care of OPAT catheters. Various techniques and cleansing agents

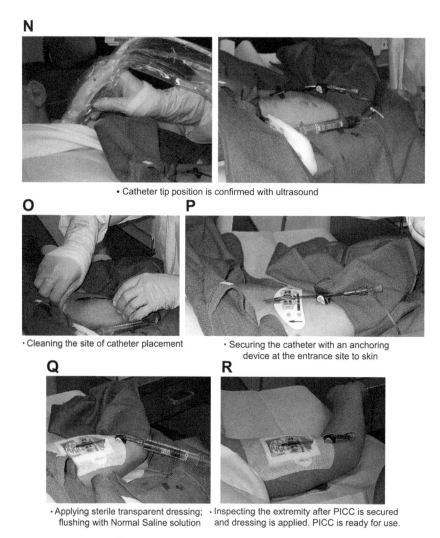

N
• Catheter tip position is confirmed with ultrasound

O   P
• Cleaning the site of catheter placement

• Securing the catheter with an anchoring
device at the entrance site to skin

Q   R
• Applying sterile transparent dressing;
flushing with Normal Saline solution

• Inspecting the extremity after PICC is secured
and dressing is applied. PICC is ready for use.

Fig. 1 (*continued*)

have been used. The old dressing is removed, observing standard precautions and avoiding contamination of the site. The OPAT nurse, then wearing sterile gloves, creates a sterile field on which to place the dressing kit. The catheter is checked for migration and the access site is inspected for discoloration, drainage, tenderness or numbness, and skin integrity. The catheter entrance site is cleaned thoroughly with friction in an outward circular fashion and the area is then allowed to dry before a new dressing is applied. The cleansing agents used may vary in their residual antimicrobial effect, from lasting for a few hours (eg, chlorhexidine gluconate, 2%) to a few minutes (eg, iodophors [povidone-iodine]) to almost no effect (eg, alcohol).

Catheters also vary regarding flushing frequency, volume and type of flushing solution, and frequency of dressing changes. Care of catheters may depend on whether they are being actively used (eg, ports). Pre-prepared flushing and dressing change kits, insertion site antimicrobial cuffs, needleless systems, and similar products have contributed markedly to the safety and reliability of outpatient vascular access systems [22].

OPAT INFUSION DEVICES

Various options for infusion devices are available for delivery of OPAT. A particular infusion device is most effective when matched with the appropriate venous access device [27,81,95,115]. Delivery of OPAT is a dynamic process with changes occurring during the course of therapy. If the venous access device is changed, the antimicrobial used or the infusion device used may need to be changed [27].

A few available options for OPAT infusion devices are described in the next sections.

Slow Intravenous Injection

Slow intravenous injection, or "IV push" is a low-tech, traditional infusion method that is regaining popularity because of reduced reimbursement for other methods and a desire to reduce the administration and supply costs where possible. However, not all antimicrobials can be safely administered through this method because some agents require longer infusion time to avoid infusion-related toxicities (eg, aminoglycosides, amphotericin B), whereas others may have irritative qualities unless diluted sufficiently (eg, vancomycin) [27,81].

The Gravity Drip System

The gravity drip system, classically used to deliver drugs in the institutional and outpatient settings, has largely been replaced by the portable infusion pump. Despite its minimal cost, the drip system is restrictive to patients because they must remain stationary during the infusion.

Infusion Pumps

Infusion (syringe) pumps are now manufactured in smaller, lighter models that are more precise, user friendly and reliable than ever before. The syringe acts as a reservoir for the antimicrobial and is loaded onto the pump. A plunger or a piston is then allowed to advance at a specified rate, infusing the drug through the patient's catheter. The patient or caregiver is trained by the OPAT team to operate the device and connect and disconnect the tubing. Syringe pumps allow the infusion of drugs at rates from 0.1 to 300 mL/h. Drug doses are usually stored as prefilled syringes in the refrigerator. The pumps may run on batteries or electric power, and some may have a spring-loaded system or an elastic band. The portability, ease of use, and reliable accuracy make syringe pumps an optimal choice for OPAT users. Additionally, the cost of using the syringe pump is usually recaptured quickly by the savings that result when compared with other infusion delivery systems [22,27].

Controlled Rate Infusion Devices (Elastometric Infusers)

This system has a pressurized reservoir that delivers the drug during deflation. These elastometric pumps, also called balloons, grenades, or baby bottles, come in various sizes (50–500 mL) and have flow rates ranging from 0.5 to 200 mL/h. As opposed to a syringe pump system, drug delivery is through a low infusion pressure mechanism, which may vary with positional changes in resistance from the patient's catheter [81] and may cause the flow rate to fluctuate by as much as 15%. These pumps are mostly disposable after drug delivery, and additional pumps (ie, doses) may easily be stored in the refrigerator to be rewarmed to room temperature before infusion to assure a uniform flow rate [22,27,81,116–119]. Elastometric infusers may be more convenient and potentially safer for certain patients because they involve less handling by the patient or caregiver [120].

Computerized Ambulatory Infusion Pumps

Sophisticated, programmable computerized infusion pumps have allowed complicated antimicrobial regimens to be delivered in the outpatient setting that were traditionally reserved for use in the hospitalized patient. These pumps allow the administration of two to four drugs simultaneously through multiple channels and at varying rates (ranging from 0.1–500 mL/h). They can be programmed to deliver medications continuously or intermittently with very minimal manipulation of the patient's catheter, thus decreasing the potential for catheter-related mechanical complications or infection. The pumps are usually powered by rechargeable or disposable batteries and they have special drug cartridges and disposable intravenous tubing sets. The more complex the function they perform, the larger, more complicated, and more costly they are [81,95].

Although precise and reliable, the programmable pump requires routine maintenance to reduce the risk of mechanical malfunction. A built-in safety mechanism to warn against potential mechanical malfunctions and allow for corrective interventions should be present. Even with these safety checks, errors in dose calculations or pump programming may occur, and therefore the OPAT team must be vigilant to detect and reduce their occurrence [1,22,27]. Recently, advances in telecommunication capabilities have allowed OPAT programs to access infusion devices remotely for monitoring and programming [27,81]. The cost of sophisticated programmable pumps may seem prohibitive, especially if not reimbursed by third-party payers [10,81,121–123]. However, reducing the need for hospitalization and the services of specialized nursing at home may actually result in overall cost savings [22].

Medication delivery systems vary in terms of cost, convenience, and reliability [27,123,124]. The challenge now, and in the future, will be to select the device that is most appropriate for the individual patient receiving OPAT.

OUTCOME MEASUREMENT AND QUALITY IMPROVEMENT

Measurement of outcome indicators and the need for quality improvement for OPAT were emphasized in the 2004 IDSA Practice Guidelines for Outpatient Parenteral Antimicrobial Therapy [1]. A well-designed outcome measurement program measures the quality and success of care delivered [125].

Traditional outcome measures for OPAT programs have focused on single retrospective indicators, such as mortality or catheter infection rates. Although these indicators are easy to measure, they do not offer information necessary to improve the quality of OPAT delivery. An active performance improvement program should evaluate the OPAT outcomes in the context of the patient's and OPAT team's goals. It must follow and measure clinical outcomes objectively, including the overall health status of the patient, clinical end points, complications associated with the vascular access device and antimicrobial agent, the patient's overall quality of life, and patient or family satisfaction [1,10,30,126].

Accrediting bodies such as the Joint Commission (formerly known as the Joint Commission on Accreditation of Healthcare Organizations [JCAHO]) and the National Committee for Quality Assurance (NCQA) require outcome measurement as part of their accreditation process of OPAT programs. In fact, the Joint Commission publishes the Comprehensive Accreditation Manual for Home Care (CAMHC) and various home care standards and performance improvement guidelines (easily accessible on the Joint Commission's Web site www.jointcommission.org) [22,126]. Most of the larger home infusion and pharmacy provider organizations have earned Joint Commission accreditation, which facilitates reimbursement by third-party payers and increases the uniformity of OPAT delivery among organizations [1,22].

OPAT providers are encouraged to participate in a registry, from which outcome data may be shared and compared with multiple similar OPAT providers. This data registry will help experts study the methods of care, drugs, or technologies and identify which are most successful [125,127]. The analysis of aggregated data may also facilitate the development of OPAT guidelines in adults and children receiving OPAT.

REIMBURSEMENT

Commercial companies, hospitals, clinics, and physicians' practices have established their own OPAT programs and facilities as the outpatient infusion industry mushroomed at a staggering pace, driven by emphasis on reducing health care cost. However, there was a significant lack of sufficient regulation, which has lead to instances of overuse and abuse and inflated charges and excessive profits. Congressional investigations and legal actions have resulted in significant consolidation of home care agencies and reduction in third-party payers' reimbursements for OPAT [1,10,16,68].

A detailed discussion of the legal, ethical, and economic aspects of OPAT is beyond the scope of this article. Although the economic dimension of OPAT delivery cannot be ignored, its monetary incentive should always be balanced with providing medical care that guarantees the best possible clinical outcome for patients.

SUMMARY

OPAT has become an expected standard of medical practice in the United States and many parts of the developed world. It requires the close cooperation of multiple team members, including patients and caregivers. It can be safe and effective while cost-saving and without compromising the outcome of therapy. Opportunities for further development of OPAT should be constantly explored in this era of advancing medical technologies. Research studies, especially in children, are needed to better answer many of the questions regarding OPAT use. Collaboration between OPAT providers and pooling of outcomes data should allow experts to learn more about the management of childhood and adult infectious diseases and the antimicrobials used to treat them.

Until medical chemists are able to produce oral antimicrobial agents that have adequate bioavailability, efficacy, and potency to provide nonparenteral alternatives to therapy, OPAT will continue to have an increasing role in the care of children with infectious diseases.

References

[1] Tice AD, Rehm SJ, Dalovisio JR, et al. Practice guidelines for outpatient parenteral antimicrobial therapy. Clin Infect Dis 2004;38:1651–72.
[2] Steinmetz D, Berkovits E, Edelstein H, et al. Home intravenous antibiotic therapy programme, 1999. J Infect 2001;42:176–80.
[3] Williams DN, Rehm SJ, Tice AD, et al. Practice guidelines for community-based parenteral anti-infective therapy. Clin Infect Dis 1997;25:787–801.
[4] Huminer D, Bishara J, Pitlik S. Home intravenous antibiotic therapy with infective endocarditis. Eur J Clin Microbiol Infect Dis 1999;18:330–4.
[5] Esposito S. Parenteral cephalosporin therapy in ambulatory care: advantages and disadvantages. Drugs 2000;59(Suppl 3):19–28.
[6] Tice A. Outpatient parenteral antimicrobial therapy as an alternative to hospitalization. Int J Clin Pract 1998;95:S4–8.
[7] Slavik RS, Jewessen PJ. Selecting antibacterials for outpatient parenteral antimicrobial therapy. Pharmacokinetic and pharmacodynamic considerations. Clin Pharmacokinet 2003;42:793–817.
[8] Rucker RW, Harrison GM. Outpatient intravenous medications in the management of cystic fibrosis. Pediatrics 1974;54:358–60.
[9] Antoniskis A, Anderson BC, Van Volkinburg EJ, et al. Feasibility of outpatient self-administration of parenteral antibiotics. West J Med 1978;128:203–6.
[10] Portez DM. Evolution of outpatient parenteral antibiotic therapy. Infect Dis Clin North Am 1998;12:827–34.
[11] Brown RB, Sands M. Outpatient intravenous antibiotic therapy. Am Fam Physician 1989;40:157–62.
[12] Leggett JE. Ambulatory use of parenteral antibacterials: contemporary perspectives. Drugs 2000;59(Suppl 3):1–8.
[13] Stiver HG, Telford GO, Mossey JM, et al. Intravenous antibiotic therapy at home. Ann Intern Med 1978;89:690–3.
[14] Gilchrist M, Franklin BD, Patel JP. An outpatient parenteral antibiotic therapy (OPAT) map to identify risks associated with an OPAT service. J Antimicrob Chemother 2008;62:177–83.

[15] Dalovisio JR, Juneau J, Baumgarten K, et al. Financial impact of a home intravenous antibiotics program on a Medicare managed care program. Clin Infect Dis 2000;30:639–42.

[16] Williams DN, Bosch D, Boots J, et al. Safety, efficacy and cost savings in an outpatient intravenous antibiotic program. Clin Ther 1993;15:169–79.

[17] Matthews PC, Conlon CP, Berendt AR, et al. Outpatient parenteral antimicrobial therapy (OPAT): is it safe for selected patients to self-administer at home? A retrospective analysis of a large cohort over 13 years. J Antimicrob Chemother 2007;60:356–62.

[18] Goodfellow AF, Wai AO, Frighetto L, et al. Quality-of-life assessment in an outpatient parenteral antibiotic program. Ann Pharmacother 2002;36:1851–5.

[19] Parker SE, Nathwani D, O'Reilly D, et al. Evaluation of the impact of non-inpatient i.v. antibiotic treatment for acute infections on the hospital, primary care services and the patient. J Antimicrob Chemother 1998;42:373–80.

[20] Gomez MM, Alvarez AM, Rathore MH. Quality of life in pediatric outpatient antibiotic therapy [abstract]. Pediatr Res 2001;49:126.

[21] Dagan R, Einhorn M. A program of outpatient parenteral antibiotic therapy for serious pediatric bacterial infections. Rev Infect Dis 1991;13(S2):S152–5.

[22] Tice AD. Handbook of outpatient parenteral antimicrobial therapy for infectious diseases. Tarrytown (NY): The Curry Rockefeller Group, LLC; 2006.

[23] Tice AD. An office model of outpatient parenteral antibiotic therapy. Rev Infect Dis 1991;13(S2):S184–188.

[24] Tice AD. Alternate site infusion: the physician-directed office-based model. J Intraven Nurs 1996;19:188–93.

[25] Jeejeebhoy KN, Zohrab WJ, Langer B, et al. Total parenteral nutrition at home for 23 months, without complication, and with good rehabilitation. Gastroenterology 1973;65:811–20.

[26] Morales JO, Von Behren L. Secondary bacterial infections in HIV-infected patients: an alternative ambulatory outpatient treatment utilizing intravenous cefotaxime. Am J Med 1994;97(Suppl 2A):9–13.

[27] Mortlock NJ, Schleis T. Outpatient parenteral antimicrobial therapy technology. Infect Dis Clin North Am 1998;12:861–78.

[28] Kunkel MJ, Tice AD, OPTIVA Study Group. Serious adverse events in outpatient parenteral antibiotic therapy: a prospective multicenter study [abstract 132]. In Program and abstracts of the 33rd Annual Meeting of the Infectious Diseases Society of America. (San Francisco), Alexandria Virginia: Infectious Diseases Society of America, 1995.

[29] Gomez M, Maraqa N, Alvarez A, et al. Complications of outpatient parenteral antibiotic therapy in childhood. Pediatr Infect Dis J 2001;20:541–3.

[30] Schultz TR, Durning S, Niewinski M, et al. A multidisciplinary approach to vascular access in children. J Spec Pediatr Nurs 2006;11:254–6.

[31] American Academy of Home Care Physicians. Home Care Credentialing Examination Information. Available at: http://www.aahcp.org/training.shtml. Accessed October 22, 2009.

[32] Infusion Nurses Society. Infusion nursing standards of practice. J Infus Nurs 2006;29(Suppl 1):S1–92.

[33] Infusion Nurses Certification Corporation Web Site. Available at: http://incc1.i4a.com/i4a/pages/index.cfm?pageid=1. Accessed October 17, 2009.

[34] American Society of Health-System Pharmacists. ASHP guidelines on the pharmacist's role in home care. Am J Health Syst Pharm 2000;57:1252–7.

[35] American Society of Health-System Pharmacists (ASHP). ASHP statement on the pharmacist's role with respect to drug delivery systems and administration devices. Am J Hosp Pharm 1993;50:1724–5.

[36] Tice AD. Bloodborne pathogen exposure and recommendations for management. J Infus Nurs 2002;25(Suppl 6):S5–9.

[37] Kaley J, Berendt AR, Snelling MJ, et al. Safe intravenous antibiotic therapy at home: experience of a UK based programme. J Antimicrob Chemother 1996;37:1023–9.

[38] Nolet BR. Patient selection in outpatient antimicrobial therapy. Infect Dis Clin North Am 1998;12:835–47.

[39] Brown RB. Selection and training of patients for outpatient intravenous antibiotic therapy. Rev Infect Dis 1991;13(Suppl 2):S147–51.

[40] Chung M, Akahoshi M. Reducing home nursing visit costs using a remote access infusion pump system. J Intraven Nurs 1999;22:309–14.

[41] DeMaio J, Schwartz L, Cooley P, et al. The application of telemedicine technology to a directly observed therapy program for tuberculosis: a pilot project. Clin Infect Dis 2001;33:2082–4.

[42] Maraqa N, Gomez M, Rathore MH. Outpatient parenteral antimicrobial therapy in osteo-articular infections in children. J Pediatr Orthop 2002;22:506–10.

[43] Goldenberg RI, Portez DM, Eron LJ, et al. Intravenous antibiotic therapy in ambulatory pediatric patients. Pediatr Infect Dis 1984;3:514–7.

[44] Gutierrez K. Continuation of antibiotic therapy for serious bacterial infections outside of the hospital. Pediatr Ann 1996;25:639–45.

[45] Leaver J, Radivan F, Patel L, et al. Home intravenous antibiotic therapy: practical aspects in children. J R Soc Med 1997;90(Suppl 31):26–33.

[46] Kinsey SE. Experience with teicoplanin in non-inpatient therapy in children with central line infections. Eur J Haematol 1998;62:S11–14.

[47] Shemesh E, Yaniv I, Drucker M, et al. Home intravenous antibiotic treatment for febrile episodes in immune-compromised pediatric patients. Med Pediatr Oncol 1998;30:95–100.

[48] Dagan R, Fliss DM, Einhorn M, et al. Outpatient management of chronic suppurative otitis media without cholesteatoma in children. Pediatr Infect Dis J 1992;11:542–6.

[49] Bradley JS, Ching DK, Phillips SE. Outpatient therapy of serious pediatric infections with ceftriaxone. Pediatr Infect Dis J 1988;7:160–4.

[50] Gilbert J, Robinson T, Littlewood JM. Home intravenous antibiotic treatment in cystic fibrosis. Pediatr Pulmonol 1988;4:84–9.

[51] Esposito S, Leone S, Noviello S, et al. Outpatient parenteral antibiotic therapy for bone and joint infections: an Italian multicenter study. J Chemother 2007;19:417–22.

[52] Zaoutis T, Localio AR, Leckerman K, et al. Prolonged intravenous therapy versus early transition to oral antimicrobial therapy for acute osteomyelitis in children. Pediatrics 2009;123:636–42.

[53] Weichert S, Sharland M, Clarke NM, et al. Acute Hematogenous osteomyelitis in children: is there any evidence for how ling we should treat? Curr Opin Infect Dis 2008;21:258–62.

[54] Bachur R, Pagon Z. Success of short-course parenteral antibiotic therapy for acute osteomyelitis of childhood. Clin Pediatr (Phila) 2007;46:30–5.

[55] Faden D, Faden HS. The high rate of adverse drug events in children receiving prolonged outpatient antibiotic therapy for osteomyelitis. Pediatr Infect Dis J 2009;28:539–41.

[56] Bradley JS. What is the appropriate treatment course for bacterial arthritis in children? Clin Infect Dis 2009;48:1211–2.

[57] Hawkshead JJ, Patel NB, Steele RW, et al. Comparative severity of pediatric osteomyelitis attributable to methicillin-resistant versus methicillin-sensitive Staphylococcus aureus. J Pediatr Orthop 2009;29:85–90.

[58] Deery H. Outpatient parenteral anti-infective therapy for skin and soft-tissue infections. Infect Dis Clin North Am 1998;12:935–49.

[59] Chapman AL, Dixon S, Andrews D, et al. Clinical efficacy and cost-effectiveness of outpatient parenteral antibiotic therapy (OPAT): a UK perspective. J Antimicrob Chemother 2009;64:1316–24.

[60] Chary A, Tice AD, Martinelli LP, et al. Experience of infectious diseases consultants with outpatient antimicrobial therapy: results of an Emerging Infections Network survey. Clin Infect Dis 2006;43:1290–5.

[61] Gerber JS, Coffin SE, Smathers SA, et al. Trends in incidence of methicillin-resistant *Staphylococcus aureus* in children's hospitals in the United States. Clin Infect Dis 2009;49: 65–71.

[62] Johnson PN, Rapp RP, Nelson CT, et al. Characterization of community-acquired *Staphylococcus aureus* infections in children. Ann Pharmacother 2007;41:1361–7.

[63] Gilchrist FJ, Lenney W. A review of the home intravenous antibiotic service available to children with cystic fibrosis. Arch Dis Child 2009;94:647.

[64] Balaguer A, González de Dios J. Home antibiotic therapy for cystic fibrosis. Cochrane Database Syst Rev 2008;16:CD001917.

[65] Termoz A, Touzet S, Bourdy S, et al. Effectiveness of home treatment for patients with cystic fibrosis: the intravenous administration of antibiotics to treat respiratory infections. Pediatr Pulmonol 2008;43:908–15.

[66] Horvais V, Touzet S, Francois S, et al. Cost of home and hospital care for patients with cystic fibrosis followed up in two reference medical centers in France. Int J Technol Assess Health Care 2006;22:525–31.

[67] Nazer D, Abdulhamid I, Thomas R, et al. Home versus hospital intravenous antibiotic therapy for acute pulmonary exacerbations in children with cystic fibrosis. Pediatr Pulmonol 2006;41:744–9.

[68] Bradley JS. Outpatient parenteral antibiotic therapy: management of serious infections. Part 1: Medical socioeconomic, and legal issues: pediatric considerations. Hosp Pract (Off Ed) 1993;28(Suppl 1):28–32.

[69] Proesmans M, DeBoeck K. Clinical Practice: treatment of childhood empyema. Eur J Pediatr 2009;168:639–45.

[70] Dimayuga E, Brown RB. Outpatient parenteral antibiotic therapy for infective endocarditis. Infect Dis Clin Pract 1995;4:468–71.

[71] Andrews MM, Reyn CF. Patient selection criteria and management guidelines for outpatient parenteral antibiotic therapy for native valve infective endocarditis. Clin Infect Dis 2001;33:203–9.

[72] Rehm SJ. Outpatient intravenous antibiotic therapy for infective endocarditis. Infect Dis Clin North Am 1998;12:879–901.

[73] Larioza J, Heung L, Girard A, et al. Management of infective endocarditis in outpatients: clinical experience with outpatient parenteral antibiotic therapy. South Med J 2009;102:575–9.

[74] Gauthier M, Chevalier I, Sterescu A, et al. Treatment of urinary tract infections among febrile young children with daily intravenous antibiotic therapy at a day treatment center. Pediatrics 2004;114:e469–76.

[75] Zorc JJ, Kiddoo DA, Shaw KN. Diagnosis and management of pediatric urinary tract infections. Clin Microbiol Rev 2005;18:417–22.

[76] Committee on Infectious Diseases. American Academy of Pediatrics. Treatment of bacterial meningitis. Pediatrics 1988;81:904–7.

[77] McCracken GH Jr, Nelson JD, Kaplan SL, et al. Consensus report: antimicrobial therapy for bacterial meningitis in infants and children. Pediatr Infect Dis J 1987;6:501–5.

[78] Kaplan SL. Serious pediatric infections. Am J Med 1990;88:185–245.

[79] Bradley JS. Outpatient antibiotic therapy. Management of serious infections. Part II: amenable infections and models of delivery. Meningitis. Hosp Pract (Off Ed) 1993; 28(Suppl 2):15–9.

[80] Waler JA, Rathore MH. Outpatient management of pediatric bacterial meningitis. Pediatr Infect Dis J 1995;14:89–92.

[81] Gilbert DN, Dworkin RJ, Raber SR, et al. Outpatient parenteral antimicrobial-drug therapy. N Engl J Med 1997;337:829–38.

[82] Neftel KA. Effect of storage of penicillin-G solutions on sensitization to penicillin-G after intravenous administration. Lancet 1982;1:986–8.

[83] O'Sullivan TL, Ruffing MJ, Lamp KC, et al. Prospective evaluation of red man syndrome in patients receiving vancomycin. J Infect Dis 1993;168:773–6.

[84] Maraqa NF, Gomez MM, Rathore MH, et al. Higher occurrence of hepatotoxicity and rash in patients treated with oxacillin compared to those treated with nafcillin and other commonly used antibiotics. Clin Infect Dis 2002;34:50–4.

[85] Bhatt-Mehta V, Schumacher RE, Faix RG, et al. Lack of vancomycin-associated nephrotoxicity in newborn infants: a case control study. Pediatrics 1999;103:e48.

[86] Sorrell TC, Collignon PJ. A prospective study of adverse reactions associated with vancomycin therapy. J Antimicrob Chemother 1985;16:235–41.

[87] Palmer-Toy DE. Therapeutic monitoring of vancomycin. Arch Pathol Lab Med 2000;124: 322–3.

[88] James CW, Guk-Turner C. Recommendations for monitoring serum vancomycin concentrations. Proc (Bayl Univ Med Cent) 2001;14:189–90.

[89] Kahyaoglu O, Akpinar M, Nolan B, et al. Vancomycin use and monitoring in pediatric patients in a community hospital. Infect Control Hosp Epidemiol 1998;19:299–301.

[90] Lau C. Transparent and gauze dressings and their effect on infection rates of central venous catheters: a review of past and current literature. J Intraven Nurs 1996;19:240–5.

[91] Pugliese G. Reducing risks of infection during vascular access. J Intraven Nurs 1997; 20(Suppl 6):S11–23.

[92] Russell PB, Kline J, Yoder MC, et al. Staphylococcal adherence to polyvinyl chloride and heparin-bonded polyurethane catheters is species dependant and enhanced by fibronectin. J Clin Microbiol 1987;25:1083–7.

[93] Schleis TG, Tice AD. Selecting infusion devices for use in ambulatory care. Am J Health Syst Pharm 1996;53:868–77.

[94] Kravitz GR. Outpatient parenteral antibiotic therapy: management of serious infections. Part 1: Medical socioeconomic, and legal issues: advances in i.v. delivery. Hosp Pract (Off Ed) 1993;28(Suppl 1):21–7.

[95] LaRue GD. Improving central placement rates of peripherally inserted catheters. J Intraven Nurs 1995;18:24–7.

[96] Hussain S, Gomez M, Wludyka P, et al. Survival times and complications of catheters used for outpatient parenteral antibiotic therapy in children. Clin Pediatr (Phila) 2007;46: 247–51.

[97] Ruebner R, Karen R, Coffin S, et al. Complications of central venous catheters used for the treatment of acute hematogenous osteomyelitis. Pediatrics 2006;117:1210–5.

[98] Gorski LA. The peripheral intravenous catheter: an appropriate yet often overlooked choice for venous access. Home Healthc Nurse 2009;27:130–2.

[99] Goodwin M, Carlson I. The peripherally inserted central catheter. J Intraven Nurs 1993;16:92–103.

[100] Wall JL, Keirstead V. Peripherally inserted central catheters. J Intraven Nurs 1995;18: 251–5.

[101] Van Winkle P, Whiffen T, Liu I. Experience using peripherally inserted central venous catheters for outpatient parenteral antibiotic therapy in children at a community hospital. Pediatr Infect Dis J 2008;27:1069–72.

[102] PowerPICC®. BARD Access Systems, Inc.Salt Lake City (UT), Avilable at: http://www.bardaccess.com/powerpicc//front.php. Accessed October 20, 2009.

[103] Knue M, Doellman D, Rabin K, et al. The efficacy and safety of blood sampling though peripherally inserted central catheter devices in children. J Infus Nurs 2005;28:30–5.

[104] Kaufman J. The interventional radiologist's role in providing and maintaining long-term central venous access. J Intraven Nurs 2001;24:S23–7.

[105] Ng PK, Ault MJ, Ellrodt AG, et al. Peripherally inserted central catheters in general medicine. Mayo Clin Proc 1997;72:225–33.

[106] Finney R, Albrink MH, Hart MG, et al. A cost-effective peripheral venous port system placed at the bedside. J Surg Res 1992;53:17–9.

[107] Stovroff MC, Totten M, Glick PL. PIC lines save money and hasten discharge in the care of children with ruptured appendicitis. J Pediatr Surg 1994;29:245–7.

[108] Thiagarajan R, Ramamoorthy C, Gettman T, et al. Survey of the use of peripherally inserted central venous catheters in children. Pediatrics 1997;99:e4.

[109] Frey A. Pediatric peripherally inserted central catheter program report: a summary of 4536 catheter days. J Intraven Nurs 1995;18:280–91.

[110] O'Grady NP, Alexander M, Dellinger EP, et al. Guidelines for the prevention of intravascular catheter-related infections. Center for Disease Control and Prevention. MMWR Morb Mortal Wkly Rep 2002;51(RR–10):1–29.

[111] Jackson D. Infection control principles and practices in the care and management of vascular access devices in the alternate care setting. J Intraven Nurs 2001;24:S28–34.

[112] Siegel JD, Rhinehart E, Jackson M, et al and the Healthcare Infection Control Practices Advisory Committee. Guideline for isolation precautions: preventing transmission of infectious agents in healthcare settings. Available at: http://www.cdc.gov/hicpac/pdf/isolation/Isolation2007.pdf. Accessed September 21, 2010.

[113] Occupational Safety and Health Administration. Revised Bloodborne Pathogens Standard. Available at: http://www.osha.gov/SLTC/bloodbornepathogens/standards.html Accessed October 20, 2009.

[114] Mermel LA, Farr BM, Sheretz RJ, et al. Guidelines for the management of intravascular catheter-related infections. J Intraven Nurs 2001;24:180–205.

[115] Tice AD. The team concept. Hosp Pract 1993;28(Suppl 1):6–10.

[116] Kaye T. Prolonged infusion times with disposable elastomeric infusion devices. Am J Hosp Pharm 1994;51:533–4.

[117] Rich DS. Evaluation of a disposable, elastomeric infusion device in the home environment. Am J Hosp Pharm 1992;49:1712–6.

[118] Coley SC, Shaw PK, Leff RD. Performance of three portable infusion-pump devices set to deliver 2 ml/hr. Am J Health Syst Pharm 1997;54:1277–80.

[119] Veal DF, Altman CE, McKinnon BT, et al. Evaluation of flow rates for six disposable infusion devices. Am J Health Syst Pharm 1995;52:500–4.

[120] Ingram PR, Sulaiman Z, Chua A, et al. Comment on: outpatient parenteral antibiotic therapy (OPAT): is it safe for selected patients to self-administer at home? A retrospective analysis of a large cohort over 13 years. J Antimicrob Chemother 2008;61:226–7.

[121] Kwan V. High-technology IV infusion devices. Am J Hosp Pharm 1989;46:320–35.

[122] New PB, Swanson GF, Bulich RG, et al. Ambulatory antibiotic infusion devices: extending the spectrum of outpatient therapies. Am J Med 1991;91:455–61.

[123] Rich D. Physicians, pharmacists, and home infusion antibiotic therapy. Am J Med. 1994;97(Suppl 1):3–8.

[124] Kappeler KH, Bridwell SW, Scheckelhoff DJ, et al. Model for evaluating costs associated with i.v. drug delivery systems. Am J Health Syst Pharm 1993;49:1478–81.

[125] Kunkel MJ. Quality assurance and outcomes in outpatient parenteral antibiotic therapy. Infect Dis Clin North Am 1998;12:1023–34.

[126] Joint Commission. 2009 Comprehensive Accreditation Manual for Home Care (CAMHC). Available at: http://www.jcrinc.com/Accreditation-Manuals/2009-CAMHC/1324/. Accessed October 19, 2009.

[127] Nathwani D, Tice AD. Ambulatory antimicrobial use: the value of an outcomes registry. J Antimicrob Chemother 2002;49:149–54.

Advances in Pediatrics 57 (2010) 247–267

ELSEVIER
MOSBY

ADVANCES IN PEDIATRICS

Current Controversies in Treatment and Prevention of Diabetic Ketoacidosis

Arleta Rewers, MD, PhD

Emergency Medicine, Department of Pediatrics, School of Medicine, University of Colorado
Denver, 13123 East 16th Avenue, B251, Aurora, CO 80045, USA

OVERVIEW OF DIABETIC KETOACIDOSIS

Pathophysiology

Common causes of diabetic ketoacidosis (DKA) include progressive β-cell failure in previously undiagnosed patients and omission or inadequate insulin dosing in established patients. Hyperglycemia develops due to impaired glucose use (lack of insulin) and increased glucose production by the liver and kidneys (excess of counterregulatory hormones). Infection, gastrointestinal illness, trauma, and stress may also precipitate DKA if the increase in counter-regulatory hormones is not matched by appropriate increase in insulin dosing. Low levels of effective circulating insulin and a concomitant increase in glucagon, catecholamines, cortisol, and growth hormone lead to catabolism of fat and protein. Lipolysis results in increased production of ketones, especially β-hydroxybutyrate (β-OHB), with the ratio between acetoacetate and β-hydroxybutyrate increased from 1:1 to about 1:10, ketonemia, and metabolic acidosis.

Definition

The American Diabetes Association (ADA) [1,2], as well as jointly the European Society for Paediatric Endocrinology (ESPE) and the Lawson Wilkins Pediatric Endocrine Society (LWPES) [3] agreed to define DKA as:

1. Hyperglycemia, ie, plasma glucose higher than 250 mg/dL or ~14 mmol/L; and
2. Venous pH <7.3 and/or bicarbonate <15 mmol/L
3. Moderate or large ketones level in urine or blood.

DKA may occur at lesser degrees of hyperglycemia. Pregnant adolescents, young or partially treated children, and those fasting during a period of insulin deficiency may have near-normal glucose levels and ketoacidosis ("euglycemic ketoacidosis").

E-mail address: rewers.arleta@tchden.org

0065-3101/10/$ – see front matter
doi:10.1016/j.yapd.2010.09.001

DKA is generally categorized by the severity of acidosis. In most laboratories, normal range for arterial pH is 7.35 to 7.45 and for venous pH 7.32 to 7.42 in adults and children older than 2 years. Currently recommended categories of severity differ slightly between adults and children (Table 1), but there is little evidence to support these differences.

Although large or moderate ketonuria is sufficient for confirmation of DKA diagnosis, measurement of whole blood β-OHB is more helpful in making treatment decisions [4,5]. Whole blood β-OHB levels of >3.0 mmol/L combined with blood glucose >250 mg/dL ($\sim$14 mmol/L) suggest the presence of DKA.

Prevalence of DKA in Type 1 and Type 2 Diabetes

Prevalence of DKA at the diagnosis of type 1 diabetes

Examples of reports on the prevalence and predictors of DKA at diagnosis around the world are presented in Table 2. The largest population-based study to date, SEARCH for Diabetes in Youth, has reported that 29% of patients with type 1 diabetes (T1D) younger than 20 years at diagnosis present with DKA [6]. In Europe, the prevalence varied from 15% to 67% [3,7] and was generally higher in populations with lower incidence of T1D. In the developing countries, 42% to 85% of T1D children present with DKA [8].

Studies in the early 2000s have suggested that the clinical severity at diagnosis of T1D in youth may be decreasing. In Colorado, the proportion of children with T1D who presented with DKA at the time of diagnosis has significantly decreased, from 38% in 1978 to 82% to 29% in 1998–2001 [9]. Similarly, the prevalence of DKA at onset decreased in Finland from 30% in 1982–1991 to 19% in 1992–2002 [10]. However, the newest reports suggest that the incidence of DKA is not decreasing, and may have increased in the current decade in United States children.

Incidence of DKA in established type 1 diabetes

The overall incidence of DKA in patients with established T1D varies from 1 to 12 per 100 person-years (Table 3) [11,12]. The incidence of DKA increases significantly with age in females, but not in males (Fig. 1) [11]. Most of the episodes of DKA beyond diagnosis are associated with insulin omission or treatment error, for example, inadequate adjustment of insulin therapy during

Table 1			
Classification of DKA severity			
Severity of DKA	ADA adults [2]	ADA children [1]	ESPE/LWPES children [3]
Severe	Arterial pH <7.0 Bicarbonate <10	Venous pH <7.1	Venous pH <7.1 Bicarbonate <5
Moderate	Arterial pH 7.0– <7.25 Bicarbonate 10– <15	Venous pH 7.1–7.2	Venous pH <7.2 Bicarbonate <10
Mild	Arterial pH 7.25–7.30 Bicarbonate 15–18	Venous pH 7.2–7.3	Venous pH <7.3 Bicarbonate <15

Table 2
Prevalence of DKA at diagnosis of diabetes

Country [Ref.]	Age	N	Completeness of record review	Study period	Definition of DKA	Prevalence of DKA (%)	Predictors
USA [6]	0–19	2824	77% Population based	2002–2004	pH <7.3 (venous) or pH <7.25 (arterial) Bicarbonate <15 or ICD-9 250.1 or medical record diagnosis	29% type 1 10% type 2	Younger age, lower family income, underinsurance, lower parental education
USA [17]	0–18	139	68% Hospital series	1995–1998	pH <7.3	38%	Younger age, lack of insurance
Europe [7] (11 countries)	0–14	1260	91% varied by center	1989–1994	pH <7.3	26%–67% (42% on average)	Area of low incidence of type 1 diabetes
Germany [55]	0–14	2121	97% Population based	1987–1997	pH <7.3 or bicarbonate <15	26%	Lower socioeconomic status
Finland [10]	0–14	585	Hospital series	1982–2001	pH <7.3 or bicarbonate ≤15	18%	Younger age
UK [56]	0–15	328	Hospital series	1987–1996	pH ≤7.25 (arterial) or bicarbonate ≤15	27%	Asian minority age less than 5 y
UK [12]	0–20	230 97	Population based	1985–1986 1990	pH <7.36 or bicarbonate <21	26% 26%	Younger age
Ireland [57]	0–14	283	72% Population based	1997–1998	pH <7.3	31%	
Kuwait [8]	0–12	103	Hospital series	2000–2003	pH <7.3	84.5	

Table 3
Incidence of DKA in children and adolescent with established type 1 diabetes

Country [Ref.]	Age group	N	Study design	Length of study	Definition of DKA	Incidence/100 person-years	Predictors
USA [11]	0–19	1243	Prospective cohort	3.5 y	DKA leading to ED visit or hospital admission	8	Female gender, age, higher HbA1c, higher insulin dose, underinsurance, psychiatric disorders
USA [18]	7–16	300	Prospective cohort	1 y	DKA leading to ED visit or hospital admission	15	Higher HbA1c
USA [58]	13–17	195	Clinical trial	7.4 y	BG >250 mg/dL, ketonuria, pH <7.3 or bicarbonate <15	4.7 conventional 2.8 intensive	NA
Sweden [59]	0–18	139	Prospective cohort	3 y	Acidosis	1.5	NA
UK [60]	1–17	135	Retrospective	6 y	pH <7.3 or bicarbonate <18	10	Female gender, family and school problems
Australia [61]	1–19	268	Retrospective	3 mo	pH <7.2 or bicarbonate <10	12	NA

Abbreviations: BG, blood glucose; ED, Emergency Department; Hb1Ac, hemoglobin A1c; NA, not available.

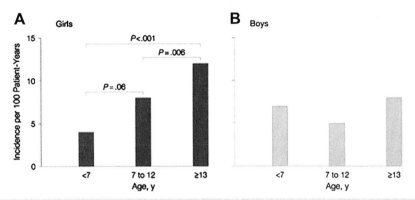

Fig. 1. Incidence of diabetic ketoacidosis by age and gender, Colorado, 1996 to 2001 (A, B). (From Rewers A, Chase HP, Mackenzie T, Walravens P, Roback M, Rewers M, et al. Predictors of acute complications in children with type 1 diabetes. JAMA 2002;287(19):2511–8. Copyright 2002 American Medical Association. All rights reserved, with permission.)

intercurrent illness or accidental interruption of continuous subcutaneous insulin infusion (insulin pump). Patients with previous episodes of DKA are at higher risk for recurrent DKA. In one study, 60% of all DKA episodes occurred in 5% of patients with recurrent events [11].

Incidence of DKA at the diagnosis of type 2 diabetes
While the conventional belief is that DKA is an uncommon presentation of type 2 diabetes, these data suggest that DKA does not help to distinguish type 1 from type 2 diabetes. The SEARCH found that 10% of type 2 diabetic youth presented in DKA [6], compared with 19% among Thai youth [13].

Incidence of DKA in established type 2 diabetes
Patients with established type 2 diabetes develop DKA or hyperglycemic hyperosmolar syndrome (HHS). Hospitalization for other medical or surgical conditions increases the risk of DKA. The number of hospitalizations for DKA among persons younger than 45 years estimated by the US National Diabetes Surveillance System increased from 37,000 (24/100,000) in 1980 to 87,000 (47/100,000) in 2003, and the number of hospital discharges with DKA diagnosis doubled from 62,000 discharges in 1980 to 115,000 in 2003.

Risk Factors for DKA at the Diagnosis of Diabetes

The prevalence of DKA at the diagnosis is significantly higher among younger children [14,15], reaching more than 50% in those younger than 2 years [16]. Lower socioeconomic status (lower family income and parental education, and less favorable health insurance creating barriers in access to care) is a powerful independent risk factor [15,17]. Low societal awareness of diabetes symptoms, such as in populations with low incidence of T1D, adds to the risk, whereas programs promoting community awareness may decrease the risk.

However, the prevalence of DKA at onset [6] and the recurrence of DKA [11] did not differ by race/ethnicity in United States youth with T1D, when controlling for the socioeconomic status. In addition, treatment with high-dose glucocorticoids, atypical antipsychotics, diazoxide, and immunosuppressive drugs have been reported to precipitate DKA in individuals not previously diagnosed with diabetes.

Risk Factors for Recurrent DKA

The risk of recurrent DKA is higher in patients with poor metabolic control [11,18]. Lower socioeconomic status and insufficient access to outpatient diabetes care are often the primary mechanism. Eating disorders, prevalent in adolescent girls, contribute to the highest risk for DKA in this group, reaching 12 per 100 patient-years. Diabetic adolescent girls often omit insulin injections to lose or maintain weight. Patients with recurrent ketoacidosis have been shown to exhibit more behavioral problems, lower social competence, and higher levels of family conflict; however, major psychiatric disorders (depression, bipolar disorder, schizophrenia) also play a role [11]. The patterns of recurrent DKA vary by age (Fig. 2). In children younger than 13 years, the risk increases with higher hemoglobin A1c (HbA1c) and with higher reported insulin dose. In older children, in addition, inadequate insurance and psychiatric disorders increase the risk of DKA [11].

Patients treated with insulin pumps are at a higher risk for DKA than their classical risk-factor profile would suggest. Undetected interruption of insulin delivery for 4 to 6 hours may be enough for DKA to ensue. Therefore, patients using insulin pumps should monitor blood glucose levels 6 to 8 times a day, and additional testing is recommended during "sick days," generally every 2 hours.

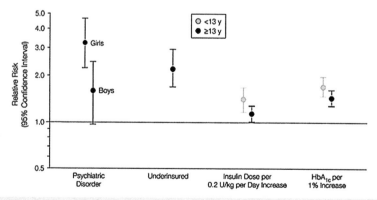

Fig. 2. Predictors of diabetic ketoacidosis in children with established diabetes, Colorado, 1996 to 2001. (*From* Rewers A, Chase HP, Mackenzie T, Walravens P, Roback M, Rewers M, et al. Predictors of acute complications in children with type 1 diabetes. JAMA 2002; 287(19):2511–8. Copyright 2002 American Medical Association. All rights reserved, with permission.)

Complications

Mortality and cerebral edema

DKA is the most common cause of death in children with T1D [19]. Cerebral edema occurs in 0.3% to 3.0% of childhood DKA cases, and is the primary fatal complication [20,21]. Less frequent causes of mortality include hypokalemia, hyperkalemia, thrombosis, other neurologic complications, sepsis, aspiration pneumonia, and pulmonary edema. Nonfatal cerebral edema is often associated with permanent neurologic deficits.

Children, in contrast to adults, may develop cerebral edema in the course of DKA. Newly diagnosed patients who are younger than 5 years, severely dehydrated, very acidotic, and very hyperosmolar are at greatest risk. The etiology of cerebral edema is only partially known. Risk factors include arterial pH <7.1 and pCO_2 <20 mm Hg in children receiving more than 50 mL/kg of fluid in the first 4 hours of treatment [22], low partial-pressure CO_2 (pCO_2) and high blood urea nitrogen (BUN) at presentation and bicarbonate treatment [21], as well as a failure of sodium concentration to increase as glucose concentration decreases. Commencement of insulin treatment before the initial rehydration bolus also may increase the risk of cerebral edema. Children with presence of subclinical cerebral edema and ventricular narrowing on magnetic resonance imaging (MRI) usually do not exhibit neurologic abnormalities [23].

Shock

Decreased vascular volume and impending circulatory collapse are features of severe DKA, and must be addressed immediately in the first several hours of therapy. Five percent albumin (10 mL/kg over 30 min) or other colloid should be given if severe shock is present or if there is still evidence of shock 1 hour after receiving saline. In patients with severe dehydration or in patients with severe mental status changes, intravascular pressure monitoring to follow hydration status is indicated.

Hyperkalemia and hypokalemia

At diagnosis of moderate to severe DKA and before initiation of intravenous (IV) fluid therapy, potassium levels are elevated in most patients. Hyperkalemia may lead to cardiac arrest, and potassium supplementation must be withheld until potassium levels decline to normal or low in effect of rehydration. Correction of acidosis and insulin replacement results in intracellular movement of K^+. Resultant hypokalemia may lead to cardiac arrhythmias, ileus, and muscular weakness. Diaphragmatic fatigue may contribute to a respiratory arrest in hyperventilating patient.

Hypoglycemia

While on a continuous IV infusion of insulin, the patient is at risk for hypoglycemia. Hourly glucose concentration checks and addition of dextrose to the IV solution when blood glucose falls to 250 mg/dL should prevent the problem.

Cost of DKA

Direct medical care charges associated with DKA represent 28% of the direct medical cost for all patients, and 56% for those with recurrent DKA [24]. In 2004, there were approximately 120,000 hospitalizations in the United States with diagnostic coding indicating DKA, and an additional 5000 were coded as "diabetic coma." Based on the Diagnostic Related Group codes in the inpatient records, the total hospital cost for DKA was estimated at $1.4 to $1.8 billion [25]. An independent analysis arrived to an estimate of the annual hospital cost of DKA in the United States also in excess of $1 billion [26]. The investigators based their estimate on an annual average of more than 100,000 hospitalizations for DKA, with an average cost of $13,000 per patient. Newly diagnosed patients may account for approximately 25% of this cost [27].

PREVENTION OF DKA

Prevention of DKA in Patients with Established Diabetes

Identification of at-risk patients

Studies to date also suggest that most, if not all, episodes of DKA beyond disease diagnosis are preventable. Risk factors, reviewed in the previous section, allow for identification of high-risk patients and targeted interventions. Patients treated with insulin pumps are at a higher risk of DKA than their classical risk-factor profile would suggest.

Education

Appropriate blood glucose monitoring. Insulin-treated patients should be educated to monitor blood glucose levels at home at least 4 times a day and those using insulin pumps 6 to 8 times a day. Additional testing is recommended during "sick days"–generally every 2 hours.

Monitoring of urine or blood ketones levels. Home measurement of ketones may greatly assist in the prevention of DKA. A combination of high blood glucose concentration (above 250 mg/dL) and elevated urine or blood ketones indicates high likelihood that DKA is present.

Ketones can be measured in urine or blood.

- Urine ketone measurements use a "dip stick" method based on a chemical reaction with acetoacetate (eg, Chemstrip from Roche; Clinistix, Ketostix, Keto-Diastix from Bayer).
- Blood β-OHB tests are available for use in the laboratory (eg, Sigma or Cobos, Roche) and home monitoring (Precision Xtra meter, Abbott MediSense). Recently Abbott/MediSense unveiled a hand-held device, the Precision Xceed Pro System, for measurement of blood glucose and β-OHB in hospitals. β-OHB monitoring using hand-held devices is as accurate as reference laboratory method, at least up to 3 mmol/L [5,28,29].

Blood ketone testing has several advantages over urine ketone testing:

- β-OHB is a better marker of ketosis than acetoacetate
- β-OHB is "real-time" whereas ketonuria is usually "old news"

- Ketonuria does not accurately reflect severity of ketonemia
- A dehydrated person may not be able to void and some people are too ill or exhausted to do the urine test
- Urine ketone strips have a short shelf life after opening.

Bedside measurement of β-OHB in blood is more sensitive (80%) in detecting ketosis than urine analysis (63%). A negative blood β-OHB test has a better negative predictive value than negative urine test in ruling out ketosis [30].

Telephone counseling including triage
Comprehensive diabetes programs and telephone services have been shown to be effective in preventing DKA. A telephone service for questions and advice, managed by a nurse diabetes educator, significantly reduces hospital admissions [31].

Early detection of mild ketosis (1.5 mmol/L >β-OHB >0.6 mmol/L) that often affects insulin-treated patients is a key to prevention of DKA. Ketosis can be handled at home, usually with telephone help from diabetes provider. A recent clinical trial has found home β-OHB monitoring effective in early detection of ketosis and prevention of DKA among T1D patients aged 3 to 22 years [4]. The frequency of blood ketone monitoring during sick days was 91%, significantly higher than among those checking only urine ketones (61%). The group monitoring blood ketones experienced significantly lower incidence of Emergency Room use or hospitalizations compared with the urine ketones monitoring group. Generally accepted algorithm for interpretation of blood β-OHB levels and treatment recommendations are summarized in Box 1.

Box 1: Algorithm for interpretation of blood β-OHB levels

Determination of β-OHB levels can guide home management of hyperglycemic crisis to avert DKA.

β-OHB <0.6 mmol/L is normal, and no action is needed

0.6–1.5 mmol/L is somewhat elevated, but usually responds quickly to oral fluids (water) and subcutaneous (SC) injection of a rapid-acting insulin in the amount of 5%–10% of the total daily dose

1.5–3.0 mmol/L marks high risk of ketoacidosis, but usually can be managed with oral fluids (water) and SC injection of a rapid-acting insulin in the amount of 10%–20% of the total daily dose. Diabetes provider or Emergency Department should be consulted.

>3.0 mmol/L is usually accompanied by acidosis. Urgent contact with diabetes provider or Emergency Department is critical.

NOTE: Urine or blood ketones are elevated in diabetic patients as a physiologic metabolic response to fasting, low carbohydrate diets (eg, Atkins diet), during prolonged exercise or pregnancy, as well as in gastroenteritis and alcohol intoxication. Blood glucose levels are normal or low in these situations and supplemental insulin is NOT indicated. Blood glucose levels must be checked and confirmed that it is above 150 mg/dL before administering insulin in patients with ketonuria or ketosis.

Reduction in health care visits and hospitalizations
Comprehensive diabetes programs including education and telephone help have reduced the rates of DKA from 15 to 60 to 5 to 6 per 100 patient-years [31–34]. Therefore, it is likely that most episodes of DKA after diagnosis could be avoided if all patients with diabetes received comprehensive diabetes health care.

Prevention of DKA at Onset of Diabetes

The role of health care professionals
Increased awareness of signs and symptoms of diabetes helps earlier diagnosis. Nearly all patients admitted with severe DKA have been seen hours or days earlier by health care providers who missed the diagnosis [35]. Diabetes should always be considered in ill children; urine and/or blood check for glucose and ketones leads to early diagnosis. Rapid confirmation and referral to an appropriate center often prevents DKA and hospitalization. Although these strategies are intuitive, programs to decrease DKA at onset need to be designed and evaluated in diverse populations and age groups. These programs should include approaches that target both the public at large and health care providers.

A growing body of evidence suggests that primary prevention of DKA in newly diagnosed children is possible and should be a major goal of diabetes care systems. The Diabetes Autoimmunity Study in Youth has demonstrated that DKA can be prevented by periodic testing for diabetes autoantibodies, HbA1c, and random blood glucose in children at genetically high risk for T1D [36]. Similarly, in the Diabetes Prevention Trial (DPT-1), awareness of increased level of risk and close biochemical monitoring made early diagnosis and prevention of DKA possible [37].

Community education
An intensive community intervention to raise awareness of the signs and symptoms of childhood diabetes among school teachers and primary care providers in a region of Italy was found to reduce the prevalence of DKA at diagnosis of type 1 disease from 83% to 13% [38]. A follow up study has shown that the campaign for DKA prevention is still effective in Parma province 8 years later, but there is also an indication that the campaign should be periodically renewed [39].

DIAGNOSIS OF DKA
Clinical Presentation
The clinical picture of DKA includes polyuria, polydipsia, and dehydration. Polyphagia is unusual and weight loss is invariably present. Abdominal pain, nausea, and vomiting are common as are signs of infection (eg, dysuria, thrush, or tachypnea that is mistaken for bronchiolitis, pneumonia) that sometimes delay proper diagnosis.

The physical examination should include vital signs (heart rate, respiratory rate, blood pressure), assessment of hydration status, and peripheral perfusion. Patients have acetone-fruity breath and, in more severe cases, Kussmaul respiration (rapid, deep, and sighing). Neurologic status worsens progressively from somnolence to coma; focal signs are present in cerebral edema.

Laboratory Tests

Initial laboratory tests include:

1. Blood glucose and blood or urine ketones. A meter glucose and urine/blood ketones concentration in an Emergency Department or office may make a diagnosis and save a life.
2. Electrolytes: sodium, potassium, calcium, phosphorus, bicarbonate, and BUN. Sodium concentrations are spuriously low in the setting of hyperglycemia and should be expressed as corrected Na = measured Na + (plasma glucose − 100)(1.6)/100
3. Blood gases including venous pH and pCO_2.
4. Serum osmolality can be measured directly or calculated as 2(Na + K) + glucose/18 + BUN/2.8 (mOsm/kg).
5. Appropriate cultures and/or urinalysis if infection is suspected.
6. If chest film is indicated, it should be delayed until hydration is normalized.
7. CT or magnetic resonance imaging of the head is not routinely indicated (see later discussion).

TREATMENT OF DKA IN EMERGENCY DEPARTMENT/HOSPITAL SETTING

Fluids

Initial bolus

The initial therapeutic step is to restore extracellular fluid volume that has been depleted, usually by 5% to 10%, through osmotic diuresis and vomiting. A less rapid fluid deficit correction with isotonic or near-isotonic solutions results in earlier reversal of acidosis [40,41].

Initial volume expansion over the first 1 to 2 hours is by accomplished by IV infusion of 10 to 20 mL/kg body weight of normal saline (0.9%) or Ringer lactate solution. The bolus may need to be repeated if the patient is severely dehydrated and/or if urine output is massive. However, the initial bolus reexpansion should never exceed 40 mL/kg of total IV fluid in the initial 4 hours of treatment.

Replacement of fluid deficit over the next 24 to 48 hours of treatment

Subsequent fluid replacement should be done with half to three-quarters normal saline (0.45%–0.67%). Potassium can be added at this time, usually at 40 mEq/L . Dehydration estimated on physical examination (5%–10% of body weight) is reversed evenly over the next 48 hours. Significant additional fluid loss after initiation of treatment is uncommon; however, additional replacement may be required for vomiting. Excessive urine output should resolve within the initial 2 to 4 hours of therapy as the hyperglycemia resolves, so replacement of urine output ("ml" for "ml") is not required.

Bolus(es) given in the first hours of treatment should be subtracted from the 24-hour totals. In addition to replacement of estimated fluid loss, the patient requires maintenance fluids calculated as shown in Table 4. Total fluid

Table 4
Calculations for fluid replacement

Body weight (kg)	24-Hour fluid maintenance requirements
Up to 10	100 mL/kg
10–20	1000 mL + 50 mL/kg over 10 kg
>20	1500 mL + 20 mL/kg over 20 kg

replacement should not exceed 4 L per square meter of body surface area per 24 h. In the severely dehydrated patient or the one with impaired mental status, monitoring fluid administration with central venous pressure and/or arterial pressure monitoring may be required.

Insulin

Insulin must be given to allow normal carbohydrate use and to stop ketogenesis. Normal glycogen and fat stores, and protein synthesis also need to be restored over time. The standard of care is "low-dose" intravenous insulin administration [42,43]. An initial intramuscular (IM) or IV insulin bolus should not be given to avoid rapid decrease in glucose levels without sufficient time given to correct the acidosis.

No insulin should be given until a blood glucose concentration has been checked at the bedside with a glucose meter and a confirmation sample sent to laboratory. It is currently recommended to start the insulin drip until well (1 hour) into the initial rehydration bolus to lower the risk of cerebral edema, but not much later. The serum glucose level falls fairly rapidly during volume reexpansion with or without insulin.

Continuous IV regular insulin is given at a dose of 0.1 unit/kg per hour. In established patients or those with mild to moderately severe DKA, this rate may need to be reduced. The aim is to have blood glucose concentration decrease by 50 to 100 mg/dL per hour. An IV insulin drip provides a relatively smooth decline in blood glucose concentration with a predictable time to expect a blood glucose at about 250 mg/dL when 5% to 10% dextrose should be added to the IV solution to keep blood glucose concentration between 150 to 250 mg/dL. Unless a patient is truly hypoglycemic, the insulin drip should not be decreased to less than 0.05 unit/kg/h as this is likely to prolong the time needed to suppress ketogenesis. IV insulin should not be discontinued until the bicarbonate is greater than 15 mmol/L or venous pH is greater than 7.30.

Rapid-acting insulin analogues hold no advantage over regular insulin in treatment of DKA. Because insulin binds to the walls of the IV tubing, the tubing should be first washed with 50 mL of the insulin solution.

Electrolytes

Potassium

Total body potassium is usually depleted by about 3 to 6 mmol/kg, but serum levels may be normal or high [44] because the intracellular K^+ moves into the extracellular space in the presence of acidosis. Vomiting may also contribute to hypokalemia. As acidosis and insulinopenia are corrected, K^+ is driven back into the cells and there is a decrease in serum K^+ despite K^+ replacements. Hyperkalemia may lead to cardiac arrest whereas hypokalemia may cause cardiac arrhythmias, ileus, and muscular weakness and cramps. Electrocardiography (ECG) monitoring is strongly recommended. Potassium must not be given as a rapid IV bolus.

Potassium must never be given IV until the serum potassium level is known. Once the serum potassium is known to be normal or low, and urine output is confirmed, all IV fluids following the initial bolus(es) should include 20 to 40 mEq/L of potassium. The replacement may be in the form of KCl, K acetate, K phosphate, or a combination of these supplements; no more than half of the potassium replacement should be given as K phosphate.

Sodium

Initial serum sodium concentration is frequently low due to urinary losses/vomiting, an osmotic dilution of extracellular solute, so that for each 100 mg/dL increase in glucose above a 100 mg/dL baseline there is an expected decrease of 1.6 mEq/L of sodium. Hyperlipidemia that displaces water may also cause serum sodium to be factitiously low.

Laboratory hyponatremia is corrected with resolution of hyperglycemia and ketonemia. Total body sodium deficit is approximately 10 mEq/kg based on a dehydration estimate of 10%. Because of the factitious sodium deficit, the sodium deficit is not usually calculated. It is important to follow the serum sodium during therapy to make certain the level is rising. Falling serum sodium may be associated with cerebral edema and impending herniation. Usually initial treatment with isotonic saline, or lactated Ringer followed by half or three-quarters normal saline, will adequately replace sodium deficit.

Phosphorus

Uncontrolled diabetes causes an increased urinary excretion of phosphorus. Serum phosphorus may, like potassium, be elevated initially in diabetic acidosis, only to decrease rapidly during therapy. Hypocalcemic tetany has occurred with excessive phosphorus administration.

Clinical problems caused by moderately low serum phosphorus are not proven, but there is some evidence that neurologic disturbances may respond to raising the serum phosphorus level when it is very low (<1 mg/dL) (normal pediatric phosphate = 3–5 mg/dL). On theoretical grounds, low phosphorus may lead to a low red cell 2,3-diphosphoglycerate, causing a shift of the 02 dissociation curve to the left, creating a relative tissue hypoxia. Treatment may be administered as K phosphate at 10 to 20 mEq/L in IV solutions as half of the total potassium administered (see Potassium section).

Calcium

Hyperglycemia also causes increased urinary calcium loss. Because of the large calcium reservoir in bone, serum calcium usually remains normal.

Acid-Base

The cause of the acidosis is primarily ketogenesis from insulinopenia. Insulin replacement reverses the acidosis. Bicarbonate therapy is not necessary even in severe DKA, and bicarbonate treatment may be an independent risk factor for cerebral edema [21]. Most of the existing evidence points against using bicarbonate therapy. In this study Glaser and colleagues [21] showed that treatment with bicarbonate was significantly associated with cerebral edema, after adjustment for other covariables. Bicarbonate therapy causes a paradoxic central nervous system (CNS) acidosis and decreases CNS oxygenation. Bicarbonate crosses the blood-brain barrier slowly, but the CO_2 formed from bicarbonate crosses rapidly into the CNS, thereby accentuating rather than reducing the CNS acidosis. The use of bicarbonate leads to a more rapid initial correction of acidosis, with resultant intracellular movement of K^+ and hypokalemia.

Osmolality

Hyperosmolality always accompanies DKA; however, it should be normalized gradually. During treatment, serum osmolality may decrease more rapidly than CNS osmolality, resulting in fluid shifts into the CNS. This process may cause life-threatening cerebral edema, thus excessive, rapid fluid administration may increase the risk for cerebral edema.

If the serum osmolality is very high (greater than 320 mOsm/kg), the elevated blood glucose and dehydration should be corrected cautiously with special attention to neurologic status. However, severe dehydration must be steadily corrected to prevent circulatory collapse. An 18 mg/dL increase in blood glucose yields a 1 mOsm increase in serum osmolality. The osmolality can be measured directly or calculated by: 2(Na + K) + glucose/18 + BUN/2.8. Measured or calculated serum osmolality should be followed if the initial osmolality is greater than 320 mOsm/kg.

HHS is different from diabetic ketoacidosis, and should not be treated as outlined in this article. Fortunately, this condition is rare in childhood. When it occurs in a pediatric patient, attention still needs to be given not to decrease the osmolality too rapidly. Children, in contrast to adults, develop cerebral edema if their rehydration is undertaken too rapidly, especially in HHS. Monitoring intravascular pressure, cardiac rhythm, and osmolality is essential for patients with HHS.

Overweight or obese children may make estimation of dehydration difficult. A measured serum osmolality should always be obtained in the overweight patient with either DKA or HHS.

Blood β-Hydroxybutyrate Levels

Acetoacetate and a small amount of acetone are measured by the urinary "dipstick" reactions as used by the clinician or laboratory; β-OHB is not measured by this method and is usually the major ketoacid in DKA. As treatment is begun, β-OHB is oxidized to acetoacetate so that ketonuria may appear to worsen initially. Urinary determinations are markedly affected by hydration status and urine output. A bedside meter, the Precision Xtra, is now available, which can be used to estimate serum β-OHB levels. Serum β-OHB levels greater than 3.0 mmol/L usually indicate severe DKA (normal <0.6 mmol/L) Serum ketones usually disappear at or about the same time the venous pH reaches a level of 7.30. Following bedside β-OHB levels may be helpful. β-OHB levels can be extremely useful, if available at home, in determining whether an ill child requires Emergency Department therapy. Repeating urine ketones is not necessary.

Bedside β-OHB testing helps to diagnose DKA in patients with known or new diabetes seen in an Emergency Department. Four studies have looked at this issue. Each used a different cut-off level for blood β-OHB. It appears that a cut-off of 2 or 3 mmol/L provides optimal combination of sensitivity and specificity and could be recommended for initial diagnosis in the Emergency Department. Hyperglycemic patients with β-OHB levels below 3 mmol/L are very unlikely to have DKA [45–48]. Data from Prisco and colleagues [49] elegantly illustrate this point. Among 118 children with newly diagnosed diabetes (Fig. 3), 28 had initial venous pH of less than 7.25. Only one of these had β-OHB of less than 2.8. It is worth noting that among children with pH greater than 7.25, about a half had β-OHB greater than 3 mmol/L and probably compensated metabolic acidosis. A recent article by the authors demonstrated a significant correlation between the bedside meter β-OHB levels and pH, bicarbonate, and pCO_2, but not blood glucose or BUN [5]. Although the initial measurement of pH, bicarbonate, and pCO_2 is warranted, real-time

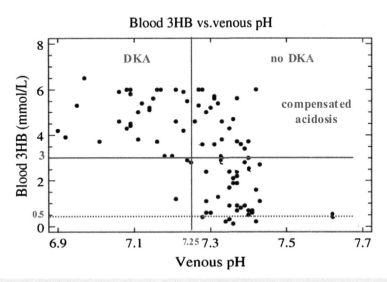

Fig. 3. Blood β-OHB versus venous pH in 118 newly diagnosed children. (*From* Prisco F, Picardi A, Iafusco D, Lorini R, Minicucci L, Martinucci ME, et al. Blood ketone bodies in patients with recent-onset type 1 diabetes (a multicenter study). Pediatr Diabetes 2006; 7(4):225; with permission.)

bedside measurement of β-OHB may replace repeat measurements of blood gases in the treatment of DKA. It also has been shown that real-time bedside measurement of β-OHB may help to optimize treatment of DKA and shorten the duration of hospitalization [49–51].

Clinical Monitoring

1. A flow sheet for fluids, insulin, vital signs (every hour until stable) and laboratory values
2. Fluid intake and output record. Urinary catheter only if the patient is unconscious. If conscious, ask patient to void every hour. In the young child, weigh the diapers hourly
3. ECG monitor for K^+ changes
4. Intravenous access for frequent blood draws when hydration allows
5. Neurologic check (pupils and sensorium) hourly for signs of cerebral edema
6. Laboratory tests: serum concentration of bicarbonate, blood glucose, K^+ every hour for 4 hours, hourly pH until pH >7.1; then every 2–4 hours until HCO_3 >15 mmol/L, and the pH is >7.3
7. Blood glucose at the bedside with each blood draw
8. Other studies (serum osmolality, calcium, phosphorus) as indicated.

Prevention/Treatment of Complications

Cerebral edema

Neurologic status should be checked at frequent and regular intervals. The patient may complain of severe headaches or have a change in mental status, arousal or behavior, incontinence, focal signs, pupillary changes, seizures, or disturbed temperature regulation hours after therapy for DKA has begun [52]. A sudden "normalization" of heart rate in appropriately tachycardic dehydrated patient is an early sign, while bradycardia, hypertension, and irregular respiration (the Cushing triad) are signs of greatly increased intracranial pressure. Most often, the patient's laboratory values are improving as she or he appears to be worsening clinically.

Early intervention before respiratory arrest is essential. Treatment includes decreasing fluids (75% maintenance fluids), giving IV mannitol (1 g/kg over 30 minutes), and elevating the head of the bed. Mannitol may need to be repeated. Normal saline (NS) 3% has also been recommended for treatment of cerebral edema in the course of DKA [53]. There are no randomized studies that compare mannitol versus 3% NS.

Dexamethasone should not be given. Also, in reversal of older recommendations, intubation and hyperventilation are not recommended unless pCO_2 is greater than 30 mm Hg or the patient is in respiratory arrest. While hypocapnea causes cerebral vasoconstriction, the patient is usually ventilating at a maximum rate and intubation may be, at least temporarily, an additional setback.

Treatment should not be delayed until after the radiographic studies have been obtained. The absence of demonstrable cerebral edema on CT scan does not preclude the diagnosis.

Medications that may alter mental status should be given with extreme caution during treatment of DKA. Agitated patients may have impending circulatory collapse or CNS catastrophe, which may be precipitated or masked by medications that alter mental status.

Hypoglycemia

Hourly glucose concentration and the addition of dextrose to the IV solution when blood glucose falls to 250 mg/dL should prevent the problem. It is appropriate to use 10% dextrose if glucose levels are less than 150 mg/dL on 5% dextrose and HCO_3 is not yet greater than 15 to 17 mmol/L, and therefore not yet appropriate to discontinue IV insulin. For acute hypoglycemia, the insulin infusion may be discontinued for 15 min, then the serum glucose rechecked and insulin restarted with a higher concentration of dextrose. If the patient can tolerate oral fluids, 2 to 4 ounces of juice may be given as well.

Transition to Subcutaneous Insulin Regimen

When ketoacidosis is resolved (β-OHB <1 mmol/L and pH >7.3 or bicarbonates >15 mmol/L), the patient is generally ready to eat. Subcutaneous insulin injections can be initiated or resumed based on appetite as well as ability to hold down food. β-OHB monitoring has been shown to help optimize the timing of switch from IV to SC. insulin [50,54].

Fluids

Whereas IV fluids can be continued (aggressive potassium replacement needed or oral fluid intake unpredictable), IV dextrose must be stopped when the insulin infusion is discontinued. IV fluids should be continued until reliable oral intake is established and the serum sodium and potassium concentration normalized.

Diet

Although detailed nutritional guidelines have been proposed, based on age and weight loss preceding DKA, in most cases the patient's appetite is the best guide. Meals, following the ADA Guidelines, usually exclude simple carbohydrates. The authors recommend an ad libitum approach with defined meals or snacks, rather than grazing. The dietary staff should determine the carbohydrate content of each meal and snack (in grams) to help develop insulin-to-carbohydrate ratio for bolus-basal insulin therapy.

Insulin

Insulin drip need not be discontinued until 30 minutes after SC insulin was given to allow sufficient time for absorption. In previously known diabetic patients the usual insulin dose is the starting point, but it often needs to be supplemented with additional rapid-acting insulin, due to insulin resistance secondary to hyperglycemia and decreased activity.

In newly diagnosed patients, the authors generally recommend basal-bolus insulin regimen. Basal insulin (Glargine, Levemir, rarely NPH) usually cover about half of daily insulin requirements with the remainder given as boluses of rapid-acting insulin analogues (Lyspro, Aspart, or glulysin, rarely regular). The total daily insulin dose varies from 0.5 to 1.5 units/kg/d, depending on factors such as age, body mass index, pubertal status, and others that are beyond the scope of this review.

An established patient must have an appointment to see their diabetes care provider in the week after treatment, so that education and changes in therapy can be given to help prevent future similar episodes. A new patient has to immediately begin education in outpatient management of diabetes.

SUMMARY

DKA is the major life-threatening complication of diabetes. DKA is theoretically preventable, but unfortunately still accounts for a large proportion of mortality, morbidity, and hospitalizations in diabetic patients, and contributes significantly to the high costs of diabetes care.

References

[1] Wolfsdorf J, Glaser N, Sperling MA. Diabetic ketoacidosis in infants, children, and adolescents: a consensus statement from the American Diabetes Association. Diabetes Care 2006;29(5):1150–9.

[2] Kitabchi AE, Umpierrez GE, Murphy MB, Kreisberg RA. Hyperglycemic crises in adult patients with diabetes: a consensus statement from the American Diabetes Association. Diabetes Care 2006;29(12):2739–48.

[3] Dunger DB, Sperling MA, Acerini CL, Bohn DJ, Daneman D, Danne TP, et al. ESPE/LWPES consensus statement on diabetic ketoacidosis in children and adolescents. Arch Dis Child 2004;89(2):188–94.

[4] Laffel LM, Wentzell K, Loughlin C, Tovar A, Moltz K, Brink S. Sick day management using blood 3-hydroxybutyrate (3-OHB) compared with urine ketone monitoring reduces hospital visits in young people with T1DM: a randomized clinical trial. Diabet Med 2006;23(3):278–84.

[5] Rewers A, McFann K, Chase HP. Bedside monitoring of blood beta-hydroxybutyrate levels in the management of diabetic ketoacidosis in children. Diabetes Technol Ther 2006;8(6):671–6.

[6] Rewers A, Klingensmith G, Davis C, Petitti DB, Pihoker C, Rodriguez B, et al. Presence of diabetic ketoacidosis at diagnosis of diabetes mellitus in youth: the Search for Diabetes in Youth Study. Pediatrics 2008;121(5):e1258–66.

[7] Levy-Marchal C, Patterson CC, Green A. Geographical variation of presentation at diagnosis of type I diabetes in children: the EURODIAB study. European and Diabetes. Diabetologia 2001;44(Suppl 3):B75–80.

[8] Abdul-Rasoul M, Habib H, Al-Khouly M. "The honeymoon phase" in children with type 1 diabetes mellitus: frequency, duration, and influential factors. Pediatr Diabetes 2006;7(2):101–7.

[9] Rewers A, Chase P, Bothner J, Hamman R, Klingensmith G. Medical care patterns at the onset of type I diabetes in Colorado children, 1978-2001. Diabetes 2003;52(Suppl 1):A62.

[10] Hekkala A, Knip M, Veijola R. Ketoacidosis at diagnosis of type 1 diabetes in children in northern Finland: temporal changes over 20 years. Diabetes Care 2007;30(4):861–6.

[11] Rewers A, Chase HP, Mackenzie T, Walravens P, Roback M, Rewers M, et al. Predictors of acute complications in children with type 1 diabetes. JAMA 2002;287(19):2511–8.

[12] Pinkey JH, Bingley PJ, Sawtell PA, Dunger DB, Gale EA. Presentation and progress of childhood diabetes mellitus: a prospective population-based study. The Bart's-Oxford Study Group. Diabetologia 1994;37(1):70–4.

[13] Likitmaskul S, Santiprabhob J, Sawathiparnich P, Numbenjapon N, Chaichanwatanakul K. Clinical pictures of type 2 diabetes in Thai children and adolescents is highly related to features of metabolic syndrome. J Med Assoc Thai 2005;88(Suppl 8):S169–75.

[14] Levy-Marchal C, Papoz L, de BC, Doutreix J, Froment V, Voirin J, et al. Clinical and laboratory features of type 1 diabetic children at the time of diagnosis. Diabet Med 1992;9(3): 279–84.

[15] Rewers A, Klingensmith G, Davis C, Petitti D, Pihoker C, Rodriguez B, et al. Diabetes ketoacidosis at onset of diabetes: the SEARCH for diabetes in Youth Study [abstract]. Diabetes 2007;54(Suppl 1):A63–4.

[16] Komulainen J, Kulmala P, Savola K, Lounamaa R, Ilonen J, Reijonen H, et al. Clinical, autoimmune, and genetic characteristics of very young children with type 1 diabetes. Childhood Diabetes in Finland (DiMe) Study Group. Diabetes Care 1999;22(12):1950–5.

[17] Mallare JT, Cordice CC, Ryan BA, Carey DE, Kreitzer PM, Frank GR. Identifying risk factors for the development of diabetic ketoacidosis in new onset type 1 diabetes mellitus. Clin Pediatr (Phila) 2003;42(7):591–7.

[18] Levine BS, Anderson BJ, Butler DA, Antisdel JE, Brackett J, Laffel LM. Predictors of glycemic control and short-term adverse outcomes in youth with type 1 diabetes. J Pediatr 2001;139(2):197–203.

[19] Edge JA, Ford-Adams ME, Dunger DB. Causes of death in children with insulin dependent diabetes 1990-96. Arch Dis Child 1999;81(4):318–23.

[20] Edge JA, Hawkins MM, Winter DL, Dunger DB. The risk and outcome of cerebral oedema developing during diabetic ketoacidosis. Arch Dis Child 2001;85(1):16–22.

[21] Glaser N, Barnett P, McCaslin I, Nelson D, Trainor J, Louie J, et al. Risk factors for cerebral edema in children with diabetic ketoacidosis. The Pediatric Emergency Medicine Collaborative Research Committee of the American Academy of Pediatrics. N Engl J Med 2001;344(4):264–9.

[22] Mahoney CP, Vlcek BW, DelAguila M. Risk factors for developing brain herniation during diabetic ketoacidosis. Pediatr Neurol 1999;21(4):721–7.

[23] Glaser NS, Wootton-Gorges SL, Buonocore MH, Marcin JP, Rewers A, Strain J, et al. Frequency of sub-clinical cerebral edema in children with diabetic ketoacidosis. Pediatr Diabetes 2006;7(2):75–80.

[24] Javor KA, Kotsanos JG, McDonald RC, Baron AD, Kesterson JG, Tierney WM. Diabetic ketoacidosis charges relative to medical charges of adult patients with type I diabetes. Diabetes Care 1997;20(3):349–54.

[25] Kim S. Burden of hospitalizations primarily due to uncontrolled diabetes: implications of inadequate primary health care in the United States. Diabetes Care 2007;30(5):1281–2.

[26] Kitabchi AE, Umpierrez GE, Murphy MB, Barrett EJ, Kreisberg RA, Malone JI, et al. Management of hyperglycemic crises in patients with diabetes. Diabetes Care 2001;24(1):131–53.

[27] Maldonado MR, Chong ER, Oehl MA, Balasubramanyam A. Economic impact of diabetic ketoacidosis in a multiethnic indigent population: analysis of costs based on the precipitating cause. Diabetes Care 2003;26(4):1265–9.

[28] Byrne HA, Tieszen KL, Hollis S, Dornan TL, New JP. Evaluation of an electrochemical sensor for measuring blood ketones. Diabetes Care 2000;23(4):500–3.

[29] Wallace TM, Meston NM, Gardner SG, Matthews DR. The hospital and home use of a 30-second hand-held blood ketone meter: guidelines for clinical practice. Diabet Med 2001;18(8):640–5.

[30] Guerci B, Benichou M, Floriot M, Bohme P, Fougnot S, Franck P, et al. Accuracy of an electrochemical sensor for measuring capillary blood ketones by fingerstick samples during metabolic deterioration after continuous subcutaneous insulin infusion interruption in type 1 diabetic patients. Diabetes Care 2003;26(4):1137–41.

[31] Hoffman WH, O'Neill P, Khoury C, Bernstein SS. Service and education for the insulin-dependent child. Diabetes Care 1978;1(5):285–8.

[32] Drozda DJ, Dawson VA, Long DJ, Freson LS, Sperling MA. Assessment of the effect of a comprehensive diabetes management program on hospital admission rates of children with diabetes mellitus. Diabetes Educ 1990;16(5):389–93.

[33] Grey M, Boland EA, Davidson M, Li J, Tamborlane WV. Coping skills training for youth with diabetes mellitus has long-lasting effects on metabolic control and quality of life. J Pediatr 2000;137(1):107–13.

[34] Svoren BM, Butler D, Levine BS, Anderson BJ, Laffel LM. Reducing acute adverse outcomes in youths with type 1 diabetes: a randomized, controlled trial. Pediatrics 2003;112(4): 914–22.

[35] Bui H, To T, Stein R, Fung K, Daneman D. Is diabetic ketoacidosis at disease onset a result of missed diagnosis? J Pediatr 2010;156(3):472–527.

[36] Barker JM, Goehrig SH, Barriga K, Hoffman M, Slover R, Eisenbarth GS, et al. Clinical characteristics of children diagnosed with type 1 diabetes through intensive screening and follow-up. Diabetes Care 2004;27(6):1399–404.

[37] Diabetes Prevention Trial–Type 1 Diabetes Study Group. Effects of insulin in relatives of patients with type 1 diabetes mellitus. N Engl J Med 2002;346(22):1685–91.

[38] Vanelli M, Chiari G, Ghizzoni L, Costi G, Giacalone T, Chiarelli F. Effectiveness of a prevention program for diabetic ketoacidosis in children. An 8-year study in schools and private practices. Diabetes Care 1999;22(1):7–9.

[39] Vanelli M, Chiari G, Lacava S, Iovane B. Campaign for diabetic ketoacidosis prevention still effective 8 years later. Diabetes Care 2007;30(4):e12.

[40] Felner EI, White PC. Improving management of diabetic ketoacidosis in children. Pediatrics 2001;108(3):735–40.

[41] Adrogue HJ, Barrero J, Eknoyan G. Salutary effects of modest fluid replacement in the treatment of adults with diabetic ketoacidosis. Use in patients without extreme volume deficit. JAMA 1989;262(15):2108–13.

[42] Burghen GA, Etteldorf JN, Fisher JN, Kitabchi AQ. Comparison of high-dose and low-dose insulin by continuous intravenous infusion in the treatment of diabetic ketoacidosis in children. Diabetes Care 1980;3(1):15–20.

[43] Kitabchi AE. Low-dose insulin therapy in diabetic ketoacidosis: fact or fiction? Diabetes Metab Rev 1989;5(4):337–63.

[44] Adrogue HJ, Lederer ED, Suki WN, Eknoyan G. Determinants of plasma potassium levels in diabetic ketoacidosis. Medicine (Baltimore) 1986;65(3):163–72.

[45] Bektas F, Eray O, Sari R, Akbas H. Point of care blood ketone testing of diabetic patients in the emergency department. Endocr Res 2004;30(3):395–402.

[46] Ham MR, Okada P, White PC. Bedside ketone determination in diabetic children with hyperglycemia and ketosis in the acute care setting. Pediatr Diabetes 2004;5(1):39–43.

[47] Naunheim R, Jang TJ, Banet G, Richmond A, McGill J. Point-of-care test identifies diabetic ketoacidosis at triage. Acad Emerg Med 2006;13(6):683–5.

[48] Harris S, Ng R, Syed H, Hillson R. Near patient blood ketone measurements and their utility in predicting diabetic ketoacidosis. Diabet Med 2005;22(2):221–4.

[49] Prisco F, Picardi A, Iafusco D, Lorini R, Minicucci L, Martinucci ME, et al. Blood ketone bodies in patients with recent-onset type 1 diabetes (a multicenter study). Pediatr Diabetes 2006;7(4):223–8.

[50] Noyes KJ, Crofton P, Bath LE, Holmes A, Stark L, Oxley CD, et al. Hydroxybutyrate near-patient testing to evaluate a new end-point for intravenous insulin therapy in the treatment of diabetic ketoacidosis in children. Pediatr Diabetes 2007;8(3):150–6.

[51] Vanelli M, Chiari G, Capuano C, Iovane B, Bernardini A, Giacalone T. The direct measurement of 3-beta-hydroxy butyrate enhances the management of diabetic ketoacidosis in children and reduces time and costs of treatment. Diabetes Nutr Metab 2003;16(5–6):312–6.

[52] Muir AB, Quisling RG, Yang MC, Rosenbloom AL. Cerebral edema in childhood diabetic ketoacidosis: natural history, radiographic findings, and early identification. Diabetes Care 2004;27(7):1541–6.

[53] Curtis JR, Bohn D, Daneman D. Use of hypertonic saline in the treatment of cerebral edema in diabetic ketoacidosis (DKA). Pediatr Diabetes 2001;2(4):191–4.

[54] Wallace TM, Matthews DR. Recent advances in the monitoring and management of diabetic ketoacidosis. QJM 2004;97(12):773–80.

[55] Neu A, Willasch A, Ehehalt S, Hub R, Ranke MB. Ketoacidosis at onset of type 1 diabetes mellitus in children—frequency and clinical presentation. Pediatr Diabetes 2003;4(2): 77–81.

[56] Alvi NS, Davies P, Kirk JM, Shaw NJ. Diabetic ketoacidosis in Asian children. Arch Dis Child 2001;85(1):60–1.

[57] Roche EF, Menon A, Gill D, Hoey H. Clinical presentation of type 1 diabetes. Pediatr Diabetes 2005;6(2):75–8.

[58] The Diabetes Control and Complications Trial Research Group. Effect of intensive diabetes treatment on the development and progression of long-term complications in adolescents with insulin- dependent diabetes mellitus: Diabetes Control and Complications Trial. Diabetes Control and Complications Trial Research Group. J Pediatr 1994;125(2):177–88.

[59] Nordfeldt S, Ludvigsson J. Adverse events in intensively treated children and adolescents with type 1 diabetes. Acta Paediatr 1999;88(11):1184–93.

[60] Smith CP, Firth D, Bennett S, Howard C, Chisholm P. Ketoacidosis occurring in newly diagnosed and established diabetic children. Acta Paediatr 1998;87(5):537–41.

[61] Thomsett M, Shield G, Batch J, Cotterill A. How well are we doing? Metabolic control in patients with diabetes. J Paediatr Child Health 1999;35(5):479–82.

Advances in Pediatrics 57 (2010) 269–286

ADVANCES IN PEDIATRICS

ELSEVIER
MOSBY

Coccidioidomycosis

Ziad M. Shehab, MD

Section of Infectious Diseases, Department of Pediatrics, Arizona Health Sciences Center, 1501 North Campbell Avenue, P.O. Box 245073, Tucson, AZ 85724-5073, USA

C occidioidomycosis is an endemic mycosis of the Southwestern United States, Northern Mexico, and parts of Central and South America that is acquired typically by inhalation of arthroconidia of the dimorphic fungus of the genus *Coccidioides*. It is responsible for an estimated 150,000 infections each year in the United States, mostly among inhabitants of or travelers to the arid or semiarid areas of the Southwestern United States and Northern Mexico, where the infection is endemic [1]. The contribution of coccidioidomycosis to respiratory illnesses is underrecognized even in areas of high endemicity [2,3]. With the increase in travel to the Southwest and the migration of people to areas of endemicity, clinicians will likely encounter this infection even outside these areas. Moreover, coccidioidal infections can reactivate in immunosuppressed hosts and thus present with clinical disease long after the individual has first encountered the organism, emphasizing the need to obtain a good travel history to assess the possible risk of infection.

The history of coccidioidomycosis begins in 1892 with the observations of Posadas in Argentina. He described a soldier with coccidioidal granuloma, a lesion thought initially to represent a tumor [4]. The next year, Rixford described a similar patient in California, with many other cases subsequently reported in California [5]. The lesions showed granulomatous inflammation with large multicellular structures initially thought to be from a protozoon, and later recognized to be fungal elements by Ophuls in 1900 [6]. The infection was thought to be rare and generally fatal in nature, and this perception did not change until the observations of Gifford [7].

As the public health officer of Kern County, California, Gifford became interested in a local disease called *San Joaquin fever* that was characterized by pulmonary findings and cutaneous lesions of erythema nodosum, a finding also present in some patients with coccidioidal granulomas. In 1938, Dickson and Gifford recognized that these two manifestations were the result of the same fungal infection [8]. Smith's important epidemiologic studies using skin testing established that coccidioidal infections were widespread in the Central California Valley and that most people who acquired the infection survived,

E-mail address: zshehab@u.arizona.edu

0065-3101/10/$ – see front matter
doi:10.1016/j.yapd.2010.08.008

with disseminated disease being the exception rather than the rule [9]. With his coworkers, he developed diagnostic tools, such as the coccidioidin skin test and serologic assays, and described the epidemiology of coccidioidomycosis, from asymptomatic infection in 60% to disseminated disease in 0.5% [10,11]. The impact of the infection in otherwise healthy individuals is not always benign, as evidenced by the experience of military trainees in the southwestern deserts during World War II [12]. In the 1960s, the introduction of amphotericin B therapy allowed for the treatment of disseminated infections; later the azoles, with miconazole followed by itraconazole and fluconazole, had a major impact on treatment of severe disease and disseminated infections.

Coccidioides is a dimorphic organism with a saprophytic phase in the environment characterized by the formation of mycelial forms, and a parasitic phase when invading tissue. The mycelia can survive in the desert soil for months to years, and multiply rapidly after a rain. During the saprophytic phase, septate branching hyphae develop, and thick-walled arthroconidia are formed along the length of the hyphae. The arthroconidia are separated by empty brittle cells allowing for their easy release into the air through wind or soil disruption.

The size of the arthroconidia (2–8 μm) allows them to reach the alveoli. In the tissues of the mammalian host, the arthroconidia start the parasitic phase of the life cycle. They develop into spherical structures, the spherules, which grow to a size of 10 to 100 μm; acquire a thick wall; and divide internally into hundreds of uninucleated endospores (2–5 μm). On rupture of the spherule, each endospore is then capable of forming a new spherule [13]. Rarely, primary infection can occur through a cutaneous portal.

Based on molecular phylogenetic methods, two species of *Coccidioides* are now recognized as causing clinically indistinguishable diseases and as having distinct geographic distribution. The California isolates have maintained the designation of *C immitis*, whereas *C posadasii* is the species that is prevalent in Arizona, Texas, Mexico, and parts of Central and South America. An overlap does not seem to occur between these endemic areas [14,15]. Outbreaks are not the result of the spread of a single clonal isolate but are caused by various genotypes, suggesting frequent genetic recombination throughout the geographic range of each species [15,16].

EPIDEMIOLOGY

The endemic area for *Coccidioides* spp is limited to the Western Hemisphere between 40° of latitude north and south. In the United States, the areas of endemicity primarily include, in Arizona, the counties of Maricopa, Pinal, and Pima, which include the cities of Phoenix and Tucson, and, in California, the counties of Kern, Tulare, and Fresno. In Mexico, endemic areas include the states of Sonora, Nuevo Leon, Coahuila, and Baja California. Coccidioidomycosis can also be found in certain areas of Argentina, Brazil, Guatemala, Honduras, Nicaragua, Paraguay, and Venezuela. These areas are characterized by arid to semiarid climates with scant rainfall and relatively few freezes.

Climate explains a large proportion of the variability in coccidioidomycosis incidence, with moist conditions allowing multiplication of the organism in the soil, followed by dry conditions leading to spore formation and dispersion under windy conditions. The dominant predictor of coccidioidomycosis in Arizona is the cumulative rainfall in the previous 7 months, average dust index, wind velocity, and severity of the drought [17]. Other factors, including human activities such as land development or biologic processes affecting interactions between *Coccidioides* and other organisms in its environment, seem to be more important in other regions [18]. Primary infections occur most commonly in the summer and fall after the rainy season. The organism can be isolated from soil typically containing an abundance of very fine sand and silt and a dearth of clay. *Coccidioides* spp can usually be found at depths of 2 to 30 cm and tends to be most abundant in rodent burrows and old American Indian ruins. The organism can persist in the soil for up to 40 years. Temperature conditions in this soil are favorable to the growth of the fungus and to decreased competition by other soil organisms [19]. In areas of endemicity, evidence of infection can also be found in various animals, including rodents, dogs, cattle, and sheep. Activities that disrupt the soil, such as archeological excavations, soil digging, and construction, result in localized epidemics [20,21]. Dust storms and earthquake activity are responsible for some epidemics [22,23].

In the United States, 95% of cases of coccidioidomycosis are reported from Arizona and California. Arizona, which reports 60% of all cases, has experienced a substantial increase in coccidioidomycosis, from a rate of 37 per 100,000 population in 1999 to 91 per 100,000 population in 2006. An increase also occurred in California between 2000 and 2006, from a rate of 2.4 to 8.0 per 100,000 population, with the most pronounced increase in the San Joaquin Valley and an associated increase in hospitalizations [24,25].

Susceptibility to primary coccidioidal infection is unaffected by age, sex, and racial background. Because the organism is acquired through the respiratory route, exposure to dust is the paramount risk factor for primary infection. Men are affected more often than women because of occupational exposure. Estimates of infection rates, which are based on the risk of infection in children, have been declining in endemic areas. Infection rates assessed through skin test reactivity have declined from approximately 10% in 1937 through 1939 to 2% in 1959, and to less than 1% thereafter among kindergarten and first-grade students who had lived all of their 5 to 7 years in Kern County, California [26]. In Tucson, Arizona, the annual risk measured through skin test conversion was estimated to be between 2% and 4% in college students [27]. Incidence rates are higher in older male children, in those living in rural areas, during wind storms, and for those with occupational exposure [9,28,29].

In contrast with susceptibility to primary infection, the frequency of dissemination varies considerably, being higher in infants [30–33], Filipinos, and African Americans, who have 10 to 170 times the risk of dissemination of non-Hispanic whites [34,35].

Genetic factors also influence the risk of dissemination, including some human leukocyte antigen (HLA) class II loci and the ABO blood group in Hispanics [36]. Men and pregnant women are more prone to disseminate their infection; sex hormones allow for the rapid maturation of spherules and release of endospores and help explain the sex- and pregnancy-related predisposition to dissemination. Immunosuppressed hosts also are at increased risk for dissemination, particularly in disorders affecting T-cell function, such as those resulting from HIV infection; cancer, and particularly Hodgkin disease; transplantation; and those requiring immunosuppression, including tumor necrosis alpha (TNF-α) inhibitors [36,37]. Half the cases in solid organ transplant recipients result from reactivation of their infection typically in the first year after transplantation. Although dissemination is common, most of these patients present with pulmonary findings [38]. In particular, patients with active coccidioidomycosis and HIV infection whose CD4 counts are lower than 250/μL are at greatly increased risk of developing severe pulmonary disease and disseminated infection [39].

PATHOGENESIS AND PATHOLOGY

Infection with *Coccidioides* spp is typically acquired through the respiratory route, with an inoculum as small as a single spore [40]. Rarely, direct inoculation can occur through puncture of the skin via a contaminated object such as a rock, cotton, hay, or cacti [41,42]. A recent report shows transmission through a bite from a cat with disseminated coccidioidomycosis [43]. In most patients, the infection remains confined to the lungs and hilar nodes. In a minority of patients (<1%), dissemination occurs outside the lungs through the lymphatics or bloodstream.

The initial cellular response consists of a polymorphonuclear cell response possibly related to chemotactic effect of endospores or complement activation by coccidioidal antigens. Tissue necrosis, spherules, and a few mononuclear cells are present at this stage of the disease, but epithelial giant cells are infrequent. The polymorphonuclear leukocytes are not effective at killing the organism at whatever stage of its life cycle, and thus cannot arrest the disease process [41]. Dendritic cells are recruited next from the peripheral circulation and are potent antigen presenting cells. Killing has been shown with natural killer cells and mononuclear leukocytes. Several studies have shown the importance of T cells in controlling the infection as measured through delayed cutaneous hypersensitivity. Skin test responses correlate well with other measures of peripheral blood lymphocyte responsiveness, such as lymphocyte transformation and cytokine production [44].

In normal hosts, the Th1 response is ultimately responsible for controlling the infection. T cells are induced to produce interferon-γ and other cytokines, with recruitment and activation of immune effector cells. As the disease progresses, cell-mediated immune defenses become defective, possibly from antigen overload, suppressor cells, immune complexes, or fungal immunosuppressive substances, resulting in an ineffective response by type 2 helper cells [45].

Recently, a primary immunodeficiency, interferon-γ receptor 1 deficiency was associated with disseminated coccidioidomycosis. This observation and the absence of reports of severe coccidioidomycosis in patients with genetic deficiencies affecting T-cell lymphocytes, such as severe combined immunodeficiency, suggest that the interleukin 12/interferon-γ axis, rather than the T cell per se, determines susceptibility to *Coccidioides* spp [46].

Disseminated coccidioidomycosis occurs relatively early, typically in the first weeks to months after initial infection. Reactivation leading to dissemination can occur later, especially in patients who are immunocompromised [38] or have HIV [39]. Dissemination typically involves the bones, meninges, lymph nodes, or soft tissues.

The pathology of fatal coccidioidomycosis indicates that the tissue reaction is mostly granulomatous and can be accompanied by elements of acute inflammation. The lesions contain abundant giant cells and histiocytes. Caseous necrosis is common, and spherules are often seen lying freely or within macrophages. Calcification is infrequent. Patients with AIDS have a higher burden of organisms and poor formation of granulomas [47].

The literature on coccidioidomycosis in young infants and children is relatively scant. Almost all cases in the first few months of life are acquired through the respiratory route and typically associated with heavy exposure to dust [32]. Most of these reported cases result in severe disease [30–32], but primary infections and even dissemination can go unrecognized [48].

Although women who acquire coccidioidal infections late in pregnancy are at increased risk of dissemination [49,50], their newborns, with few exceptions, are born without evidence of infection even when the placenta is involved [48]. In the few infants with apparent perinatal transmission, the mothers had coccidioidal endometritis, and the likely source of infection was inhaled or ingested amniotic fluid [51]. However, placental infection does not necessarily imply fetal or neonatal infection [48].

Although dissemination of coccidioidomycosis is frequent in immunosuppressed individuals with T-cell defects who have resided in endemic areas, specific immunologic deficits in other high-risk populations, such as Filipinos, have not been elucidated. Patients with disseminated disease frequently show evidence of impaired cell-mediated immunity [45,52], especially when extensive disease is involved. Patients with disseminated disease often have a lack of response to skin test antigens without having generalized anergy. Their responses to in vitro stimulation of their lymphocytes to coccidioidal antigens are depressed [45]. Patients with disseminated disease who have a positive coccidioidal skin test also exhibit responses to lymphocyte stimulation that are comparable to those of healthy individuals who have recovered from primary infection. A return of specific and nonspecific cell-mediated immunity can be seen in individuals recovered from severe disseminated disease [52]. Children with coccidioidomycosis are thought to have responses similar to those reported in adults, but their immunologic responses have not been well characterized.

CLINICAL MANIFESTATIONS
Primary Infections
Primary coccidioidal infections are asymptomatic or may manifest as a mild upper respiratory tract infection in 60% of immunocompetent individuals. A flu-like illness lasting 1 to 2 days occurs in another 25%, and the remainder have more significant lower respiratory tract disease, including pneumonia that may be lobar, pleural effusions, or, occasionally, pericarditis [40]. When exposure to dust is more intense, such as during heavy military exercises, the attack rate and proportion of symptomatic infections may be high [34]. The disease may present like bacterial pneumonia or sepsis [53,54]. In endemic areas such as Tucson and Phoenix, Arizona, up to 29% of individuals presenting with community acquired pneumonia have evidence of coccidioidal infection when serologic studies are used routinely [2,3]. However, only 2% to 13% of ambulatory patients with community-acquired pneumonia get tested for coccidioidomycosis, even in endemic areas [55]. The more common presentation is that of a subacute pneumonia, which is self-limited. Some patients will develop more complicated pulmonary infections and even extrapulmonary disease. These patients are more likely to be unrecognized, especially in areas that are not endemic for coccidioidomycosis, leading to delays in diagnosis and extensive work-ups if the possibility of coccidioidomycosis is not considered [56].

The usual incubation period is 10 to 16 days but may range from less than 1 week to a month. Among young adults, 77% will present with fatigue, 64% with cough, 53% with chest pain, and 17% with dyspnea. Fever occurs in 56%, whereas headaches, myalgias, and arthralgias are present in 22% each [57]. The chest pain is often pleuritic and can be severe, and may be followed by vague symptoms of chest pain that can persist for months [40]. In infants, stridor may be a symptom of primary infection of subglottic tissues or the epiglottis [58,59].

Two types of rashes are observed in coccidioidomycosis: 1) reactive rashes that contain no live organism, such as erythema nodosum, erythema multiforme, generalized rashes, Sweet syndrome, and reactive interstitial granulomatous dermatitis, and 2) lesions in which the organism is found in the cutaneous tissues on biopsy and that result from hematogenous dissemination to the skin. Reactive rashes are common in symptomatic children [28,42].

Erythema nodosum is the most characteristic reactive cutaneous lesion of coccidioidomycosis. It presents typically as erythematous, painful, tender lesions usually on the lower extremities that appear 1 to 3 weeks after the onset of illness. It is four times more common in adult women than men, but this difference is not observed in children [9]. It is infrequent in African Americans, Hispanics, and Filipinos.

Erythema nodosum is associated with a vigorous immune response, and these patients are at lower risk for disseminated disease. Erythema multiforme–like lesions can also be seen early in the course of the infection, and are more common in children. An acute exanthem, *toxic erythema*, is also described with acute coccidioidomycosis and presents early, typically preceding or occurring within 48 hours of the onset of symptoms. The lesions can be macular, papular, urticarial, morbilliform, or target-like; may be pruritic; last for several weeks, and are sometimes followed by palmar desquamation. Rare cases of Sweet syndrome and interstitial granulomatous dermatitis have also been reported [42]. These reactive skin manifestations may occur in diseases such as group A ß-hemolytic streptococcal infections, tuberculosis, histoplasmosis, and inflammatory bowel disease, but their presence in an endemic area almost always signifies coccidioidomycosis.

Acute coccidioidomycosis can also be associated with arthralgias or arthritis, hence the name *desert rheumatism*. These findings are generally transient and do not signify dissemination, and it is presumed that spherules are not present in the joint.

Primary cutaneous coccidioidomycosis is rare. Most cases are reported in laboratory workers, but some have been reported in children [41]. The lesion occurs at a site of skin trauma and develops 1 to 3 weeks after the initial inoculation. It is usually accompanied by regional lymphadenitis. The process resolves spontaneously over 2 to 3 months. In children, progressive and prolonged infection may occur and may require antifungal therapy [41,42].

The radiologic findings of primary coccidioidomycosis are nonspecific [41,60,61]. Bronchopneumonia, often with hilar adenopathy, is the most common finding; segmental or lobar infiltrates and nodular or patchy infiltrates can also occur. Pleural effusions occur in up to 15% of hospitalized patients and are usually sterile [62,63]. The radiographic changes resolve in 90% to 95% of symptomatic patients and typically do not require antifungal therapy, although the resolution can be slow in some. Nodules, cavities, bronchiectasis and calcification may be residua from pulmonary infiltrates [64]. The cavities are thin-walled and asymptomatic, and often resolve spontaneously but, rarely, lead to the development of an empyema or pyopneumothorax, which are more likely to occur in immunosuppressed hosts or those with diabetes. Nodules and cavities that are typically single, well-circumscribed, and less than 6 cm in diameter occur in 5% of patients with coccidioidal pneumonia. A miliary pattern is sometimes seen, typically in immunocompromised individuals such as those with AIDS, and suggests hematogenous dissemination [65]. Endobronchial or endotracheal lesions can sometimes be seen on endoscopy [66].

In neonates, focal consolidation and diffuse nodular densities associated with nonspecific symptoms and minimal clinical evidence of lower respiratory infection can be seen but are not specific for coccidioidomycosis at this age [66,67].

DISSEMINATED INFECTIONS
Skin Disease
Cutaneous dissemination may begin several weeks to a month after the initial infection and occurs through hematogenous spread from the lungs. The rash may consist of papules, nodules, verrucous plaques, abscesses, pustules, and sinus tracts. They may be single or multiple and may remain chronic after

other manifestations of coccidioidomycosis have resolved. Verrucous granuloma at the nasolabial fold is the most common form of disseminated cutaneous disease. The lesions may mimic those caused by other endemic mycoses, tuberculosis, actinomycetes, or syphilis [42].

BONE AND JOINT DISEASE

Bone involvement occurs through hematogenous spread and is often multifocal, with 20% involving two bones, 10% three bones, and another 10% four or more bones. The bones most frequently involved are the tibia, vertebrae, skull, metatarsals, and metacarpals. The infection results in chronic osteomyelitis, which often drains in the soft tissues and may form fistulae to the overlying skin [68–70]. Radiologically, the lesions are lytic.

Vertebral osteomyelitis can involve all parts of the vertebra, with relative sparing of the disk. Spread of vertebral infection leading to meningitis or paravertebral infection is a serious concern. Coccidioidal arthritis can have a waxing and waning course and typically involves large joints. It may also result from direct inoculation of the joint, such as with a cactus spine, or may be associated with adjacent osteomyelitis [71].

MENINGITIS

Central nervous system involvement occurs through lymphohematogenous spread from the lungs, and presents soon after to up to 6 months after pulmonary infection. It may be part of widespread dissemination or may be the only manifestation of disseminated coccidioidal infection [72–74]. The most common presenting symptom is that of headache, which may manifest early with a picture of aseptic meningitis, or a few weeks to a few months later, when the headache is typically the result of hydrocephalus. Other common symptoms are sluggishness, ataxia, vomiting, and altered mental status. Meningeal signs are often absent, and the patient may present with focal neurologic deficits, most commonly cranial nerve palsies, as a result of basilar involvement of the meninges and the granulomatous nature of the infection. Parenchymal and spinal cord abscesses can also occur [75,76]. Vasculitis may be manifested by infarction and stroke-like presentations, which may be abrupt in onset [76,77]. The cerebrospinal fluid (CSF) shows a mononuclear cell pleocytosis, usually 100 to 500 cells/mm [3], with a range of few cells to greater than 10,000, with an elevated protein level and a somewhat decreased glucose level [74,78].

Early on, polymorphonuclear cell predominance is not unusual. The presence of eosinophils in the CSF suggests the diagnosis of coccidioidal meningitis but is of no prognostic significance. The spinal fluid findings differ depending on the source of CSF sampled. The findings tend to be most accentuated in the lumbar fluid and milder in the cisternal and ventricular CSF. Before the availability of amphotericin B, coccidioidal meningitis was uniformly fatal within 2 years, and the average survival of children was only 5.5 months. Death from coccidioidal meningitis is now a rare event and mostly associated with vascular complications or severe hydrocephalus [79]. Meningitis can be a potentially devastating complication during pregnancy [73].

COCCIDIOIDOMYCOSIS IN PREGNANCY

Early studies show that pregnant women who acquire coccidioidomycosis are at high risk of dissemination and death, especially when the disease occurs in the third trimester. More recent population-based studies indicate that coccidioidal infections are not frequent during pregnancy but are still associated with a significant rate of complications, especially when acquired during the third trimester or soon after delivery [38]. The risk of dissemination varies widely among different studies, but all point to an increased rate of dissemination compared with the general population. The increase observed during the third trimester is presumed to be the result of pregnancy-induced immunosuppression and high hormonal levels, which have been shown in vitro to stimulate the growth and maturation of spherules. The presence of erythema nodosum is associated with a lower risk of dissemination [51,80].

COCCIDIOIDOMYCOSIS IN THE IMMUNOCOMPROMISED HOST

Disease in the immunocompromised host can result from primary infection or reactivation of an old infection. The highest risk for morbidity and mortality is in patients with decreased T-cell function. For recipients of solid organ transplants, the highest risk is in the first year after transplantation, but they remain at risk for reactivation later, albeit at a lower level. The risk is increased for those with a recent history of coccidioidomycosis or those with a positive serology at transplantation. Dissemination occurs in 75% of these individuals and their mortality is high (29%). Multifocal disease is common. These patients are more likely to experience progression, especially when undergoing immunosuppressive regimens to combat acute rejection or with the chronic use of high-dose corticosteroids because of their effect on the development of host cell-mediated immune responses. If at all possible, coccidioidomycosis must be controlled by chemotherapy long before the transplant occurs. Donor-derived coccidioidomycosis has rarely been documented [38].

The clinical presentation of coccidioidomycosis in patients with AIDS has changed dramatically since the introduction of highly active antiretroviral therapy (HAART). In the 1980s in Tucson, 25% of a cohort of patients followed over 3.5 years developed coccidioidomycosis [81]. Among these patients, symptomatic disease was associated with a CD4 count of less than 250 cells/μL and the diagnosis of AIDS, and only half of the cases reported were from endemic areas. Patients in endemic areas typically present with primary infection, whereas those in nonendemic areas tend to experience reactivation of old infection [39].

A dramatic decrease in the incidence of symptomatic disease with the advent of HAART was shown in Southern Arizona [82]. The disease frequently presented with severe pneumonia and diffuse "reticulonodular" infiltrates on chest radiograph, findings that were associated with a high mortality. Primary coccidioidal infection in individuals with HIV now presents in a manner similar to that in patients without HIV infection most commonly with community acquired pneumonia involving cough, fever, and a focal pulmonary infiltrate. Patients may present with coccidioidal seropositivity without evidence of clinical disease, and these patients are more likely to have a normal CD4 count and undetectable viral loads. In a recent report, Masannat and Ampel [39,82] show that the incidence of symptomatic coccidioidomycosis has decreased significantly over the past decade. Severity of coccidioidomycosis was inversely related to CD4 counts and overall treatment and control of HIV infection.

DIAGNOSIS

Coccidioidal pneumonia is underdiagnosed even in areas of endemicity [2,3]. The diagnosis is made in endemic areas by having a high index of suspicion for the disease and by obtaining the appropriate diagnostic studies. In nonendemic areas, obtaining an appropriate travel history is critical for diagnosis. Respiratory infection may present in a manner similar to community-acquired pneumonias such as bacterial, viral, or mycoplasmal pneumonia; pulmonary tuberculosis; or fungal pneumonia such as Histoplasma, and may result from a very brief exposure in an endemic area [24].

HEMATOLOGIC FINDINGS

Hematologic findings in primary coccidioidal pneumonia are nonspecific and may include leukocytosis, eosinophilia, and an elevated erythrocyte sedimentation rate [13]. Eosinophilia is common and marked eosinophilia may indicate dissemination [83]. The diagnosis is established through serologic studies, cultures, and histology.

SEROLOGY

The serologic response may consist of IgM or IgG antibodies but may be absent in immunocompromised patients. The IgM antibody, also known as *tube precipitin* (TP) is present in 50% of patients after 1 week and in 90% of patients after 3 weeks from onset of symptoms. This antibody resolves rapidly, with only 10% of patients with uncomplicated infection yielding a positive serology after 5 months [84]. IgM has been recognized occasionally in the cord blood of newborns whose mothers had detectable antibody, but these newborns did not exhibit any evidence of disease [85]. The IgG antibody, also known as complement fixation (CF) antibody, presents later, becoming positive at 2 to 28 weeks, and can remain positive for 6 to 8 months. It is more commonly detected in symptomatic patients and is present in 50% to 90% of individuals by 3 months after onset of symptoms.

An IgM or IgG response is demonstrable in 90% of patients with symptomatic infection [13,85]. The magnitude of the IgG antibody response correlates with the severity of infection and the likelihood of dissemination [86]. Titers of 1:32 or greater correlate with extrapulmonary infection and are present in 61% of these patients, compared with fewer than 5% of those without dissemination.

Serology alone is not sufficient to support the diagnosis of disseminated coccidioidomycosis. Some patients with severe pulmonary disease or pleural disease can develop high titers, whereas patients with dissemination, especially to single sites, or those with hematogenous spread of infection often have lower titers [13,71]. Patients with HIV infection can have extensive disease with low or undetectable antibody titers, as can bone marrow transplant recipients. Conversely, some patients will remain seropositive without evidence of disease [40,85].

The serologic assays are performed using one of three techniques: enzyme immunoassay (EIA), immunodiffusion (ID), or complement fixation (CF). The CF test has been important in the understanding of coccidioidal epidemiology, but it is difficult to perform and is now rarely used because of the better sensitivity of the ID and EIA assays. An EIA is available for the detection of IgG and IgM and is rapid and more sensitive than ID or CF, but is not quantitative. However, the IgM assay can yield false-positives and must be confirmed if the clinical picture is not compatible. In a recent study, Blair and Currier [87] did not observe any false-positive IgM anticoccidioidal serologies in a series of 706 EIAs, of which 28 had isolated IgM seropositivity. The ID assay requires 3 days before negative tests can be reported, but can be made into a quantitative assay. The value of serologic assays of the pleural or synovial fluid is not established.

Coccidioidal meningitis is diagnosed based on a positive CSF serology or culture. The serology can be positive also because of an adjacent vertebral osteomyelitis or epidural abscess. In a serologic evaluation of patients with coccidioidal meningitis, serology was positive in 82%, with 83% of the patients having a positive EIA, 71% a positive ID, and only 56% a positive CF. Although a positive test is helpful in establishing the diagnosis, a negative test does not rule out coccidioidomycosis [13].

ANTIGEN DETECTION

Recently, antigenuria was detected by a Histoplasma EIA [88]. A Coccidioides EIA, which detects coccidioidal galactomannan, has since been described with an improved sensitivity of 71% in patients with more severe forms of coccidioidomycosis [89]. The role of this assay remains to be determined.

SKIN TESTING

Intradermal skin testing with coccidioidin or with spherulin has been used as an epidemiologic tool. However, these antigens have not been commercially available for the past decade.

CULTURE AND ISOLATION

Coccidioides spp can be grown on various media, including routine bacteriologic, fungal, or *Legionella* media. Specimens likely to contain other organisms should be plated on selective media because the organism competes poorly with other bacteria and fungi. Growth is usually apparent in 4 to 5 days. The colonies are white buff but may have various colors as they age. The typical initial description of the colony is that of a nonpigmented mold. Confirmation at the genus level is achieved through the use of a molecular genetic probe. Identification at the species level is not phenotypically possible, and molecular methods that are not generally available are needed to separate *C immitis* from *C posadasii*. The yield of coccidioidal organisms on specimens submitted for fungal culture is highest for respiratory tract specimens (8.3%) and lowest for blood cultures (0.4%), in which it is associated with severe disease. CSF cultures also have a low yield (0.9%) [13].

Arthroconidia can easily be aerosolized and cause a hazard to the laboratory worker. Biosafety Level 2 practices are required for handling these agents, and *Coccidioides* spp is considered to be a select agent of bioterrorism by the United States.

HISTOPATHOLOGY

Identification of endospore-containing spherules in infected material is diagnostic of coccidioidomycosis. This evaluation can performed using a potassium hydroxide (KOH) smear, a fluorescent calcofluor white (CFW) stain, or histopathologic stains with Grocott's methenamine silver (GMS), hematoxylin and eosin (H&E), or periodic acid Schiff (PAS) stains. The CFW stain has the best sensitivity, with 22% of specimens resulting in a positive culture, whereas the GMS stain is the most sensitive in histopathologic preparations. Spherules containing endospores are seen in giant cells and microabscesses. Mycelia may occasionally be seen in the CSF, especially in patients with a drainage tube such as a ventriculoperitoneal shunt, in skin lesions, and in the lung at the boundaries of old cavitary lesions. Molecular probes for detecting organisms in clinical specimens and polymerase chain reaction assays are not available for diagnosing coccidioidomycosis [13].

Except for in individuals with primary cutaneous disease, identification of spherules outside the pulmonary cavity indicates disseminated disease and biopsies may be very useful, especially in individuals whose complement fixation titer is borderline or negative.

TREATMENT
Primary Infection
Coccidioidomycosis is a self-limited illness in more than 90% of children. In a few of these children, antifungal therapy may be indicated to alleviate the severity of the infection or help prevent dissemination in those with elevated coccidioidal antibody titers. Selection of patients for therapy of primary uncomplicated infection remains controversial. In adults, approximately one-half of patients with symptomatic primary pulmonary coccidioidomycosis were treated with antifungal therapy largely based on clinical severity [90]. Severe infection in adults is usually associated with weight loss of more than 10%, night sweats lasting longer than 3 weeks, bilateral pulmonary infiltrates or infiltrates that

encompass more than one-half of one lung, prominent or persistent hilar adenopathy, a CF titer of greater than 1:16, inability to work, or symptoms that last more than 2 months [1]. These data are not available in children.

Pregnant women and women who acquire their primary coccidioidal infection soon after delivery are at high risk of severe disease and should be considered for treatment. Treatment of pregnant women should be with amphotericin B because of the teratogenic effects of fluconazole and possibly the other azoles [91]. Persons of Filipino or African American ancestry should also be considered for treatment because of their increased risk of dissemination.

The course of therapy generally lasts 3 to 6 months. Bilateral reticulonodular infiltrates or miliary patterns on chest radiograph suggest underlying immunosuppression or a high inoculum size and are an indication for therapy. These patients are typically treated with amphotericin B if hypoxia is present or clinical deterioration is rapid. In general, amphotericin B yields a faster response than azoles in severely ill patients [1]. An azole can then be substituted a few weeks later as the patient is convalescing. Therapy should be continued for at least 1 year, followed by secondary prophylaxis. Immunosuppressed patients, such as those with AIDS, who have undergone organ transplantation, taking high-dose steroids, or receiving tumor necrosis factor (TNF)-α inhibitors, are considered to warrant antifungal therapy. Similarly, therapy should also be considered in those who are likely to handle coccidioidal infections less well, such as those with diabetes or cardiovascular conditions [1]. Stable pulmonary solitary nodules do not require antifungal therapy, and asymptomatic pulmonary cavities typically do not either. These cavities usually have a benign course and evidence of benefit of therapy is lacking. If the cavity persists for more than 2 years, is enlarging, or is subpleural in location, resection can be considered to obviate later complications.

Therapy with azoles should be considered for patients with chest discomfort, superinfection, or hemoptysis. Alternatively, surgical resection of the cavity can be considered for those with recurrent problems. Pyopneumothorax results from rupture of a cavity in the pleural space and is best treated with decortications and lobectomy. For patients with coexisting diseases such as diabetes, the approach often includes antifungal therapy in addition to surgical approaches. Treatment of this form of disease is surgical with or without adjunctive antifungal therapy. Treatment options for those with a poor or slow response involve a switch to a different azole, the use of an azole at a higher dose, or the use of amphotericin B [1].

Patients with fibrocavitary disease are typically treated with an azole for at least 1 year. Surgical resections may be beneficial in refractory lesions or cases of severe hemoptysis [1].

Disseminated Infection
Nonmeningeal dissemination
Therapy is usually initiated with an azole, typically fluconazole or itraconazole. In adults, the dose used in clinical trials has been 400 mg/d for either drug.

Recently, some experts have advocated the use of much higher doses, such as up to 2000 mg/d of fluconazole or 800 mg/d of itraconazole. Lipid amphotericin B formulations are commonly used but have not been studied in coccidioidal disease. Combination therapy with an azole and amphotericin B has not been studied and concerns exist about the possibility of antagonism. In the only comparative study of itraconazole and fluconazole, itraconazole showed a trend for higher activity, especially in skeletal infections. This benefit must be weighed against its higher cost, dietary restrictions, and erratic bioavailability of itraconazole in children. Surgery should be considered for large or enlarging abscesses, bony sequestration, instability of the spine, or impingement on critical organs or tissues [1].

Meningitis

Fluconazole is the preferred therapy for coccidioidal meningitis. It is typically initiated at a dose of 12 mg/kg/d. The dose that has been studied in adults is 400 mg/d, although some experts would start at a dose of 15 to 23 mg/kg/d in children and 800 to 1200 mg/d in adults [73]. Therapy is continued for a lifetime because of the high rate of relapse among patients treated with azoles [92]. Amphotericin B has been associated with a significant improvement in survival but is associated with significant side effects, and its intrathecal administration can be complicated by headache, nausea, vomiting, chills and fever, arachnoiditis, and sometimes paralysis, seizures, and coma. The symptoms of arachnoiditis can be similar to those of relapse.

The role of voriconazole and posaconazole remains to be defined. A few case reports suggest the efficacy of voriconazole in patients with disseminated coccidioidomycosis, including meningitis, who have been switched to voriconazole because of toxicity or intolerance of other drugs or by physician choice [93]. Posaconazole, which is structurally related to itraconazole, has had good results in a murine model of coccidioidomycosis, and small nonrandomized clinical trials suggest that it may be useful in patients for whom azole therapy failed [94].

Prevention

Prevention of coccidioidomycosis relies primarily on limiting exposure, such as through environmental dust abatement programs. Vaccines that would boost cell-mediated immune responses are desirable. A trial of killed spherule vaccine has been inconclusive. Multiple candidate vaccines are being evaluated in animal models and seem to be promising. Recombinant peptides, synthetic peptides, and adjuvants such as recombinant interleukin-12 are being investigated as possible vaccines [52].

References

[1] Galgiani JN, Ampel NM, Blair JE, et al. Coccidioidomycosis. Clin Infect Dis 2005;41: 1217–23.
[2] Valdivia L, Nix D, Wright M, et al. Coccidioidomycosis as a common cause of community-acquired pneumonia. Emerg Infect Dis 2006;12:958–62.

[3] Kim MM, Blair JE, Carey EJ, et al. Coccidioidal pneumonia, Phoenix, Arizona, USA, 2000–2004. Emerg Infect Dis 2009;15(3):397–401.

[4] Posadas A. Un Nuevo caso de micosis fungoidea con posrospemias. An Cir Med Argent 1892;15:585–97.

[5] Rixford E, Gilchrist TC. Two cases of protozoan (coccidioidal) infection of the skin and other organs. Johns Hopkins Hosp Rep 1896;10:209–68.

[6] Ophüls W, Moffitt HC. A new pathogenic mould formerly described as a protozoan (Coccidioides immitis pyogenes): preliminary report. Philadelphia Med J 1900;5:1471–2.

[7] Gifford MA, Buss WC, Douds RJ. Annual report: Kern County Department of Public Health for the fiscal year July 1, 1936 to June 30, 1937. Kern County Department of Public Health 1937:47–52.

[8] Dickson EC, Gifford MA. Coccidioides infection (coccidioidomycosis). ii. The primary type of infection. Arch Intern Med 1938;62:853–71.

[9] Smith CE. Epidemiology of acute coccidioidomycosis with erythema nodosum ("San Joaquin" or "Valley Fever". Am J Public Health 1940;30:600–11.

[10] Galgiani JN. Coccidioidomycosis: changing perceptions and creating opportunities for its control. Ann N Y Acad Sci 2007;1111:1–18.

[11] Hirschmann JV. The early history of coccidioidomycosis: 1892–1945. Clin Infect Dis 2007;44:1202–7.

[12] Crum-Cianflone NF. Coccidioidomycosis in the U.S. Military: a review. Ann N Y Acad Sci 2007;1111:112–21.

[13] Saubolle MA, McKellar PP, Sussland D. Epidemiologic, clinical, and diagnostic aspect of coccidioidomycosis. J Clin Microbiol 2007;45(1):26–30.

[14] Fisher M, Koenig G, White T, et al. Molecular and phenotypic description of Coccidioides posadasii sp. nov. previously recognized as the non-California population of Coccidioides immitis. Mycol Soc Am 2002;94:73–84.

[15] Barker BM, Jewell KA, Kroken S, et al. The population biology of Coccidioides. Epidemiologic implications for disease outbreak. Ann N Y Acad Sci 2007;1111:147–63.

[16] Fisher M, Koenig G, White T, et al. Pathogenic clones versus environmentally driven population increase: analysis of an epidemic of the human fungal pathogen Coccidioides immitis. J Clin Microbiol 2000;38(2):807–13.

[17] Comrie AC, Glueck MF. Assessment of climate-coccidioidomycosis model: model sensitivity for assessing climatologic effects on the risk of acquiring coccidioidomycosis. Ann N Y Acad Sci 2007;1111:83–95.

[18] Talamantes J, Behseta S, Zender CS. Fluctuations in climate and incidence of coccidioidomycosis in Kern County, California—a review. Ann N Y Acad Sci 2007;1111:73–82.

[19] Fisher FS, Bultman MW, Johnson SM, et al. Coccidioides niches and habitat parameters in the southwestern United States—a matter of scale. Ann N Y Acad Sci 2007;1111:47–72.

[20] Winn WA, Levine HB, Broderick JE, et al. A localized epidemic of coccidioidal infection: Primary coccidioidomycosis occurring in a group of ten children infected in a backyard playground in the S Joaquin Valley of California. N Engl J Med 1963;268:867–70.

[21] Centers for Disease Control and Prevention. Coccidioidomycosis in workers at an archeological site—Dinosaur National Monument, Utah, June–July 2001. MMWR 2001;50:1005–8.

[22] Smith CE, Beard RR, Rosenberger HG, et al. Effect of season and dust control on coccidioidomycosis. JAMA 1946;132:833–8.

[23] Centers for Disease Control and Prevention. Coccidioidomycosis following the Northridge Earthquake–California, 1994. MMWR 1994;43:164–5.

[24] Sunenshine RH, Anderson S, Erhart L, et al. Public Health surveillance for coccidioidomycosis in Arizona. Ann N Y Acad Sci 2007;1111:96–102.

[25] Centers for Disease Control and Prevention. Increase in coccidioidomycosis—California 2000–2007. MMWR 2009;58(5):105–9.

[26] Larwood TR. Coccidioidin skin testing in Kern County, California: decrease in infection rate over 58 years. Clin Infect Dis 2000;30:612–3.
[27] Kerrick SS, Lundergan LL, Galgiani JN. Coccidioidomycosis at a university health service. Am Rev Respir Dis 1985;131:100–2.
[28] Richardson HB Jr, Anderson JA, McKay BM. Acute pulmonary coccidioidomycosis in children. J Pediatr 1967;70:376–82.
[29] Roberts PL, Lisciandro RC. A community epidemic of coccidioidomycosis. Am Rev Respir Dis 1967;96:766–72.
[30] Cohen R. Coccidioidomycosis: case studies in children. Arch Pediatr 1949;66:241–65.
[31] Christian JR, Sarre SG, Peers JH, et al. Pulmonary coccidioidomycosis in a twenty-one-day-old infant. Am J Dis Child 1956;92:66–73.
[32] Hyatt HW Sr. Coccidioidomycosis in a 3-week-old infant. Am J Dis Child 1963;105:93–8.
[33] Sievers ML. Disseminated coccidioidomycosis among southwestern American Indians. Am Rev Respir Dis 1974;109:602–12.
[34] Crum NF, Lederman ER, Stafford CM, et al. Coccidioidomycosis: a descriptive survey of a re-emerging disease. Clinical characteristics and emerging controversies. Medicine (Baltimore) 2004;83:149–75.
[35] Louie L, Ng R, Hajjeh R, et al. Influence of host genetic factors on the severity of coccidioidomycosis. Emerg Infect Dis 1999;5:672–80.
[36] Bergstrom L, Yocum DE, Ampel NM, et al. Increased risk of coccidioidomycosis in patients treated with tumor necrosis factor α antagonists. Arthritis Rheum 2004;50:1959–66.
[37] Mertz LE, Blair JE. Coccidioidomycosis in rheumatology patients. Incidence and potential risk factors. Ann N Y Acad Sci 2007;1111:343–57.
[38] Blair JE. Coccidioidomycosis in patients who have undergone transplantation. Ann N Y Acad Sci 2007;1111:365–76.
[39] Ampel NM. Coccidioidomycosis in persons infected with HIV type 1. Clin Infect Dis 2005;41:1174–8.
[40] Galgiani JN. Coccidioidomycosis. West J Med 1993;159:153–71.
[41] O'Brien JJ, Gilsdorf JR. Primary cutaneous coccidioidomycosis in childhood. Pediatr Infect Dis 1986;5:485–6.
[42] DiCaudo DJ. Coccidioidomycosis: a review and update. J Am Acad Dermatol 2006;55:929–42.
[43] Gaidici A, Saubolle MA. Transmission of coccidioidomycosis to a human via a cat bite. J Clin Microbiol 2009;47(2):505–6.
[44] Ampel NM, Bejarano GC, Salas SD, et al. In vitro assessment of cellular immunity in human coccidioidomycosis: relationship between dermal hypersensitivity, lymphocyte transformation, and lymphokine production by peripheral blood mononuclear cells from healthy adults. J Infect Dis 1992;165:710–5.
[45] Cox RA, Magee MM. Coccidioidomycosis: host response and vaccine development. Clin Microbiol Rev 2004;17:804–39.
[46] Vinh DC, Masannat F, Dzioba RB, et al. Refractory disseminated coccidioidomycosis and mycobacteriosis in interferon-γ receptor 1 deficiency. Clin Infect Dis 2009;49:e62–5.
[47] Graham AR, Sobonya RE, Bronnimann DA, et al. Quantitative pathology of coccidioidomycosis in acquired immunodeficiency syndrome. Hum Pathol 1988;19:800–6.
[48] Arnold CA, Rakheja D, Arnold MA, et al. Unsuspected, disseminated coccidioidomycosis without maternofetal morbidity diagnosed by placental examination: case report and review of the literature. Clin Infect Dis 2008;48:e119–23.
[49] Wack EE, Ampel NM, Galgiani JN, et al. Coccidioidomycosis during pregnancy: an analysis of ten cases among 47,120 pregnancies. Chest 1988;94:376–9.
[50] Crum NF, Ballon-Landa G. Coccidioidomycosis in pregnancy: case report and review of the literature. Am J Med 2006;199:e11–7.
[51] Spinello IM, Johnson RH, Baqi S. Coccidioidomycosis and pregnancy—a review. Ann N Y Acad Sci 2007;1111:358–64.

[52] Ampel NM. The complex immunology of human coccidioidomycosis. Ann N Y Acad Sci 2007;1111:245–58.

[53] Lopez AM, Williams PL, Ampel NM. Acute pulmonary coccidioidomycosis mimicking bacterial pneumonia and septic shock: a report of two cases. Am J Med 1993;95:236–9.

[54] Arsura AL, Bellinghausen PL, Kilgore WB, et al. Septic shock in coccidioidomycosis. Crit Care Med 1998;26:62–5.

[55] Chang DC, Anderson S, Wannemuehler K, et al. Testing for coccidioidomycosis among patients with community-acquired pneumonia. Emerg Infect Dis 2008;14(7):1053–9.

[56] Desai SA, Minai OA, Gordon SM, et al. Coccidioidomycosis in non-endemic areas: a case series. Respir Med 2001;95:305–9.

[57] Tom PF, Long TJ, Fitzpatrick SB. Coccidioidomycosis in adolescents presenting as chest pain. J Adolesc Health Care 1987;8:365–71.

[58] Gardner S, Seilheimer D, Catlin F, et al. Subglottic coccidioidomycosis presenting with persistent stridor. Pediatrics 1980;66:623–5.

[59] Hajare S, Rakusan TA, Kalia A, et al. Laryngeal coccidioidomycosis causing airway obstruction. Pediatr Infect Dis 1989;8:54–6.

[60] Child DC, Newell JD, Bjelland JC, et al. Radiographic findings of pulmonary coccidioidomycosis in neonates and infants. Am J Roentgenol 1985;145:261–3.

[61] Greendyke WH, Resnick DL, Harvey WC. The varied roentgen manifestations of primary coccidioidomycosis. Am J Roentgenol Radium Ther Nucl Med 1970;109:491–9.

[62] Lonky SA, Catanzaro A, Moser KM, et al. Acute coccidioidal pleural effusion. Am Rev Respir Dis 1976;114:681–8.

[63] Merchant M, Romero AO, Libke RD, et al. Pleural effusion in hospitalized patients with coccidioidomycosis. Respir Med 2008;102:537–40.

[64] Birsner JW. The roentgen aspects of five hundred cases of pulmonary coccidioidomycosis. Am J Roentgenol Radium Ther Nucl Med 1954;72:556–73.

[65] Arsura EL, Kilgore WB. Miliary coccidioidomycosis in the immunocompetent. Chest 2000;117:404–9.

[66] Polesky A, Kirsch CM, Snyder LS, et al. Airway coccidioidomycosis—report of cases and review. Clin Infect Dis 1999;28:1273–80.

[67] Bernstein DI, Tipton JR, Schott PF, et al. Coccidioidomycosis in a neonate: maternal-infant transmission. J Pediatr 1981;99:752–4.

[68] Bisla RS, Taber TH Jr. Coccidioidomycosis of bone and joints. Clin Orthop 1976;121:196–204.

[69] Deresinski SC. Coccidioidomycosis of bone and joints. In: Stevens DA, editor. Coccidioidomycosis: a text. New York: Plenum Medical; 1980. p. 195–224.

[70] Dennis JL, Hansen AE. Coccidioidomycosis in children. Pediatrics 1954;14:481–94.

[71] Adam RD, Elliott SP, Tojlanovic MS. The spectrum and presentation of disseminated coccidioidomycosis. Am J Med 2009;122:770–7.

[72] Bouza E, Dreyer JS, Hewitt WL, et al. Coccidioidal meningitis: an analysis of thirty-one cases and review of the literature. Medicine 1981;60:139–72.

[73] Johnson RH, Einstein HE. Coccidioidal meningitis. Clin Infect Dis 2006;42:103–7.

[74] Shehab ZM, Britton H, Dunn JH. Imidazole therapy of coccidioidal meningitis in children. Pediatr Infect Dis J 1988;7:40–4.

[75] Mischel PS, Vinters HV. Coccidioidomycosis of the central nervous system: neuropathological and vasculopathic manifestations and clinical correlates. Clin Infect Dis 1995;20:400–5.

[76] Erly WK, Bellon RJ, Seeger JF, et al. MR imaging of acute coccidioidal meningitis. Am J Neuroradiol 1999;20:509–14.

[77] Williams PL, Johnson R, Pappagianis D, et al. Vasculitic and encephalitic complications associated with *Coccidioides immitis* infection of the central nervous system in humans: report of 10 cases and review. Clin Infect Dis 1992;14:673–82.

[78] Caudill RG, Smith CE, Reinarz JA. Coccidioidal meningitis: a diagnostic challenge. Am J Med 1970;49:360–5.

[79] Arsura EL, Johnson R, Penrose J, et al. Neuroimaging as a guide to predict outcome for patients with coccidioidal meningitis. Clin Infect Dis 2005;40:624–7.

[80] Arsura EL, Kilgore WB, Ratnayake SN. Erythema nodosum in pregnant patients with coccidioidomycosis. Clin Infect Dis 1998;27:1201–3.

[81] Bronnimann D, Adam RD, Galgiani JN, et al. Coccidioidomycosis in the acquired immunodeficiency syndrome. Ann Intern Med 1987;106:372–9.

[82] Masannat FY, Ampel NM. Coccidioidomycosis in patients with HIV-1 infection in the era of potent antiretroviral therapy. Clin Infect Dis 2010;50:1–7.

[83] Harley WB, Blaser MJ. Disseminated coccidioidomycosis associated with extreme eosinophilia. Clin Infect Dis 1994;18:627–9.

[84] Smith CE, Saito MT, Simons SA. Pattern of 39,500 serologic tests in coccidioidomycosis. JAMA 1956;160:546–52.

[85] Pappagianis D, Zimmer DL. Serology of coccidioidomycosis. Clin Microbiol Rev 1990;3:247–68.

[86] Smith CE, Saito MT, Beard RR, et al. Serological tests in the diagnosis and prognosis of coccidioidomycosis. Am J Hyg 1950;52:1–21.

[87] Blair JE, Currier JT. Significance of isolated positive IgM serologic results by enzyme immunoassay for coccidioidomycosis. Mycopathologia 2008;166:77–82.

[88] Kuberski T, Myers R, Wheat LJ, et al. Diagnosis of coccidioidomycosis using cross reaction with a Histoplasma antigen. Clin Infect Dis 2007;44:e50–4.

[89] Durkin M, Connolly P, Kuberski T, et al. Diagnosis of coccidioidomycosis with use of the Coccidioides antigen immunoassay. Clin Infect Dis 2008;47:e69–73.

[90] Ampel NM, Giblin A, Mourani JP, et al. Factors and outcomes associated with the decision to treat primary pulmonary coccidioidomycosis. Clin Infect Dis 2009;48:172–8.

[91] Aleck KA, Bartley DL. Multiple malformations syndrome following fluconazole use in pregnancy: report of an additional patient. Am J Med Genet 1997;72:253–6.

[92] Dewsnup DH, Galgiani JN, Graybill JR, et al. Is it ever safe to stop azole therapy for Coccidioides immitis meningitis? Ann Intern Med 1996;124:305–10.

[93] Freifeld A, Proia L, Andres D, et al. Voriconazole use for endemic fungal infections. Antimicrobial Agents Chemother 2009;53(4):1648–51.

[94] Ampel NM. Coccidioidomycosis: a review of recent advances. Clin Chest Med 2009;30:241–51.

Advances in Pediatrics 57 (2010) 287–294

ADVANCES IN PEDIATRICS

Advances in the Care and Treatment of Children with Hemophilia

Marilyn J. Manco-Johnson, MD

Department of Pediatrics, Hemophilia and Thrombosis Center, The Children's Hospital, University of Colorado Denver, Building 500, 13001 East, 17th Place, Room WG109, Anschutz Medical Campus, Aurora, CO 80045-0507, USA

H emophilia A and B are rare bleeding disorders caused by genetic deficiencies in plasma clotting factors VIII and IX, respectively. With the availability of virus-inactivated recombinant and plasma derived coagulation factor concentrates, life expectancy for children affected with these severe chronic disorders has increased from early adolescence a century ago to essentially normal today. Over the past 10 years, rapid advances have been made in the care of children with hemophilia. These advances can be attributed to the establishment of national patient databases, translational research, derivation of evidence from specific pediatric randomized clinical trials, and translation of molecular engineering from the bench to the clinic.

NATIONAL DATABASES
The development of national databases has been essential to aggregating observations that provide information about the natural history of hemophilia and predictors of outcomes. Owing to the low prevalence and phenotypic heterogeneity of hemophilia, advances in knowledge from single-center studies are limited. The US Centers for Disease Control and Prevention (CDC) first conducted a pilot 6-state surveillance study of hemophilia outcomes from 1993 to 1995, which determined reduced mortality rates ($P = .002$) in persons receiving care from the federally funded network of specialized clinics dedicated to multidisciplinary comprehensive care of hemophilia [1]. Based on the success of this demonstration project, the CDC initiated a prospective national data collection project for hemophilia called the Universal Data Collection (UDC) Study in 1997. This database now includes up to 13 years of annual data entered on a cohort of 24,000 patients with congenital bleeding disorders, including more than 17,000 persons with hemophilia [2]. The UDC database has recently published data on the presentation of hemophilia in a cohort of

E-mail address: marilyn.manco-johnson@ucdenver.edu

0065-3101/10/$ – see front matter
doi:10.1016/j.yapd.2010.08.007

more than 404 newborns and children, as shown in Table 1 [3]. In the US cohort, most newborns were diagnosed in the first month of life and the sites of hemorrhage included circumcision, head bleeds (of which half were intracranial) and heel sticks. Infants presenting beyond the first 6 months of life primarily manifest head injuries (with only 8% being intracranial) and mouth and joint bleeding. This prospective database has generated invaluable data on complications in persons with rare congenital bleeding disorders, including bleeding symptoms, inhibitor formation, and joint limitation of motion [4–6].

European registries have also contributed to the understanding of the natural history of hemophilia. The Italian Association of Hemophilia Centers recently reported mortality rates and life expectancy in their cohort of 443 persons with hemophilia who died between 1990 and 2007. In the cohort data between 2000 and 2007, after excluding mortality related to hepatitis C and AIDS, the life expectancy of persons with hemophilia overlapped that of the general population [7].

The presence of inhibitors is one of the most difficult and costly complications of hemophilia. Approximately 25% of persons with severe factor VIII deficiency develop inhibitory IgG antibodies after exposure to replacement therapy with factor VIII; the rate of antibody formation against factor IX is lower at 1% to 4%. Many of these inhibitors are low titer or transient and do not generally cause major long-term morbidity. However, 10% of children with severe factor VIII deficiency develop persistent high-titer antibodies that limit the ability to replace factor VIII. Children with high-titer inhibitors develop poorly controlled hemorrhages that result in crippling arthropathy at a young age and a higher rate of life- and limb-threatening hemorrhages and hospitalizations. Recent discoveries have helped elucidate the mystery of inhibitor development in hemophilia. Predisposition to inhibitor formation has been related to the type of gene mutation, with large deletions, gene inversions, and nonsense mutations conveying a high risk for inhibitor formation and small deletions or insertions as well as missense mutations predicting a low inhibitor risk [8]. The location of missense mutation also influences inhibitor risk. Missense mutations affecting molecular sites that are critical for protein interactions convey a higher inhibitor risk than similar mutations in more neutral regions of the factor VIII molecule. A recent publication described 2 nonsynonymous single nucleotide polymorphisms in the factor VIII gene of African Americans, which differ from the predominant genotype in whites from whom recombinant factor VIII and most plasma donations have been derived [9]. This minimal molecular difference could explain the higher rate of inhibitor formation in African American children after the infusion of factor VIII. In addition to factor VIII mutation, polymorphisms related to cytokines that regulate the immune response have been associated with inhibitor risk [10]. Environmental factors also influence inhibitor formation. In the CANAL (Concerted Action on Neutralizing Antibodies in severe hemophilia A) study, including 366 consecutively born infants with severe hemophilia A from the Netherlands, early factor VIII exposure of high dose and duration and surgery

Table 1
Sites of first bleeding event by hemophilia type and severity

	Hemophilia type			Hemophilia severity		
	All N = 404[a]	A N = 331	B N = 73	Severe N = 265	Moderate N = 91	Mild N = 47
Sites of first bleed (%)						
Circumcision	27.4	28.4	23.2	23.5	34	37.8
Head (Percentage of Intracranial[b])	19.0 (36.4)	17.2 (38.6)	27.3 (30.0)	19.4 (46.2)	16.5 (6.7)	20 (33.3)
Oral mucosa	9.6	7.9	17.7	8.6	11	13.3
Joint	6.2	6.6	4.0	6.4	7.7	2.2
Heel stick	5.9	7.0	1.2	7.8	2.2	2.2
IM injection	4.0	3.6	5.3	4.5	4.4	0
Soft tissue	6.9	7.0	6.7	7.8	5.5	4.4
Venipuncture	2.5	2.4	2.6	2.6	3.3	0
Other	11.4	12.7	5.3	11.6	11	11.2
Unknown	7.1	7.2	6.7	7.8	4.4	8.9

Abbreviations: IM, intramuscular; N, number of participants.

[a] Age at first bleed was unknown for 10 infants with a bleed.

[b] Percentage of infants whose initial bleeding site was a head bleed.

Data from Kulkarni R, Soucie JM, Lusher J, et al. Sites of initial bleeding episodes, mode of delivery and age of diagnosis in babies with haemophilia diagnosed before the age of 2 years: a report from The Centers for Disease Control and Prevention's (CDC) Universal Data Collection (UDC) project. Haemophilia 2009;15:1281–90.

as the indication for first treatment were significantly associated with clinically relevant inhibitor formation, as shown in Table 2 [11]. In contrast, early administration of regular preventive infusions of factor VIII, known as prophylaxis, showed a trend toward decreased inhibitor risk. A validated inhibitor risk score derived from the CANAL cohort study improved a priori risk stratification for early inhibitor formation [12]. Although these data need to be confirmed in a larger prospective clinical trial, the implications of such findings would be to use conservative doses of factor VIII for replacement when needed, to avoid elective surgery, and to prevent severe bleeding episodes that require longer-duration replacement by providing early prophylaxis.

Inclusion of Children in Randomized Clinical Trials

Until recently, the pediatric age has been a general exclusion criterion from participation in human research, and children with hemophilia suffered from the lack of specific pediatric data. Observational data from Malmo, Sweden, indicated that prophylaxis with moderate dose (ie, 25–35 IU/kg) frequent (every other day to thrice weekly) infusions of factor VIII to maintain a trough of factor VIII plasma activity of greater than or equal to 1% was successful in the prevention of joint damage in young children with severe hemophilia. This treatment regimen requires 3000 to 6000 units per kilogram per year of factor VIII replacement at a conservative cost of US $1 per unit. In a recent clinical trial in the United States, 65 children younger than 30 months of age were randomized to either 25 U/kg of recombinant factor VIII given every other day by intravenous infusion or treatment with recombinant factor VIII (using liberal dosing) only at the time of clinically apparent bleeding events [13]. All children underwent normal joint imaging by magnetic resonance imaging and plain radiography as eligibility criteria for study entry. The primary end point was maintenance of normal bone and cartilage in all 6 index joints (both elbows, knees, and ankles) tested by the same imaging techniques at study exit at age 6 years. In this randomized clinical trial, bone and cartilage were preserved in all 6 index joints in 93% of children receiving prophylaxis in comparison to 55% treated at the time of joint hemorrhage (Table 3) [13]. Based on this level I evidence, prophylaxis was established as the treatment of choice for all children with hemophilia, with recommendations for starting

Table 2
Environmental risk factors for high-titer inhibitor development

Risk factor	Adjusted RR (95% CI)	P value
Dose greater than 50 IU/kg	3.0 (1.3–6.9)	.01
Duration at first treatment episode 5 d or more	4.1 (2.4–7.0)	<.0001
Surgical procedure as an indication for first treatment	3.2 (1.6–6.7)	.002
Regular prophylaxis	0.5 (0.2–1.0)	.05

Abbreviations: CI, confidence interval; RR, relative risk.
Data from Gouw SC, van der Bom JG, van den Berg HM. Treatment-related risk factors of inhibitor development in previously untreated patients with hemophilia A: the CANAL cohort. Blood 2007;109:4648–54.

Table 3
Primary results from the joint outcome study

Variable	Prophylaxis (N = 32)	Enhanced episodic therapy (N = 33)	P value
MRI findings			
Number of participants with primary outcome data	27	29	.73
Number of participants with joint damage	2 (7%)	13 (45%)	.002
Number of participants without joint damage	25 (93)	16 (55)	
Radiographic findings			
Number of participants with primary outcome data	28	27	.73
Number of participants with joint damage	1 (4%)	5 (19%)	.10
Number of participants without joint damage	27 (96%)	22 (81%)	
Number of days in study			.95
Mean	1497	1490	
Total	47,895	49,179	
Reported number of factor VIII infusions			<.001
Mean	653 ± 246	187 ± 100	
Total	20,896	6176	
Reported number of factor VIII units infused			<.001
Mean	352,793 ± 150,454	113,237 ± 65,494	
Total	11,289,372	3,736,807	
Joint hemorrhages (number/participant/y)			<.001
Mean	0.63 ± 1.35	4.89 ± 3.57	
Median	0.20	4.35	
Total hemorrhages (number/participant/y)			<.001
Mean	3.27 ± 6.24	17.69 ± 9.25	
Median	1.15	17.13	

Plus-minus values are means ± SD. The data on magnetic resonance imaging and radiographic findings include interim-analysis data for children who were removed from the study because of early joint failure.

Abbreviation: MRI, magnetic resonance imaging.

Data from Manco-Johnson MJ, Abshire TC, Shapiro AD, et al. Recombinant factor VIII for the prevention of joint disease in children with severe hemophilia: prophylaxis compared with episodic treatment. N Engl J Med 2007;357:535–44.

therapy before the onset of recurrent joint hemorrhage. However, 80% of children with hemophilia, worldwide, have little or no access to replacement factor VIII, and the World Health Organization lists this replacement factor as a priority for hemophilia care in developing countries.

A second randomized clinical trial of hemophilia therapies, specifically for children, is the international Sippet Study, which is currently enrolling subjects [14]. Based on uncontrolled observational studies, it was reported that inhibitor risk appeared decreased in patients treated with factor VIII in combination with the von Willebrand factor (vWF), as found in some plasma-derived products [15]. The role of the vWF in the stabilization of factor VIII in plasma has been well characterized. In the absence of vWF, the plasma half-life of factor VIII decreases from 12 to 2 hours, and patients with severe (type 3) von Willebrand disease generally manifest plasma levels of factor VIII less than or equal to 5% of the normal level. A murine model of hemophilia as well as in vitro experiments support decreased immunogenicity of factor VIII when preincubated with vWF [15,16].

Newer Treatment Products

A remaining limitation to the implementation of preventive therapies for young children with hemophilia, besides cost, is the need for relatively frequent intravenous infusions. Proteins, including factors VIII and IX, are degraded by stomach acid and digestive enzymes and have not been produced in a form that is amenable to absorption after oral administration. Factor VIII is a large molecule (molecular weight [MW] approximately 200 kDa) and is not absorbed from subcutaneous injection sites. Factor IX is a moderate-sized protein (MW approximately 56 kDa); subcutaneous factor IX is absorbed into the blood stream but with an approximately 5% efficiency. The half-life of factors VIII and IX are decreased in infants and young children younger than 6 years owing to an age-related increased volume of distribution and accelerated plasma clearance. Maintenance of a small amount of clotting protein activity in the plasma requires infusions of factor VIII every 2 to 3 days and infusions of factor IX every 2 to 4 days. Frequent peripheral venipuncture is difficult in young children, and the chronic use of indwelling venous access devices in children with hemophilia is fraught with problems [17]. For these reasons, the care for children with hemophilia would be greatly advanced with the availability of a longer-acting preparation of replacement protein.

Recently, multiple approaches have been taken to increase the effective halflife of factors VIII and IX after infusion. One approach has been to noncovalently associate factor VIII with liposomes conjugated with polyethylene glycol. In a phase I/II study of a product that is under development by Bayer HealthCare (Leverkusen, Germany), adults experienced cessation of spontaneous bleeding for 10 to 13 days after an infusion of commercial, recombinant, fulllength factor VIII after incubation with pegylated liposomes [18]. Animal and in vitro studies determined prolonged association of factor VIII with pegylated liposomes on the surfaces of platelets and monocytes, although the apparent plasma half-life was not prolonged [19,20]. A phase III study constructed to show the noninferiority of once-weekly prophylaxis with the novel product compared with the thrice-weekly prophylaxis with native recombinant factor VIII is in process [21]. This trial is a landmark in the quest to improve factor VIII replacement therapy. Using another approach, directly pegylated liposomes have been shown to bind noncovalently but with high affinity to the external liposome surface and to prolong the plasma survival of factor VIII [22]. A similar pegylation technique has been applied to prolong the circulatory half-life and hemostatic effects of recombinant activated factor VII, a bypassing agent used to treat bleeding events in persons with hemophilia and inhibitory antibodies [23]. Other designer coagulation proteins are being developed by fusion with plasma proteins that are known to prolong circulating half-life. A fusion molecule of factor IX with a monomeric Fc fragment increases functional half-life up to 4-fold than the native factor IX protein [24]. The type of molecular engineering typified by these examples is likely to revolutionize the treatment of patients with genetic bleeding disorders.

SUMMARY

Hemophilia is advancing rapidly on many fronts. Improvements in therapies and outcomes can be attributed to innovations in research methodologies ranging from inclusion of children in randomized clinical trials, creative design of registries, and clinical/translational studies, to molecular engineering and large-scale expression of modified recombinant proteins. Although the future therapeutic landscape of hemophilia cannot be precisely predicted, continued improvement in medical outcomes, acceptable treatment schedules, and patient quality of life are likely outcomes.

References

[1] Soucie JM, Nuss R, Evatt B, et al. Mortality among males with hemophilia: relations with source of medical care. Blood 2000;96:437–42.

[2] Available at: www.cdc.gov/ncbddd/hbd/hemophilia.htm. Accessed March 9, 2010.

[3] Kulkarni R, Soucie JM, Lusher J, et al. Sites of initial bleeding episodes, mode of delivery and age of diagnosis in babies with haemophilia diagnosed before the age of 2 years: a report from The Centers for Disease Control and Prevention's (CDC) Universal Data Collection (UDC) project. Haemophilia 2009;15:1281–90.

[4] Metjian AD, Wang C, Sood SL, et al. Bleeding symptoms and laboratory correlation in patients with severe von Willebrand disease. Haemophilia 2009;15:918–25.

[5] Kempton CL, Soucie JM, Abshire TC. Incidence of inhibitors in a cohort of 838 males with hemophilia A previously treated with factor VIII concentrates. J Thromb Haemost 2006;4: 2576–81.

[6] Soucie JM, Cianfrini C, Janco RL, et al. Joint range-of-motion limitations among young males with hemophilia: prevalence and risk factors. Blood 2004;103:2467–73.

[7] Tagliaferri A, Rivolta GF, Iorio A, et al. Mortality and causes of death in Italian persons with haemophilia, 1990–2007. Haemophilia 2010;16:437–46.

[8] Gouw SC, van den Berg HM. The multifactorial etiology of inhibitor development in hemophilia: genetics and environment. Semin Thromb Hemost 2009;35:723–34.

[9] Viel K, Ameri A, Abshire TC, et al. Inhibitors of factor VIII in black patients with hemophilia. N Engl J Med 2009;360:1618–27.

[10] Pavlova A, Delev D, LaCroix-Desmazes S, et al. Impact of polymorphisms of the major histo-compatibility complex class II, interleukin-10, tumor necrosis factor-α and cytotoxic T-lymphocyte antigen-4 genes on inhibitor development in severe hemophilia A. J Thromb Haemost 2009;7:2006–15.

[11] Gouw SC, van der Bom JG, van den Berg HM. Treatment-related risk factors of inhibitor development in previously untreated patients with hemophilia A: the CANAL cohort. Blood 2007;109:4648–54.

[12] Ter Avest PC, Fischer K, Mancuso ME, et al. Risk stratification for inhibitor development at first treatment for severe hemophilia A: a tool for clinical practice. J Thromb Haemost 2008;6:2048–54.

[13] Manco-Johnson MJ, Abshire TC, Shapiro AD, et al. Recombinant factor VIII for the prevention of joint disease in children with severe hemophilia: prophylaxis compared with episodic treatment. N Engl J Med 2007;357:535–44.

[14] Mannucci PM, Gringeri A, Peyvandi F, et al. Factor VIII products and inhibitor development: the SIPPET study (survey of inhibitors in plasma-product exposed toddlers). Haemophilia 2007;13:65–8.

[15] Kaveri S, Gringeri A, Heisel-Kurth M, et al. Inhibitors in haemophilia A: the role of VWF/ FVIII concentrates. Haemophilia 2009;15:587–91.

[16] Delignat S, Dasgupta S, André S, et al. Comparison of the immunogenicity of different therapeutic preparations of human factor VIII in the murine model of hemophilia A. Haematologica 2007;15:587–91.

[17] Ewenstein BM, Valentino LA, Jouneycake JM, et al. Consensus recommendations for use of central venous devices in haemophilia. Haemophilia 2004;10:1–20.

[18] Spira J, Plyushch OP, Andreeva TA, et al. Prolonged bleeding-free period following prophylactic infusion of recombinant factor VIII reconstituted with pegylated liposomes. Blood 2006;108:3668–73.

[19] Pan J, Liu T, Kim JY, et al. Enhanced efficacy of recombinant FVIII in noncovalent complex with PEGylated liposome in hemophilia A mice. Thromb Haemost 2009;114:2802–11.

[20] Jeon JY, Hwang SY, Cho SH, et al. Effect of cholesterol content on affinity and stability of factor VIII and annexin V binding to a liposomal bilayer membrane. Chem Phys Lipids 2010;163:335–40.

[21] DiMinno G, Cerbone AM, Coppola A, et al. Longer-acting factor VIII to overcome limitations in haemophilia management: the PEGylated liposomes formulation issue. Haemophilia 2010;16(Suppl 1):2–6.

[22] Yatuv R, Dayan I, Carmel-Goren L, et al. Enhancement of factor VIIa haemostatic efficacy by formulation with PEGylated liposomes. Haemophilia 2008;(14):476–83.

[23] Mei B, Pan C, Jiang H, et al. Rational design of a fully active, long-acting PEGylated factor VIII for hemophilia A treatment. Blood 2010;116:270–9.

[24] Peters RT, Low SC, Kamphaus GD, et al. Prolonged activity of factor IX as a monomeric Fc fusion protein. Blood 2010;115:2057–64.

Advances in Pediatrics 57 (2010) 295–313

ADVANCES IN PEDIATRICS

ELSEVIER
MOSBY

Bridging Mental Health and Medical Care in Underserved Pediatric Populations: Three Integrative Models

Arturo Brito, MD, MPH[a], Adrian J. Khaw, MD[b],
Gladys Campa, LMHC[b], Anai Cuadra, PhD[b],
Sharon Joseph, MD[c,d], Lourdes Rigual-Lynch, PhD[c,d],
Alina Olteanu, MD, PhD[e], Alan Shapiro, MD[c,d],
Roy Grant, MA[a],*

[a]Children's Health Fund, 215 West 125th Street, New York, NY 10027, USA
[b]University of Miami Miller School of Medicine, Department of Pediatrics, Miami, FL 33101, USA
[c]Children's Hospital at Montefiore Medical Center, Bronx, New York, NY 10467, USA
[d]Albert Einstein College of Medicine, Department of Pediatrics, New York, NY 10461, USA
[e]Section of Community Pediatrics and Global Health, Department of Pediatrics, Tulane University
School of Medicine, New Orleans, LA 70112, USA

I n pediatric primary care, the term mental health should be taken to include child and family psychosocial needs across a wide spectrum. Mental illness therefore includes developmental, behavioral, emotional, and cognitive dysfunction. Quantifying the number of children with a mental illness can be challenging. Even within a narrow definition limited to psychiatric disorders, there is wide variation in prevalence estimates because of differing methodologies and criteria used (eg, screening or clinical diagnosis, different screening instruments, who makes the diagnoses and whether diagnoses are ascertained by chart review or parent report, and whether diagnoses reflect current symptoms or a prior lifetime diagnosis). A published review of 52 articles found prevalence estimates ranging from 1% to 51%, with a median of 18% [1]. The most frequently cited prevalence rate for child and adolescent psychiatric disorders is 20%, from the Surgeon General's mental health report (1999) [2]. This figure, derived from a federal survey that only included children and youths 9 to 17 years of age, indicates that at least 8.4 million children have a diagnosable psychiatric condition, including 4.3 million with a disability (ie, a condition that impairs daily functioning at home, school, and community), of whom an estimated 2 million have severe functional impairments [3].

Although this number of children with psychiatric illness is impressive, it does not include diagnosed preschool-age children or young children who

*Corresponding author. E-mail address: rgrant@chfund.org

0065-3101/10/$ – see front matter
doi:10.1016/j.yapd.2010.08.001

developmentally do not meet criteria for a psychiatric diagnosis despite atypical social-emotional functioning. Pediatric primary care providers (PCPs) are in the ideal position to identify and begin the process of managing mental health illness early in its course. However, pediatric PCPs often lack the necessary tools and means to do so consistently and effectively. Often PCPs work within systems that themselves may be barriers. Moreover, pediatric PCPs providing care to the medically underserved confront even greater challenges to meeting their patients' needs because these populations generally have higher rates of mental illness and even fewer community resources compared with the general pediatric population. An enhanced medical home has previously been described as a means to address these often complex needs of the medically underserved [4]. This model includes an integrative approach to care between medical and mental health providers.

This article discusses integrative pediatric and mental health care, differentiating it from other types of collaborative care, and provides 3 examples of how this integrative model is currently being applied to 3 distinct medically underserved populations of the country: homeless children in New York City, immigrant children in South Florida, and children affected by Hurricane Katrina in New Orleans. These 3 populations are currently being served by programs supported by Children's Health Fund (CHF), a national nonprofit organization focused on medically underserved pediatric populations and their families through the use of innovative strategies to deliver that care, most notably the use of mobile clinics.

THE ROLE OF THE PEDIATRIC PCP

In pediatrics, the term mental health may be used to encompass the range of psychosocial issues presented in primary care, such as emotional and behavioral problems, developmental delay, and problems families have coping with their circumstances, including poverty [5]. There has been a trend toward an increased level of psychosocial need presented by pediatric primary care patients, with the rate tripling between 1979 and 1996 [6]. The role of the pediatric PCP has evolved accordingly to include a greater emphasis on identification of child and family needs [7], ongoing developmental surveillance and screening [8], and the identification and management of mental health problems [9].

However, success with the early identification of mental health needs in the primary care setting has fallen short. Federal data show that, in 2007, only 2.5% of infants and toddlers who were age eligible for an Early Intervention (EI) program received services [10]. EI programs provide services for developmental delays, including social-emotional problems, as well as disorders for infants and toddlers from birth to 36 months of age, at no cost or low cost to families. However, federal survey data from the Early Childhood Longitudinal Study, Birth Cohort, indicate that 13% of toddlers aged 9 to 24 months have delays that should make them eligible for EI services [11].

This suggests a failure to identify and treat early developmental delays in the primary care setting. Data from various sources show that children are not routinely screened for developmental problems in primary care using any type of standardized, evidence-based instruments. However, when formal screening is carried out, it is often targeted toward children who are already suspected of having a delay [12,13].

There has been a dramatic increase in the availability of standardized screening instruments for use in primary care designed to identify young children with social-emotional problems. These instruments can be used in combination with a first-level developmental surveillance or screening tool to identify young children at risk of developmental problems, with the social-emotional screening instrument used based on risk [14]. Screening for developmental delay and referring for EI services may also contribute to primary prevention of behavioral and emotional problems of childhood, because developmental delays place the child at heightened risk of later psychiatric disorders [15]. For instance, 3-year-old children with developmental delays are up to 4 times more likely than young children without delays to show signs of a behavior problem (based on a standardized measure, the Child Behavior Checklist). These behavior problems increase parental stress, which further heightens the child's risk of emotional problems [16]. National Health Interview Survey data show that 18% of school-age children (5–17 years old) have a functional deficit that affects their learning (sensory, motor, cognitive, or emotional/behavioral). The highest percentage (10%) had a reported emotional or behavioral problem [17,18]. Depression is a serious psychiatric disorder that is increasingly prevalent among adolescents. Lifetime prevalence for adolescent depression is as high as 20% [19].

HIGH-RISK POPULATIONS

Mental illness prevalence rates are notably higher in high-risk populations [20]. Children in homeless families have a higher rate of acute and chronic illness and psychosocial problems compared with other pediatric populations, and often do not have a regular source of care [21]. In one study of homeless school-age children, more than half (57%) had current symptoms consistent with clinically diagnosed depression [22]. Children in homeless families are exposed to more stress than low-income children in community housing, as well as more interruptions of their school placement because of their transient housing situation. This profile is consistent with homeless children also showing a higher rate of behavior problems [23]. Often their needs are not identified in a timely fashion and, as such, they do not receive necessary services. In a study of children and youths in Los Angeles homeless shelters, nearly half (45%) had learning problems consistent with special education placement, and most had never received any needed services [24].

Compared with other low-income families, domestic violence is more common among homeless families (35% vs 16% in 1 study) [25]. Mothers in homeless family shelters show high rates of depression and of trauma-related psychiatric disorders including posttraumatic stress disorder [26]. In comparing the mental status of homeless mothers in 2003 with those in shelters a decade previously, investigators found that the prevalence of these conditions had increased [27]. In another study of homeless children in New York City shelters, about one-third (34%) had been exposed to domestic violence and 30% of children and youths from 12 months to 19 years of age had a diagnosed psychiatric or developmental disorder. Virtually none of these children and youths received any intervention before becoming patients of a comprehensive health care for the homeless program, the New York Children's Health Project (NYCHP) [28].

Latino children, especially if poor and/or not born in the United States, often have difficulty accessing health care. They are often uninsured even when eligible for a public insurance program such as Medicaid [29,30]. Financial access barriers may be exacerbated by immigration, cultural, language, and geographic issues [31]. Transportation may also be a significant barrier to care for children living in rural communities [32]. Immigrant children of parents without documented citizenship are 5 times more likely than other children to lack a usual source of care, and are also more likely to be in poor health than other children [33]. Access to mental health care is even more problematic [34]. Studies have found that 60% to nearly 80% of Latino children with mental health problems do not access needed care [35].

Multiple data sources show that children exposed to a disaster have increased rates of mental health problems, and that these problems persist for years after the event. For example, after Hurricane Andrew in South Florida in 1992, high rates of posttraumatic stress symptoms were found among school-age children nearly 2 years later [36]. Three weeks after the terror attacks of 9/11/01 in New York City, survey data show that 36% of children citywide were reported by their parents as having 3 or more new signs of psychological distress. Two years after this disaster, nearly 1 in every 4 children (23%) continued to show multiple signs of distress. The highest rates were in the city's lowest income boroughs and among African American and Hispanic children. A related study of available postdisaster mental health services found that services were least available in these high-risk communities where mental health care need was greatest [37].

In the aftermath of Hurricane Katrina in New Orleans, a disaster in which the most affected community was poor and predominantly African American, persistent mental health needs were found among children and families, many of whom had protracted periods of displacement from home following evacuation from the flooded city. A prospective longitudinal study of displaced children and families in shelters found that nearly half of parents reported that their child had a new psychiatric symptom 6 months after the hurricane [38]. This rate did not substantially abate 2 years after the disaster, and increased levels of hurricane-related mental health disability and poor academic performance continued to be reported by parents 3 years after the disaster [39].

MENTAL HEALTH SERVICE GAPS

Overall, only an estimated 1 in every 4 children in need of mental health services gets the necessary interventions [20], with at least 6.5 million remaining unserved [2,40]. The problem of unmet mental health need is even greater for preschool-age children [41]. This lack of service reflects the long-standing shortage of child and adolescent mental health professionals. After the Surgeon General's report, former President Bush's New Freedom Commission on Mental Health confirmed the inadequate supply of child and adolescent mental health professionals [42]. To illustrate this shortage, in Florida in 2001, there were only 255 child psychiatrists for a child and adolescent population (birth to 17 years of age) of 3.6 million. Before Hurricane Katrina made landfall in Louisiana, there were 81 child psychiatrists for a population of 1.2 million children and adolescents. Overall, mental health professionals are poorly distributed, with the greatest shortages found in low-income inner-city urban and rural communities, where the need is by far the greatest [43,44]. There are also significant racial and ethnic disparities in access to mental health care, with minority children and youths having lower use of outpatient mental health treatment [45,46].

The outlook for an adequate supply of child and adolescent mental health professionals remains bleak. In their joint statement in 2009, the American Academy of Pediatrics (AAP) and American Academy of Child & Adolescent Psychiatry noted that there has been a steady decline in the number of positions in child psychiatry residency programs. There has also been a concurrent increase in the management of mental health disorders by primary care pediatricians, with about one-fourth of children (4–17 years of age) who receive mental health care other than psychotropic medication being seen by a general medical practitioner. However, systemic problems complicate the pediatrician's role in treating mental health conditions. These problems include restrictions on reimbursement for management of subclinical psychosocial problems that do not meet diagnostic criteria; lack of reimbursement for necessary collateral contacts with parents, teachers and others involved in the pediatric patient's care; and restrictions on third-party reimbursement to PCPs for visits with a patient who has a primary mental health diagnosis [47].

Collaborative models to bring together primary care pediatricians and mental health care professionals have emerged as a strategy to improve child mental health access. Consultation and referral are best facilitated when the pediatric practice has on-site mental health care (colocation of services) [48].

COLLABORATIVE STRATEGIES TO ADDRESS MENTAL HEALTH–RELATED ILLNESS IN THE PEDIATRIC PRIMARY CARE SETTING

There are 3 basic models of collaboration in which pediatric PCPs formally consult with, and refer patients to, mental health providers: (1) external consultation, (2) colocation, and (3) integration. External consultation models can vary widely, and are generally used when resources do not permit mental health services within the primary care setting, the clinic's mental health caseload is not large enough to warrant hiring permanent staff, or patients' mental health needs are beyond the capacity (volume) or specific skills set (specialization) of existing mental health providers. The colocation model adds the advantage of medical and mental health providers working within the same structural setting. However, colocation does not necessarily translate into integrated care, and services may not be an improvement compared with the more traditional external consultation model (ie, referrals from primary care to a mental health provider via the completion of a form and provision of instructions for making an appointment) [49].

The most comprehensive model, the integrative model, refers to a system in which primary and mental health care providers work together to identify the most appropriate screening and management tools for their patient population and clinic setting, as well as to develop protocols for their collaborative use and for their bidirectional and ongoing communication about patient needs and progress [49]. This communication includes the development of a system for sharing relevant components of patients' medical and mental health records, whether paper or electronic. Ultimately, the integrative model allows PCPs serving medically underserved populations to focus more on the biomedical needs of patients, while mental health professionals address their patients' psychosocial concerns. In contrast, PCPs working in isolation frequently spend valuable time addressing both types of needs, slowing clinical flow.

Collaborative models have been shown to result in higher satisfaction among PCPs, more comfort addressing psychiatric disorders, and greater adherence to evidence-based standards of care [50]; however, data on their efficacy are limited. To the extent that outcome data are available, they generally are disease-specific and limited to adult populations. Integration of care from psychologists and pediatric PCPs improves access to mental health, but there continues to be insufficient empirical evidence to support their apparent clinical and cost benefits [51]. In one randomized controlled trial limited to white, middle-class adults with major depression, participants receiving a multifaceted intervention, including alternating visits between PCPs and psychiatrists, had increased adherence to adequate dosages of antidepressant medication, rated quality of care more often as good to excellent, and were more likely to rate antidepressant medications as helping somewhat or a great deal compared with the group receiving usual care only from the PCP [52]. The integrated team discussed here included PCPs who received extra mental health training before the trial and psychologists who were physically located in the primary care office and available for consultation.

In a review of 42 studies that were conducted to assess the effects of on-site mental health workers delivering psychotherapy and psychosocial interventions in primary care settings on the clinical behavior PCPs, having on-site mental health workers decreased the PCP's need for external consultation and referral around mental health issues and to prescribe psychotropic medication for their patients [53]. There have also been several randomized controlled trials conducted within the Veterans Administration (VA) system to determine the efficacy of the integrative model [54,55]. In one study, integration of mental health care providers in a VA primary care clinic resulted in increased patient and provider satisfaction as well as fewer referrals to external mental health specialists [55]. In another study, a primary care team was specifically integrated into a VA mental health center. Compared with control patients who received usual PCP care, these integrated care patients were more likely to visit their PCP and receive preventive care and, as such, reported both higher satisfaction with care and better physical health status [56].

In the pediatric population, the external consultation model has been shown to be effective in managing attention-deficit/hyperactivity disorder (ADHD). In one study in which psychologists did not meet or interact with patients but were responsible for helping pediatricians with diagnostic and treatment decisions, scoring and interpreting behavioral ratings, and creating medication titration and maintenance plans, there was a significant decrease of patients' ADHD-related symptoms [56].

In another collaborative model, psychologists were colocated on-site at a large pediatric primary care clinic in New York City and focused on young children to 36 months of age. This model facilitated the screening of all infants and toddlers for developmental and social-emotional problems and improved the ability of primary pediatric care staff to identify developmental problems and to provide more effective anticipatory guidance. Parents of young pediatric patients reported that the PCPs were more responsive to their specific concerns, a change consistent with the medical home model. The on-site presence of a psychologist specializing in infant-toddler care also allowed for immediate, short-term intervention. In addition, the psychologist served as a direct link between the primary care clinic and a larger developmental/learning disability clinic, which facilitated referral to more comprehensive services for patients with more serious, longer-term needs. The psychologists also regularly educated pediatric PCPs about infant mental health and development [57].

Another study conducted in North Carolina looked at 3 different colocation models between pediatric primary care facilities and mental health providers: (1) a community mental health center employee was out-stationed in a private pediatric practice, (2) a mental health provider was employed by a pediatric practice, and (3) an independent mental health practice was located on the same floor as a pediatric practice. This study was conducted by interviewing patients and providers, and focused primarily on process outcomes. All 3 models resulted in improved perceived quality of care by patients and increased comfort among physicians in diagnosing and treating behavioral health disorders, such as medication management. Pediatricians and mental health providers in all 3 models reported satisfaction with colocation and increased patient follow-through with mental health referrals. Communication between pediatricians and mental health providers to coordinate care for shared patients was also improved. The colocation model was especially effective in reducing patient concerns about stigma associated with mental health care [58].

THE PEDIATRIC MEDICAL HOME MODEL

The AAP advocates that all children have a medical home in which health care is accessible, continuous, comprehensive, family-centered, coordinated, compassionate, and culturally effective. In their definition of the pediatric medical home, the AAP emphasizes that it is not simply a physical place but, more importantly, an approach to care by an experienced and dedicated primary health care team [59]. Having a pediatric medical home has been shown to reduce both nonurgent emergency department use and hospitalizations [60]. However, children in medical homes with mental health–related illness are more likely to have unmet health care needs than those with biomedical illness. In a cross-sectional analysis of National Survey of Children's Health 2003 survey data, the proportion of children in medical homes was the same, but children with ADHD were more likely to have unmet health care needs than children with asthma [61].

Medically underserved children, with heightened health risks associated by socioeconomic, geographic, and psychosocial factors, frequently have multiple and complex health care needs. They are best served in an enhanced medical home model that provides more comprehensive care than the core medical home [4]. This model includes the components of the traditional medical home as defined by the AAP and adds the following attributes:

- The capacity to spend more time than typical at pediatric visits
- The ability to provide evidence-based and -informed care to manage chronic conditions beyond what would be expected from a PCP
- The provision of health education that is concordant with the dominant language, culture, and health literacy level of the patient and family
- Facilitated access to pediatric subspecialists, including dentists, with coordination at the primary care site
- The incorporation of health information technology to effectively improve access to care
- The integration of pediatric subspecialty services, including mental health care.

The CHF, a nonprofit organization established in 1987, supports a national network of 25 programs and affiliates that use a fleet of 50 mobile medical, dental, and mental health clinics in 16 states and the District of Columbia. In 2008, the national network provided 206,491 encounters (in this article, encounters refers to an aggregate number that includes discrete medical, mental health, oral health, health education, case management, screening/testing, nutrition, and immunization activities) to an estimated 65,000 patients at more than 200 different community- and school-linked sites. Populations served by the mobile clinics are generally of low income and from minority backgrounds. Services are free of charge to patients, comprehensive, and consistent with the traditional medical home model.

Previous studies have documented the efficacy of mobile health clinics in the early identification, prevention, and management of specific illnesses [62,63];

the reduction of unnecessary emergency department use [64]; and the overall reduction in health care costs, particularly when targeting medically underserved populations [65].

To more effectively address the needs of underserved populations served by mobile clinics, CHF programs integrate medical and mental health services. Medical and mental health clinicians work together to choose the most appropriate mental health screening tools for their patient population and develop protocols for making and prioritizing referrals to mental health providers and related services, both on and off site, when problems are identified. Once a referral has been made, medical and mental health providers continue to communicate about patient status regularly via scheduled meetings and through sharing pertinent parts of the respective medical records. In an effort to lessen the stigma of accessing mental health services, and to increase the likelihood of adherence to mental health appointments, medical providers routinely introduce patients and their families to mental health providers who are also available for on-the-spot consultations. Box 1 shows how CHF mobile clinic programs meet the 7 requisite components of the traditional pediatric medical home and integrate mental health services.

MOBILE CLINIC–BASED INTEGRATIVE APPROACHES

Three of CHF's national network programs and corresponding case histories are described later, highlighting aspects of how the integration of medical and mental health services more effectively serves 3 distinct medically underserved populations: homeless children in New York City, immigrant children in South Florida, and postdisaster-affected children in New Orleans.

NYCHP

Since 1987, CHF's flagship program, the NYCHP, based at Montefiore Medical Center and the Albert Einstein College of Medicine's Department of Pediatrics, has been addressing the health care needs of homeless children, youths, and adults in New York City. In 2008, 3 mobile medical clinics visited 13 homeless sites, including 9 family shelters, a shelter and drop-in center for homeless youths, and 2 domestic violence shelters, providing 12,757 encounters, in which 2483 were mental health visits. Forty-eight percent of this population self-identified as being Hispanic and 48% as African American.

The NYCHP mental health team is led by a clinical psychologist and includes 2 licensed clinical social workers and an outreach worker. A mental health provider is present at most primary care sites. Sites that cannot accommodate a mental health provider because of logistics send patients to the home office of the NYCHP where they receive care. The entire mental health team is both bilingual (English/Spanish) and multicultural.

With homeless populations, medical providers have a small window of opportunity in which to intervene because families tend to shuttle though the system rapidly and frequently. In spite of this, of the 60 to 75 monthly referrals

Box 1: How CHF mobile clinic programs meet the 7 requisite components of the traditional pediatric medical home and integrate mental health services

1. Accessible. Mobile clinics bring care directly to communities where medically underserved pediatric populations reside, reducing transportation barriers. No one is turned away based on ability to pay. Medical and mental health clinicians are available by phone when not at the service site.

2. Continuous. Many medical and mental health providers on mobile clinics have been at their specific projects for years and have been providing health care to their patients from infancy through adolescence and into young adulthood, after which they help transition their care to patient-centered medical homes.

3. Comprehensive. Primary care and mental health providers on mobile clinics are well trained in all aspects of pediatric health care. Each program is based at an academic medical center/children's hospital or a federally qualified health center ensuring that other aspects of care such as subspecialty and inpatient care may be accessed when needed. Preventive care, including the provision of immunizations, growth and developmental assessments, age-appropriate screenings, and anticipatory guidance, is prioritized with the AAP/Bright Futures schedule of recommendations as the guide [66]. Case managers ensure that families are well informed and have access to needed programs that help meet their psychosocial needs, such as EI; Women, Infants, and Children; Medicaid; and Children's Health Insurance programs.

4. Family centered. Mobile clinics visit community or school sites on a regularly scheduled basis with the same team members, giving patients and their families the opportunity to develop trusting and long-lasting relationships. Care is provided in the context of the patient's family, involving them in the decision making and care coordination processes. The physical structure of the mobile clinics provides a more intimate feeling and is less intimidating than larger environments of hospital-based or public health clinics.

5. Coordinated. Medically underserved children often face multiple barriers to accessing subspecialty care, including insurance problems, transportation restrictions, and psychosocial issues [4]. The Referral Management Initiative, a special initiative of CHF, is designed to facilitate timely scheduling of pediatric subspecialty appointments, coordinate appointments with available transportation and make transport services available if needed, help patients navigate medical center complexes, and integrate medical records from the specialist into the primary care and mental health records. This initiative has previously been demonstrated to significantly increase adherence with specialty appointments for homeless children and families [67].

6. Compassionate. The well-being of the child is the priority. Mobile clinic staff are sensitive to the psychosocial circumstances facing families, and care is provided in a nonjudgmental manner.

7. Culturally effective. Providers, in many cases from similar cultural and ethnic backgrounds as their patients, respect the varied cultural backgrounds, beliefs, and approaches to health care. Each provider communicates in the patient's preferred language, using a translator when necessary. In collaboration with its national network, CHF produces low-literacy and culturally sensitive health educational materials for use by the projects [68].

that medical providers of the NYCHP made to the mental health team in 2008, 75% received assessment/treatment services, a significantly higher rate than for general, nonhomeless populations [69].

Since 1988 the NYCHP has used an electronic health records system (EHR) developed in collaboration with CHF and others from the national network. The current system is designed to address the needs of medically underserved pediatric populations in the community setting. The psychosocial history is comprehensive and includes elements relevant to homeless populations. The system is organized on the notion of a comprehensive patient-centered pediatric medical home and allows for time-efficient sharing of pertinent health information between medical and mental health providers. The system also facilitates more effective communication with shelter staff to help families access needed community resources. Smart Forms, which facilitate the entry and retrieval of clinical content, are also included in the EHR and are routinely used by providers to screen children and their caregivers. Examples include the 2- and 9-item Patient Health Questionnaires (PHQ-2 and PHQ-9), Center for Epidemiologic Studies Depression Scale (CES-D), and the Pediatric Symptom Checklist.

The NYCHP protocol for the identification and management of developmental delays is rigorous because of the higher incidence in homeless populations [28]. When a developmental delay is suspected, the medical and mental health providers jointly make an initial assessment, meet with the child's caregiver(s) to review results, provide anticipatory guidance, and answer questions regarding the findings. When referrals are needed, they may include the Early Intervention Program (EI), Committee on Preschool Education, Committee on Special Education, and accessible mental health clinics for conditions that may require long-term care. Case managers and family health workers guide families through the referral process, providing transportation services, and facilitating communication with outside referral sources when necessary. The mental health team also screens for maternal depression, which has the benefit of both engaging the parent in care and potentially preventing or ameliorating the developmental effects of maternal depression on the child. A representative case study is shown in Box 2.

South Florida Children's Health Project

The South Florida Children's Health Project (SFCHP), established in 1992 and based at the University of Miami Miller School of Medicine Department of Pediatrics, addresses the health care needs of an almost exclusively uninsured pediatric population (birth to 21 years of age) through the use of a mobile medical clinic. In 2008, the mobile medical clinic visited 11 schools/day care centers and 7 community centers in 8 different regions of Miami-Dade County, providing 7974 encounters, of which 697 were mental health visits. Only 3% of this population had Medicaid, with the reminder being uninsured (97%). Sixty-nine percent self-identified as being Hispanic and 20% as being Haitian.

The population served by the SFCHP has income at or less than the federal poverty level, limited English language proficiency, and is generally unaware of

Box 2: Case study #1*

Ms Q. is a 23-year-old woman with a long history of major depression, insomnia, and being underweight. Her medical history includes strabismus and severe scoliosis. Her social history is significant for a childhood of cycling in and out of foster care homes and eventually being raised by her maternal grandparents. She is in the homeless shelter with her 3-year-old daughter and 1-year-old son. Her daughter has a history of sleepwalking, temper tantrums, and speech delay. Her son presents with irritability, unspecified developmental delays, and constant crying. Ms Q. and the 2 children are referred to the mental health team. As Ms Q. tells her history, she starts crying and states that "her mother didn't want her because she is damaged" and "it hurts." Ms Q. requires help in opening her public assistance case because she does not have all of the required documents.

She is subsequently referred to a psychiatrist, prescribed psychotropic medication, and receives individual counseling. Because of scoliosis and associated chronic pain, arrangements are made for an aide to regularly visit her home to assist with daily tasks. Her daughter is referred for preschool special education evaluation and services. Her son is referred to the EI program for comprehensive developmental evaluation. He is subsequently diagnosed with autism spectrum disorder and begins to receive appropriate services.

Almost a year later, Ms Q is in permanent housing, continues to have a home attendant, and receives ongoing assistance from a case worker from a community agency. Her daughter is enrolled in a Head Start program, receiving speech and language services, and her 1-year-old son is receiving intensive home-based EI services.

*This and the following are not actual patient case histories but are representative of patients and families seen by these programs.

resources available in the community. These factors are often compounded in this community by fear about immigration issues and further limitation of access to medical care and contributions to health disparities. The SFCHP health care team includes medical and mental health providers who provide culturally and linguistically competent services.

More than 1 in 5 children in Florida was uninsured before the recession of 2008, with 120,000 uninsured children residing in Miami-Dade County [70,71]. There has been an increase of demand for health care services in the county partly as a result of the steady influx of disenfranchised families from other parts of the country, the continuing influx of immigrants, and health provider shortages. Many families live in rural areas without public transportation or any other means to get to health providers.

The SFCHP has an on-site mental health team that includes a full-time social worker/mental health counselor and a part-time clinical psychologist. These 2 mental health specialists work in collaboration with the medical team that comprises 2 pediatricians, a nurse practitioner, a medical assistant, and resident physicians and students. The mental health team provides mental health screenings, consultation with the medical team, individual and family counseling/therapy, parenting training, school advocacy, psychoeducational assessments, and referrals to community-based mental health agencies if long-term, intensive treatment is indicated. The mental health team also contributes to the training of the residents and medical students by consulting with them about mental health and psychosocial issues that are of particular importance to the population served. The mental health team also helps families navigate a large public medical system and access low-cost and/or free visits with medical specialists and rehabilitation services (ie, physical and occupational therapies), and makes sure that families are informed about community resources to address everyday needs and to enhance psychosocial support.

All children receive standardized developmental and behavioral screening at their routine well-care visits. Either the Parents Evaluation of Developmental Status (PEDS), a parent report developmental screening instrument, or the Guidelines for Adolescent Preventive Services (GAPS) surveys is used for this particular screen, according to the age of the child. A complete physical examination and appropriate laboratory tests are completed to rule out medical causes. Depending on the needs of the child and family, the referral process to mental health/social work services is initiated through a consult form explaining the reason for referral, which includes a brief description of medical, behavioral, developmental or psychological symptoms. Also, one of the medical team members explains the reason for referral face to face with the mental health specialist when appropriate.

If time allows, the mental health team meets with the patient and the family to gather more information and to further assess the situation on the same day as the referral. In addition, cases that are critical, such as those with previous or present concerns about abuse, domestic violence, suicidality, major depression or anxiety, and severe developmental delays are prioritized and followed on the same day as the referral. Otherwise, parents are provided with a copy of the consult form, briefly meet a member of the mental health team, are instructed to complete and mail behavioral questionnaires such as the Behavioral Assessment System for Children (BASC) and/or ADHD Rating Scale-IV when appropriate, and receive a letter explaining the mental health referral process. The mental health team follows up within a week of referral and/or receipt of these questionnaires.

In 2008, about 1 child in 5 (21%) screened by the SFCHP in well child visits received a mental health or developmental referral. The most common primary symptoms among the patients referred were learning difficulty (18%), ADHD symptoms (16%), developmental delay (16%), behavioral problems (15%), adjustment issues (11%), and depressive symptoms (8%). Other symptoms included anxiety (4%), conduct/oppositional disorder (4%), parental conflict (4%), medical condition (2%), and abuse/neglect (2%).

Although mobile clinics are an atypical service modality, services adhere to the highest professional standards, including protection of patient privacy for mental health services. For families receiving care from community-based agencies, parents report back to the medical and mental health team on their compliance with following through with the referrals, barriers accessing these outside services, progress made through the services received, and need for additional referrals. The trust established during the medical visits and initial contact with a mental health provider as an integrated part of a medical team encourages these families to continue to communicate about their various issues of concern. A representative case study is shown in Box 3.

New Orleans Children's Health Project

The New Orleans Children's Health Project (NOCHP), based at Tulane University School of Medicine Department of Pediatrics, was established in 2006 to address the ongoing health care needs of the community in the aftermath of Hurricane Katrina. NOCHP operates out of 2 mobile clinics. One offers pediatric primary care services and the other, referred to as the Community Support and Resiliency Unit (CSRU), provides children and their families with mental health and case management services. In 2008, the mobile clinics visited 4 schools in communities devastated by Hurricane Katrina that experienced continued limited health care access on a regular schedule and provided 6953 encounters, including 3750 mental health encounters (including collateral contacts with teachers, parents, and other community-based providers). Most of the patients were either insured through Medicaid/Comprehensive Health Insurance Plan (60%) or uninsured (40%). Fifty percent self-identified as being African American and 30% as being Hispanic.

Recognizing that depression may present as physical symptoms or co-occur with medical illnesses and that early detection and management is key to minimizing lifelong effects, an adolescent depression screening project was developed by medical and mental health staff of the NOCHP. A review of patient information data collected for the beginning of 2008 revealed that medical

---

Box 3: Case study #2

Juan is a 9-year-old boy from Colombia. At the time of referral, he had been living in Miami for 6 months and was reported to be failing in school. Multiple teachers have complained that he will not stop talking and disrupting the class. At home, his mother states that he has to be constantly reminded to perform household chores and scolded for fighting with his sister. This behavior had also occurred in Colombia, but was never addressed. He was referred to our team by a school counselor.

After a medical history and physical examination to rule out medical causes, Juan's mother and 2 teachers were given BASC and ADHD Rating Scale-IV forms to evaluate his behavior at home and at school, respectively. The pediatrician summarized the patient's story to the on-site psychologist, who scored the BASC forms. The evaluations resulted in Juan being diagnosed with ADHD. At an information interview with Juan's mother, it was agreed that behavioral therapy would be started. The psychologist then discussed the diagnosis and treatment plan with the referring pediatrician. After 1 month, Juan's mother noticed a small improvement in his symptoms, but agreed that he may benefit more from a daily medication trial. Juan is followed monthly in collaboration with the on-site psychologist and the pediatrician and has shown great progress both in school and at home.

providers of NOCHP did not routinely screen for depression or, if they provided a screening, did not document having done so. In collaboration with the mental health providers of NOCHP and consistent with US Pediatric Task Force Preventive Guidelines [19], a depression screening protocol was developed and implemented. All patients 11 years of age or older accessing the mobile medical clinic were to be screened using the PHQ-2; patients with a positive PHQ-2 screen were to have a PHQ-9; and all patients who screened positive on the PHQ-9 questionnaire were referred to the CSRU for depression evaluation and management.

Of the initial 19 patients screened, 8 (42%) had positive findings: 5 patients with symptoms consistent with mild depression, 2 with moderate depression, and 1 with severe depression. As per protocol, all 8 were referred to the CSRU, but only 1 followed up. Based on this result, medical and mental health staff revaluated and revised the protocol, bringing it more in line with the Guidelines for Adolescent Depression in Primary Care tool kit [72] and adding a suicide screening question for patients who screened positive for depression on the PHQ-9. Only moderate and severely depressed patients were referred for mental health services. The mildly depressed patients were managed by the pediatrician, received written self-care information, including a depression information handout developed by the mental health staff, and were scheduled for a 1-month follow-up appointment with the pediatrician. In a 12 month period, 107 patients aged 11 to 18 years were screened for depression. Of these, 30 patients (28%) screened positive on the PHQ-9, indicating that they were experiencing symptoms consistent with a diagnosis of depression at the time of screening. More than half of these patients were either African American or Hispanic.

As part of the quality improvement incentive program of the Louisiana Public Health Institute in collaboration with the National Committee for Quality Assurance, the NOCHP clinic was recently awarded recognition as a medical home, one of the first mobile programs in the country to be awarded this designation.

A representative case study is shown in Box 4.

Box 4: Case study #3

Pam is a 12-year-old girl referred by her school to the mobile medical clinic for immunizations. The pediatrician completed a full checkup because she had not had one for several years. During the visit, the patient completed the depression screening and GAPS questionnaires, as per protocol, revealing a long history of suicidal ideation. She was immediately referred to the mental health team for further evaluation and was diagnosed with major depressive disorder and initiated on antidepressant medication. Subsequently, Pam was admitted to a collaborating psychiatric inpatient facility for further management. After discharge from the inpatient facility, she continued to be treated at its outpatient psychiatric clinic and was reported to be doing well, functioning at a high level in school and with family.

SUMMARY

There is a long-standing shortage of child and adolescent mental health professionals in the United States, which contributes to serious problems accessing care for children in need of services. Several strategies have emerged in response to this situation, including expanding the role of pediatric PCPs to better identify and manage psychosocial problems. Collaborative efforts to integrate mental health and pediatric primary care is another strategy for addressing access to mental health services. These efforts are consistent with the medical home model of care, which emphasizes comprehensive, coordinated, continuous, and family-centered services. The enhanced medical home model is designed for medically underserved populations and adds facilitated access to mental health and other needed specialty services. The integrative mental health-primary care model is a crucial part of the enhanced medical home model. It functions in a way that is practical and amenable to families, and facilitates communication between medical and mental health providers. Families and children are able to receive needed mental health and psychosocial services immediately on-site, eliminating many barriers that frequently interfere with access to mental health services. These barriers may include transportation problems, difficulty finding a provider, language limitations, and the stigma that some families perceive regarding mental health care. As such, the integrated team approach described here may serve as a model for others working with similar underserved populations.

References

[1] Roberts RE, Attkisson CC, Rosenblatt A. Prevalence of psychopathology among children and adolescents. Am J Psychiatry 1998;155:715–25.

[2] U.S. Department of Health and Human Services. Mental health: a report of the Surgeon General. Rockville (MD): US Department of Health and Human Services, Substance Abuse and Mental Health Services Administration, National Institutes of Health, National Institute of Mental Health; 1999.

[3] Applying data from US Census Bureau, Census 2000.

[4] Brito A, Grant R, Overholt S, et al. The enhanced medical home: the pediatric standard of care for medically underserved children. Adv Pediatr 2008;55:9–28.

[5] Hagan JH Jr. The new morbidity: where the rubber hits the road or the practitioner's guide to the new morbidity. Pediatrics 2001;108:1206–10.

[6] Kelleher KJ, McInerny TK, Gardner WP, et al. Increasing identification of psychosocial problems: 1979–1996. Pediatrics 2000;105:1313–21.

[7] Coleman WL, Howard BJ. Family-focused behavioral pediatrics: clinical techniques for primary care. Pediatr Rev 1995;16:448–55.

[8] American Academy of Pediatrics Council on Children with Disabilities. Policy statement. Identifying infants and young children with developmental disorders in the medical home: an algorithm for developmental surveillance and screening. Pediatrics 2006;118:405–20.

[9] American Academy of Pediatrics. Policy statement – the future of pediatrics: mental health competencies for pediatric primary care. Pediatrics 2009;124:410–21.

[10] U.S. Education Department. Office of Special Education Programs Data Accountability Center. Individuals with Disabilities Education Act (IDEA) Data, Part C (2007), Table 8-1. Available at: http://www.ideadata.org/arc_toc9.asp#partcCC. Accessed December 16, 2009.

[11] Rosenberg SA, Zhang D, Robinson CC. Prevalence of developmental delays and partic-ipation in early intervention services for young children. Pediatrics 2008;121(6): e1503–9.

[12] Halfon N, Regalado M, Sareen H, et al. Assessing development in the pediatric office. Pedi-atrics 2004;113:1926–33.

[13] Sices L, Feudtner C, McLaughlin J, et al. How do primary care physicians identify young chil-dren with developmental delays? A national survey. J Dev Behav Pediatr 2003;24:409–17.

[14] Carter AS, Briggs-Gowan MJ, Ornstein Davis N. Assessment of young children's social-emotional development and psychopathology: recent advances and recommendations for practice. J Child Psychol Psychiatry 2004;45:109–34.

[15] Feldman MA, Hancok CL, Rielly N, et al. Behavior problems in young children with or at risk for developmental delay. J Child Fam Stud 2000;9:247–61.

[16] Baker BL, Blacher J, Crnic KA, et al. Behavior problems and parenting stress in families of three-year-old children with and without developmental delays. Am J Ment Retard 2002;107:433–44.

[17] Pastor PN, Reuben CA, Loeb M. Functional difficulties among school-age children: United States, 2001–2007. Natl Health Stat Report 2009;19. Available at: http://www.cdc.gov/nchs/data/nhsr/nhsr019.pdf. Accessed December 16, 2009.

[18] Available at: http://www.brightfutures.org/mentalhealth/pdf/professionals/ped_sympton_chklst.pdf. Accessed December 16, 2009.

[19] Williams SB, O'Connor EA, Eder M, et al. Screening for child and adolescent depression in primary care settings: a systematic evidence review for the US Preventive Services Task Force. Pediatrics 2009;123(4):e716–35.

[20] US Public Health Service. Report of the Surgeon General's Conference on Children's Mental Health: a National Action Agenda. Washington, DC: Department of Health and Human Services; 2000. Available at: http://www.surgeongeneral.gov/topics/cmh/cmhreport.pdf. Accessed January 4, 2010.

[21] Weinreb L, Goldbert R, Bassuk E, et al. Determinants of health and service use patterns in homeless and low-income housed children. Pediatrics 1998;102:554–62.

[22] Menke EM. The mental health of homeless school-age children. J Child Adolesc Psychiatr Nurs 1998;11:87–98.

[23] Masten AS, Miliotis D, Graham-Bermann SA, et al. Children in homeless families: risks to mental health and development. J Consult Clin Psychol 1993;61:335–43.

[24] Zima BT, Gussing R, Forness SR, et al. Sheltered homeless children: their eligibility and unmet need for special education evaluations. Am J Public Health 1997;87:236–40.

[25] Wood D, Valez B, Hayashi T, et al. Homeless and housed families in Los Angeles: a study comparing demographic and family function characteristics. Am J Public Health 1990;80:1049–52.

[26] Bassuk EL, Buckner JC, Perloff JN, et al. Prevalence of mental health and substance use disor-ders among homeless and low-income housed mothers. Am J Psychiatry 1998;155:1561–4.

[27] Weinreb LF, Buckner JC, Williams V, et al. A comparison of the health and mental status of homeless mothers in Worcester, Mass: 1993 and 2003. Am J Public Health 2006;96: 1444–8.

[28] Grant R, Shapiro A, Joseph S, et al. The health of homeless children revisited. Adv Pediatr 2007;54:173–87.

[29] Granados G, Puvvula J, Berman N, et al. Health care for Latino children: impact of child and parental birthplace on insurance status and access to health services. Am J Public Health 2001;91:1806–7.

[30] Kincheloe J, Frates J, Brown ER. Determinants of children's participation in California's Medicaid and SCHIP programs. Health Serv Res 2007;42:847–66.

[31] American Academy of Pediatrics, Committee on Community Health Services. Policy State-ment. Providing care for immigrant, homeless, and migrant children. Pediatrics 2005;115: 1095–100.

[32] Gentry K, Quandt SA, Davis SW, et al. Child healthcare in two farmworker populations. J Community Health 2007;32:419–31.

[33] Hill I, Dubay L, Kenney GM, et al. Improving coverage and access for immigrant Latino children: the Los Angeles Healthy Kids Program. Health Aff 2008;27:550–9.

[34] Kataoka SH, Stein BD, Jaycox LH, et al. A school-based mental health program for traumatized Latino immigrant children. J Am Acad Child Adolesc Psychiatry 2003;42:311–8.

[35] Lopez C, Dewey Bergren M, Painter SG. Latino disparities in child mental health services. J Child Adolesc Psychiatr Nurs 2008;21:137–45.

[36] Shaw JA, Applegate B, Shorr C. Twenty-one month follow-up study of school-age children exposed to Hurricane Andrew. J Am Acad Child Adolesc Psychiatry 1996;35(3):359–64.

[37] Garrett AL, Grant R, Madrid P, et al. Children and megadisasters: lessons learned in the new millennium. Adv Pediatr 2007;54:189–214.

[38] Abramson D, Garfield R. On the edge: children and families displaced by hurricanes Katrina and Rita face a looming medical and mental health crisis. Available at: http://www.ncdp.mailman.columbia.edu/files/On_the_Edge_Executive_Summary.pdf. Accessed December 16, 2009.

[39] Abramson D, Stehling-Ariza T, Garfield R, et al. Prevalence and predictors of mental health distress post-Katrina: findings from the Gulf Coast Child and Family Health Study. Disaster Med Public Health Prep 2008;2:77–86.

[40] InCrisis.org. The prevalence of mental health and addictive disorders. Available at: http://www.incrisis.org/Articles/PrevalenceMHProblems.htm. Accessed December 16, 2009.

[41] Kataoka SH, Zhang L, Wells KB. Unmet need for mental health care among U.S. children: variation with ethnicity and insurance status. Am J Psychiatry 2002;159:1548–55.

[42] Koppelman J. The provider system for children's mental health: workforce capacity and effective treatment. National Health Policy Forum Issue Brief No. 801. 2004. Available at: http://www.nhpf.org/library/issue-briefs/IB801_ChildMHProvider_10-26-04.pdf. Accessed January 4, 2010.

[43] Thomas CR, Holzer CE III. The continuing shortage of child and adolescent psychiatrists. J Am Acad Child Adolesc Psychiatry 2006;45:1023–31.

[44] Campbell CD, Kearns LA, Patchin S. Psychological needs and resources as perceived by rural and urban psychologists. Prof Psychol Res Pr 2006;37:45–50.

[45] Witt WP, Kasper JD, Riley AW. Mental health services use among school-age children with disabilities: the role of sociodemographics, functional limitations, family burdens, and care coordination. Health Serv Res 2003;38:1441–66.

[46] Garland AF, Lau AS, Yeh M, et al. Racial and ethnic differences in utilization of mental health services among high-risk youth. Am J Psychiatry 2005;162:1336–43.

[47] American Academy of Pediatrics and American Academy of Child & Adolescent Psychiatrists. Improving mental health services in primary care: reducing administrative and financial barriers to access and collaboration. Pediatrics 2009;123:1248–51. Available at: http://www.aacap.org/galleries/LegislativeAction/Final%20Background%20paper%203-09.pdf. Accessed January 4, 2010.

[48] Guevara JP, Greenbaum PE, Shera D, et al. Survey of mental health consultation and referral among primary care pediatricians. Acad Pediatr 2009;9:123–7.

[49] National Institute for Health Care Management Foundation [NICHM]. Strategies to support the integration of mental health into pediatric primary care. Issue Paper. August 2009. Available at: http://nihcm.org/pdf/PediatricMH-FINAL.pdf. Accessed January 4, 2010.

[50] Upshur C, Weinreb L. A survey of primary care provider attitudes and behaviors regarding treatment of adult depression: what changes after a collaborative care intervention? Prim Care Companion J Clin Psychiatry 2008;10:182–6.

[51] Kubiszyn T. Integrating health and mental health services in schools: psychologists collaborating with primary care providers. Clin Psychol Rev 1999;99:179–98.

[52] Katon W, Von Korff VM, Lin E, et al. Collaborative management to achieve treatment guidelines. JAMA 1995;273(13):1026–31.

[53] Harkness EF, Bower PJ. On-site mental health workers delivering psychological therapy and psychosocial interventions to patients in primary care: effects on the professional practice of primary care providers. Cochrane Database Syst Rev 2009;1:CD000532. DOI: 10.1002/14651858.CD000532.pub2.

[54] Felker BL, Barnes RF, Greenberg DM, et al. Preliminary outcomes from an integrated mental health primary care team. Psychiatr Serv 2004;55(4):442–4.

[55] Druss BG, Rohrbaugh RM, Levinson CM, et al. Integrated medical care for patients with serious psychiatric illness. Arch Gen Psychiatry 2001;58:861–8.

[56] Epstein JN, Rabiner D, Johnson DE, et al. Improving attention-deficit/hyperactivity disorder treatment outcomes through the use of a collaborative consultation treatment service by community-based pediatricians. Arch Gen Psychiatry 2007;161(9): 835–40.

[57] Briggs RD, Racine AD, Chinitz S. Preventive pediatric mental health care: a co-location model. Infant Ment Health J 2007;28(5):481–95.

[58] Williams J, Shore SE, Foy JM. Co-location of mental health professionals in primary care settings: three North Carolina Models. Clin Pediatr 2006;45(537):543.

[59] American Academy of Pediatrics Policy Statement. The medical home. Pediatrics 2002;110:184–6.

[60] Starfield B, Shi L. The medical home, access to care, and insurance: a review of evidence. Pediatrics 2004;113(5):1493–8.

[61] Toomey SL, Finkelstein J, Kuhlthau K. Does connection to primary care matter for children with attention-deficit/hyperactivity disorder? Pediatrics 2008;122:368–74.

[62] Liao O, Morphew T, Amaro S, et al. The Breathmobile: a novel comprehensive school-based mobile asthma care clinic for urban underprivileged children. J Sch Health 2006;76: 313–9.

[63] Brody BL, Roch-Levecq A, Klonoff-Cohen HS, et al. Refractive errors in low-income preschoolers. Ophthalmic Epidemiol 2007;14:223–9.

[64] Patel B, Sheridan P, Detjen P, et al. Success of a comprehensive school-based asthma intervention on clinical markers and resource utilization for inner-city children with asthma in Chicago: the mobile C.A.R.E. Foundation's asthma management program. J Asthma 2007;44:113–8.

[65] Oriol NE, Cote PJ, Vavasis AP, et al. Calculating the return on investment of mobile healthcare. BMC Med 2009;7:27. Available at: http://www.biomedcentral.com/content/pdf/1741-7015-7-27.pdf. Accessed January 4, 2010.

[66] Hagan JF, Shaw JS, Duncan PM. Bright futures: guidelines for health supervision of infants, children and adolescents. Available at: http://www.brightfutures.org/mentalhealth/pdf/professionals/ped_sympton_chklst.pdf. Accessed December 16, 2009.

[67] Redlener I, Grant R, Krol DM. Beyond primary care: ensuring access to subspecialists, special services, and health care systems for medically underserved children. Adv Pediatr 2005;52:9–22.

[68] Health education materials and a comprehensive list of developmental screening tools for use in pediatric primary care are available at Children's Health Fund website. Available at: http://www.childrenshealthfund.org/.

[69] Kessler RC, Olfson M, Berglund PA. Patterns and predictors of treatment contact after first onset of psychiatric disorders. Am J Psychiatry 1998;155:62–9.

[70] Kaiser Family Foundation. State health facts. Florida. Available at: http://www.statehealthfacts.org/profileind.jsp?ind=134&cat=3&rgn=11. Accessed January 8, 2010.

[71] Miami-Dade County. FY 2005-06 Children and Families Budget and Resource Allocation Report. Available at: http://www.miamidade.gov/budget/FY2005-06/PDF/ch_condition.pdf. Accessed January 8, 2010.

[72] Cheung AH, Zuckerbrot RA, Jensen PS, et al. Guidelines for Adolescent Depression in Primary Care (GLAD-PC): II. Treatment and ongoing management. Pediatrics 2007;120(5):e1313–26.

Advances in Pediatrics 57 (2010) 315–329

ADVANCES IN PEDIATRICS

ELSEVIER
MOSBY

Ketosis and the Ketogenic Diet, 2010: Advances in Treating Epilepsy and Other Disorders

John M. Freeman, MD*, Eric H. Kossoff, MD

Neurology and Pediatrics, Johns Hopkins Medical Institutions, Baltimore, MD, USA

S ince the authors' 1997 review of the ketogenic diet in *Advances in Pediatrics*, a remarkable increase has been seen in interest in its use, in reports of its effectiveness, and in studies of how the diet works. Although used primarily for treating seizures in children, the diet has also been shown to be useful in treating intractable seizures in adults, and possibly for treating other nonepileptic conditions, such as brain tumors, Alzheimer's disease, and diabetes.

The ketogenic diet is a high-fat, adequate protein, low-carbohydrate diet designed to produce ketosis through mimicking the metabolic changes of starvation. It is carefully calculated to be nutritionally adequate for each individual, providing 90% of needed calories as fat, a minimum of 1 g/kg of protein, and minimal carbohydrates. The ratio of fats to protein and carbohydrate is classically 4:1. The diet and its cousins—the modified Atkins diet, the medium chain triglyceride (MCT) diet, and the low glycemic index treatment—have provided substantial advances in the treatment of childhood seizures. However, because of myths and misunderstandings about the benefits and side effects of the diet, and because of the lack of trained physicians and dieticians to provide the diet, it is used too infrequently. This report summarizes progress made during the past decade and provides information about both the diet's documented usefulness in childhood epilepsy and its potential uses in other conditions. A considerably fuller discussion of the classic ketogenic diet and its implementation are provided elsewhere [1–3].

The ketogenic diet only should be undertaken only under the medical supervision of a physician and a dietician knowledgeable in its management.

Many myths and misconceptions exist about the ketogenic diet, such as:

1. The ketosis of starvation and of the ketogenic diet is dangerous and similar to the ketoacidosis of diabetes.
2. High-fat diets are unpalatable and difficult to calculate and prepare.

*Corresponding author. 1026 Rolandvue Road, Baltimore, MD 21204.
E-mail address: jfreeman@jhmi.edu

0065-3101/10/$ – see front matter
doi:10.1016/j.yapd.2010.08.003

3. High-fat diets should not be used in infants and young children.
4. High-fat diets will make one fat.
5. The ketogenic diet will cause atherosclerosis.
6. The ketogenic diet is bad for a child's health.
7. The ketogenic diet should only be used when all anticonvulsants have failed.

MYTH #1. THE KETOSIS OF STARVATION AND OF THE KETOGENIC DIET IS DANGEROUS AND SIMILAR TO THE KETOACIDOSIS OF DIABETES

The ketogenic diet and its accompanying ketosis are not dangerous. Many physicians are confused about ketosis and ketonemia and believe, based on their knowledge of diabetic ketoacidosis, that ketosis is an ominous and pathologic state. However, ketosis is a human survival mechanism and different from the pathologic state associated with diabetes known as *diabetic ketoacidosis.*

Ketosis

Ketosis is a survival mechanism during prolonged starvation or lack of carbohydrate ingestion. Fat metabolism and its by-product ketone bodies are essential mechanisms for survival in animals and humans. Early humans were hunter–gatherers and, for continued energy, depended on the protein and fat acquired by hunting. They used stored fat for energy until their next successful hunt, because their carbohydrate ingestion was opportunistic [4–6]. Not until agriculture began did grain and carbohydrates become a stable source of energy. Perhaps because of this change in nutrition, the ability to use fats as a primary energy source remains an underused human trait.

Fasting

During fasting, the primary source of carbohydrate reserve is glycogen, but glycogen stores provide only a 12- to 14-hour energy reserve [4]. When fasting is more prolonged, muscle protein begins to break down, using gluconeogenesis to provide needed energy. The resulting muscle weakness would have been a substantial disadvantage to hunter–gathers.

During more prolonged fasting or during starvation, the principal source of stored human energy is the fat stored in adipose tissue. Body fat is readily metabolized by the liver to form ketone bodies (acetone, acetoacetate, and ß-hydroxybutyric acid), and these water-soluble compounds gain easy access to the central nervous system. As blood concentrations of ketone bodies increase, their metabolism by the brain displaces its glucose use and spares muscle protein [5,6]. Normal-weight individuals can survive for 2 months and obese individuals even a full year on stored fat burned as ketone bodies. The accompanying ketosis is in marked contrast to the ketoacidosis of diabetics.

Diabetic Ketoacidosis

In contrast to starvation or deprivation of carbohydrate, diabetic ketoacidosis is caused by a deficiency of insulin. This deficiency causes the body to metabolize triglycerides and muscle protein instead of glucose for energy. Lack of insulin also produces an excess of glucagon and stimulates the synthesis of the ketone bodies normally inhibited by the insulin, resulting in a rapid and large increase in ketone bodies. In addition, the hyperglycemia caused by insulin deficiency produces an osmotic diuresis, leading to marked urinary losses of water and electrolytes. In contrast, the slow initiation of a ketogenic diet avoids these side effects.

The ketosis of the diabetic, which makes diabetic ketoacidosis a life-threatening emergency, is only a sign of the multiple metabolic changes occurring in a person with diabetes who lacks insulin. Its potential lethality is from the combination of ketosis, hyperglycemia, loss of potassium, and dehydration, and the rapidity with which they occur.

MYTH # 2. THE KETOGENIC DIET IS UNPALATABLE AND DIFFICULT TO CALCULATE AND PREPARE

High-fat diets are not unpalatable nor are the meals difficult to calculate and prepare. Because the high-fat ketogenic diet is considered unpalatable by some parents and physicians (but not often by children), the MCT diet, the modified Atkins diet, and the low glycemic index treatment have been developed. At Hopkins the classic diet has only occasionally been found to be unpalatable to children. It seems to be well tolerated when it is useful in controlling seizures or permitting a decrease in medication toxicity; the diet is burdensome when either seizures are not markedly decreased or medications and their side effects are not substantially reduced. If, after a several-week trial, an individual finds the diet unpalatable, using the modified Atkins diet may improve compliance while maintaining benefits of the diet. Alternatively, the diet can be stopped and further medication trials continued.

Adolescents and adults are sometimes started on the modified Atkins diet and switched to the classic ketogenic diet if the Atkins diet it is not sufficiently effective.

Many recipes are available on the Internet and using the KetoCalculator (www.ketocalculator.com), and culture-specific diets have been designed to appeal to a wide variety of cultures and tastes. The diet can also be successfully used for families of children who are vegetarian, but it is nearly impossible for those who are vegan (lacto-ovo-vegetarian).

MYTH # 3. THE KETOGENIC DIET IS DANGEROUS IN INFANTS AND YOUNG CHILDREN

Infants and young children can and do thrive on a properly calculated ketogenic diet. It is widely misbelieved that the brain uses only glucose for fuel, that ketosis cannot be achieved during the first weeks or months of life, and that nutrition of the very young could be adversely affected by the ketogenic diet. For these reasons it is misbelieved that the ketogenic diet should not be used in the newborn or during the first 2 years of life. However, the newborn brain avidly uses ketone bodies and during fetal life uses them for myelin synthesis. The ketogenic diet clearly is mandatory in infants presenting with seizures caused by congenital deficiency of glucose transport (GLUT-1 deficiency) and pyruvate dehydrogenase complex deficiency. The diet is also effective, and may be the preferred treatment, in infantile myoclonic epilepsies, such as West, Dravet, and Lennox-Gastaut syndromes.

For these reasons, and with the ready availability of multiple ketogenic diet infant formulas (eg, KetoCal, Ross Carbohydrate Free), the infant population is one of the most rapidly growing age groups on the ketogenic diet.

The high-fat ketogenic diet also may be worthy of study in the asphyxiated newborn for treating cortical damage and ensuing seizures [5]. Recent evidence also suggests it may be helpful for recently worsening seizures and status epilepticus [6].

When used in infants and young children, growth and weight gain should be carefully monitored [7,8]. Evidence shows that children younger than 2 years on the diet may grow less well than older children, and the ketogenic diet ratio and ketosis may need to be adjusted [9]. Dyslipidemia is significantly less common in infants receiving an all-liquid ketogenic diet than in those on the diet receiving solid foods [8].

MYTH # 4. THE HIGH-FAT KETOGENIC DIET WILL MAKE ONE FAT

Obesity is caused by the intake of excess calories from whatever source, not the ingestion of fat. Properly administered, the caloric intake of the ketogenic diet is carefully calculated and monitored. If the child is gaining or losing weight disproportionate to growth, calories can be adjusted appropriately. The current epidemic of obesity has been reviewed by Taubes [10], who believes the obesity epidemic is from society's high intake of less satisfying and more rapidly metabolized carbohydrates and the avoidance of more appetite-suppressing dietary fat. The ketogenic diet, the Atkins diet, and other low-carbohydrate diets increasingly are being used to treat obesity [11].

MYTH # 5. THE HIGH-FAT KETOGENIC DIET WILL CAUSE SIGNIFICANT HYPERCHOLESTEROLEMIA AND ATHEROSCLEROSIS

Studies have shown that children on the ketogenic diet experience only a modest (eg, 20%) increase in lipids and cholesterol, and that elevation seems to decrease spontaneously with time [12]. No evidence shows a long-term effect of the diet on atherosclerosis, and children followed up for several years after discontinuing the ketogenic diet experienced normalization of their serum lipid values without reports of heart disease [13]. The increase of lipids also seems to be less in children receiving ketogenic diet formulas.

MYTH #6. THE KETOGENIC DIET IS BAD FOR THE CHILD'S HEALTH

Hypoproteinemia, infections, and death from cardiomyopathy or pancreatitis have been reported occasionally in children on the diet, but the relationship of each of these alleged complications to the diet is unclear. The diet is often used as a last resort in very fragile children with uncontrolled seizures, and it is notable that the authors had two deaths that occurred on the day the child was about to begin the diet. Complications can and do occur in children on the ketogenic and modified Atkins diets and are discussed later in this article. Fortunately, most are both preventable and treatable without the need for diet discontinuation.

MYTH #7. THE KETOGENIC DIET SHOULD ONLY BE USED AS A LAST RESORT

Many neurologists claim that the ketogenic diet is so restrictive that it should only be used when all medications have failed. Families often disagree and approximately half would have tried the diet first if given the opportunity [13]. For most children with epilepsy, the authors recommend attempting control with one or at most two medications, appropriately used before using the ketogenic diet.

Evidence shows that the ketogenic diet works best for infantile spasms if used before 1 year of age and before multiple anticonvulsants have been tried [14]. The authors are routinely using the diet as a first-line treatment for infantile spasms, and 62% of these infants have become spasm-free within 2 weeks [15]. The diet may also be a reasonable first-line treatment for Doose syndrome (myoclonic-astatic epilepsy) [16].

HISTORY OF THE KETOGENIC DIET

In the early 1920s, at a time when only bromides and phenobarbital were available as anticonvulsants, Dr Hugh Conklin, an osteopathic physician, erroneously thought epilepsy was the result of intoxication from the Peyer patches of the intestine. He hypothesized that episodic fasting would reduce this intoxication and found that fasting of children for as long as 25 days produced remarkable immediate- and long-term seizure control. Reported at the American Medical Association (AMA) convention in 1921, the success of fasting led others to note that the metabolic effects of fasting could be mimicked by a diet high in fat and restricted in carbohydrate. This regimen became, and remains, the standard ketogenic diet (a more complete description of the origin of the diet is found elsewhere[1,17].)

The diet was found to be effective and was widely used during the 1920s and '30s, until the discovery of phenytoin (Dilantin) in 1939. With the subsequent discovery of other useful anticonvulsants, the more laborious diet was used less frequently, and fewer physicians and dieticians remained familiar with it.

In the early 1990s, a child named Charlie Abrahams began to have intractable myoclonic seizures. Charlie was seen by multiple physicians and subjected to multiple procedures and medications without benefit. His father, Hollywood producer Jim Abrahams, found reference to the authors use of the ketogenic diet and brought Charlie to Johns Hopkins in 1993, where the diet brought his seizures under control in only a few days.

Upset about the lack of awareness of the ketogenic diet, Abrahams created the Charlie Foundation to make others aware of its effectiveness. The foundation funded a multicenter study of the diet and the first edition of *The Epilepsy Diet Treatment: An Introduction to the Ketogenic Diet* [1]. NBC's Dateline and the made-for-TV film "First Do No Harm," starring Meryl Streep, further disseminated the information in 1997. Since 1994, the number of articles about the diet referenced in PubMed has increased from 6 to 8 per year to more than 200 per year [17]. The diet is now available in more than 50 countries [18] and may also be cost-effective in developing countries where modern medications may be expensive or unavailable [19]. Nonetheless, it remains underused today, partially because of the lack of dietetic support, and is still considered by many neurologists to be the treatment of last resort. Medications, even if less effective, are easier to prescribe.

USE OF THE KETOGENIC DIET
Initiation of the Diet
Fasting allows more rapid development of ketosis and therefore more rapid seizure control. Although classically the diet was initiated after a multiday in-hospital fast, recently it has been started after fasting for only 3 days, or even with little or no fasting. At Hopkins the diet is now started typically with a 24-hour fast unless the child is believed to be too medically fragile [20]. The authors find that hospitalization during the initiation of the diet allows careful observation of the fasting child, and permits the dietician to provide more complete instruction to the parents. Gradual introduction of calories of the diet over several days also allows the patient to adjust slowly to the increasing ketosis and the high fat content of the diet, reduces vomiting, and allows the diet to be effective more quickly [21]. Initiation of the diet and its subsequent fine-tuning are more fully discussed in the authors' book [1].

When to Use the Diet
The ketogenic diet is mandatory as the initial management of GLUT-1 deficiency and pyruvate dehydrogenase deficiency, and may also be considered a first-line treatment for infantile spasms, myoclonic seizures, tuberous sclerosis, myoclonic-astatic epilepsy (Doose syndrome), Dravet syndrome, Rett syndrome, and Lennox-Gastaut syndrome, each of which is often refractory to medication. Although rarely used as the first treatment for other seizure disorders (Fig. 1), the diet should be considered when the child's seizures are difficult to control (ie, uncontrolled after the use of two properly administered anticonvulsant medications). The diet is effective as formula-only (KetoCal) in small infants and in gastrostomy or tube-fed patients. Recent studies suggest the diet may be a useful adjunct in the treatment of refractory status epilepticus in adults and children [22] and after brain injury [23].

Management of Seizures

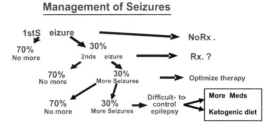

Fig. 1. Management of seizures.

EFFECTIVENESS OF THE KETOGENIC DIET FOR CHILDHOOD EPILEPSY

Numerous studies have documented that the diet is both effective and tolerable if after a trial of 3 weeks [21] the number of seizures decreases substantially or the toxicity of medications is decreased. A study of 150 patients followed up over 3 to 6 years [24] documented that 83 of the children (55%) initiating the diet remained on it for at least 1 year. Their outcomes are shown in Table 1. Children benefiting are kept on the diet for an arbitrary 2 years, and many remain seizure-free when the diet is discontinued, even without anticonvulsant medication. Although most studies of the diet have been uncontrolled, two

Table 1
Outcome of 150 children started on the classic ketogenic diet

Number	At onset 150	At 12 mo 83	At 3–6 y Same 83
Seizure-free	0	11	11 off diet, 9 off medications Seizure-free: 8 >90% seizure-free: 2
90%–99% seizure-free	0	30	23 off diet, 9 off medications Seizure-free: 10 90%–99% seizure-free: 13
50%–90% seizure-free	0	34	26 off diet, 11 off medications Seizure-free: 2 90%–99% seizure-free: 6 50%–90% seizure-free: 15
<50% seizure-free	150	8	All off diet >90% seizure-free: none 50%–90% seizure-free: 4 <50% seizure-free: 4

Data from Hemingway C, Freeman JM, Pillas DJ, et al. The ketogenic diet: a 3–6 year follow-up of 150 children prospectively enrolled. Pediatrics 2001;108:898–905.

recent randomized controlled studies have further documented its effectiveness in seizure control [25–28].

NEWER ALTERNATIVE KETOGENIC-TYPE DIETS
Since "rediscovery" of the classic ketogenic diet's efficacy, several modifications have been developed and seem useful. With the exception of the modified Atkins diet, however, few controlled studies of its relative effectiveness have been performed.

The Modified Atkins Diet
Started as an outpatient treatment without a fasting period, the modified Atkins diet [20] is more liberal, and allegedly more palatable, than the classic ketogenic diet. For the modified Atkins diet, the authors restrict carbohydrates to 10 g/d (15–20 g/d for adults) and encourage high-fat foods without protein, caloric, or fluid restrictions. Although the classic ketogenic diet has a high ratio of fat to protein and carbohydrate of 4:1 or 3:1, the modified Atkins diet is approximately 1:1, and standard (nonketogenic) diets are 0.3:1. Now, after nearly 8 years of use, the modified Atkins diet's effectiveness has been documented in 13 publications. Results are similar to those of the classic ketogenic diet: 43% of patients have had greater than 50% seizure reduction and 14 (11%) became seizure-free. The modified Atkins diet may be valuable in developing countries where limited dietitian support is available [19]. It is of growing interest for adults with epilepsy not traditionally offered the ketogenic diet.

Medium Chain Triglyceride Diet
MCTs are liquid fats and more ketogenic than the long chain fats of the classic ketogenic diet. The MCT diet was introduced by Huttenlocher to allow a more palatable and more varied diet, and seems to be as effective as the classic ketogenic diet in controlling seizures [29–31]. However, many find the MCT diet causes more gastrointestinal side effects (bloating, cramps, vomiting, and diarrhea) and is therefore used less frequently. At Hopkins the authors often add MCT oil to the classic ketogenic diets to relieve a child's constipation and reduce elevated cholesterol (when present).

The Low Glycemic Index Treatment
Some carbohydrates raise blood glucose more than others. This effect is related to particle size, starch structure, fiber content, and other factors. Pfeifer and colleagues [32] have found that by using low glycemic index foods, a ketogenic-like diet may be as effective, more palatable, and better tolerated than the classic ketogenic diet [33]. They state that half of their 60 patients continued on the low glycemic index treatment for 6 months, and 60% of these had a greater than 50% reduction in seizures, whereas 38% had a greater than 90% reduction. The relative usefulness of this approach requires additional studies.

MANAGEMENT OF CHILDREN ON THE KETOGENIC DIET
Weight Gain and Weight Loss
Children (particularly those <2 years of age) on the diet should be carefully monitored for excessive weight gain or loss [7]. In general, weight gain is intentionally limited by caloric restriction to the amount appropriate to linear growth. The caloric intake should be adjusted if excessive gain or loss occurs. Small decreases in caloric intake have been found to improve seizure control when the child is gaining weight disproportionate to growth.

Growth
Although children grow in length on the diet, the rate of growth may be somewhat slower than normal. This pattern is most notable in young children and merits close observation [7,34].

COMPLICATIONS OF THE KETOGENIC DIET
Vitamin and Mineral Deficiency
The ketogenic diet is deficient in the water-soluble vitamins thiamin (vitamin B_1), riboflavin (vitamin B_2), niacin, vitamin B_6, folate, vitamin B_{12}, biotin, and pantothenic acid, and they **must** be supplemented in a sugar-free form.

Mineral supplementation may also be provided, although symptomatic deficiency of zinc, selenium, and calcium is rare.

Kidney Stones
Calcium oxalate or uric acid kidney stones have been reported to occur in 13% to 20% of children on the classic ketogenic diet [35]. The calcium oxalate stones are a result of the hypercalciuria secondary to bone demineralization, increased calcium excretion by the kidney, and acidosis. Stones can be prevented by the prophylactic or therapeutic administration of potassium citrate [36]. The urine of children on the diet should be checked periodically for elevated calcium to creatinine ratio and for microscopic hematuria, an indication of kidney stones.

Lipids
It is widely misbelieved that a high-fat diet will lead to dramatically elevated lipids and atherosclerosis. One study [12] documented an increase in cholesterol and other lipids and lipoproteins after 6 months on the ketogenic diet, but this dyslipidemia was only slightly higher than the acceptable range, and decreased when measured in the same children at 12 and 24 months on the diet. Because few children remain on the diet more than 2 years, the significance of the elevations in causing future atherosclerosis is unclear and should be weighed against the diet's benefits [8,13].

Gastrointestinal Symptoms
Vomiting is common during initiation of the diet because of the ketosis but disappears as the individual becomes tolerant of the lipids and the ketonemia. If severe, vomiting can be controlled with a small amount of glucose. Constipation also is common on the diet and may be relieved with Miralax or the addition of small amounts of MCT oil.

CLINICAL CONTROVERSIES REGARDING THE KETOGENIC DIET

At this stage in use of the ketogenic diet and its variations, many different opinions exist regarding its implementation and supplementation [37]. Hospital admission for initiation of the diet is used at most centers but not by all. Although we have found hospitalization useful, it may not be mandatory or even necessary. Fasting before initiation of the diet was once thought to be mandatory but has now been shortened or even abandoned. Studies indicate, however, that seizures may improve more rapidly after fasting [21].

Specific ratios of fat to protein and carbohydrate on the diet remain variable [38]. The classic diet is four parts fat to one part protein and carbohydrate. A ratio of 3:1 is used in young children and adolescents. However, some children experience seizure control with the newer diets using lower ratios of fat to protein and carbohydrates. A minority of children may require higher ratios for seizure control.

Ketosis itself, once considered the secret of the diet, may not be mandatory or related to seizure control. Fluid restriction once was considered mandatory, but no scientific evidence supports it. Calorie restriction has been shown to be important for seizure control in some animal models, but no careful studies have been done in humans. However, in those on the ketogenic diet with less than optimal control, further restriction of calories has often been useful. The diet's use in children with surgically resectable static lesions causing the seizures is also controversial, but the diet sometimes is successful in controlling their seizures and thus avoiding surgery [39].

Carnitine supplementation of the diet is used by some centers, but the need for this expensive supplement and its usefulness are undocumented [40]. When children on the diet appeared weak or failing to thrive on the diet, the authors have attempted carnitine supplementation but rarely found it useful. Supplementation of the diet with multivitamins and calcium is used by all, but supplementation with zinc, selenium, some vitamins (vitamin D), citrate, and laxatives remains variable.

As with most teachings about the diet, the details of its use remain more of an art than a science. Implementation and management of the diet, therefore, requires supervision by a knowledgeable dietician.

BASIC SCIENCE AND THE DIET

How do Ketogenic Diets Control Seizures and Epilepsy?

The large number of recent clinical studies documenting the efficacy of the ketogenic diet in controlling seizures and epilepsy in childhood has stimulated a flurry of basic science activity to find the diet's mechanisms of action. These studies were the subject of a recent international symposium summarized in *Epilepsia* [41]. Despite all of this activity, only limited information is available on the diet's mechanisms.

What is know is that acidosis is not the answer. Ketosis may be a partial answer, but diets such as the modified Atkins diet and the low glycemic index diet may be effective without producing ketosis. Glucose restriction and calorie restriction have anticonvulsant and antiepileptic effects documented in animal models, but whether this is how the diet exerts its anticonvulsant effects is unclear. Clinical evidence indicates that glucose administration and excess calories may negate the efficacy of the diet. Thus, glucose restriction seems to be an important ingredient of a successful diet, but again, the mechanism through which glucose exerts its effects is unclear.

The inhibitory effects of γ-aminobutyric acid (GABA) underlie the mechanisms of many anticonvulsant medications, but little evidence shows that the ketogenic diet's effects are mediated through this mechanism. Leptin, which regulates energy intake and expenditure, may be increased in rats fed a ketogenic diet. If and how leptin affects seizures and epilepsy is currently unknown.

Acetone, acetoacetate, increased energy stores, increased levels of glutathione, and increases in polyunsaturated fatty acids have each been proposed as mechanisms for the diet's effectiveness, but studies have been inconclusive.

THE FUTURE OF THE KETOGENIC DIET

The ketogenic diet is effective in controlling many different types of seizures in children—as effective, perhaps more effective, than current anticonvulsant medications. It has fewer cognitive side effects and perhaps longer-lasting antiepileptic effects than current anticonvulsant medications and may have a positive disease-modifying (perhaps even a curative) effect in some children. As the diet's mechanisms of action have come to be understood, perhaps some of the mechanisms underlying epilepsy will begin to be understood. Perhaps that knowledge can then be encapsulated in a pill [42].

The ketogenic diet may also have more wide-ranging usefulness than just for epilepsy [43].

THE KETOGENIC DIET FOR BRAIN TUMORS AND OTHER TUMORS

Animal models [44] and anecdotal human studies indicate that the ketogenic diet may be useful in the treatment of brain tumors. Cancerous cells require glucose for survival and are unable to use ketones for energy. Normal brain cells readily metabolize ketones for energy. In 1995, Nebeling and colleagues [44] treated two children who had nonresectable gliomas with the ketogenic diet. Both had remarkable tumor regression and long-term survival. Seyfried and colleagues [45] documented tumor regression in rat brain tumor models with use of the calorie-restricted ketogenic diet. Anecdotes from patients with cancer placed on the ketogenic diet support these reports [46]. The authors are unaware of any series of human brain tumors treated with a caloric-restricted ketogenic diet, although this treatment should have minimal side effects and could be studied as an adjunct to standard brain tumor protocols.

Glucose transport and ketone metabolism also may play a role in the treatment of other cancers. The glycolysis inhibitor 3-bromopyruvate preferentially suppressed the growth of colon cancer cells, suggesting that glucose deprivation is useful in blocking their growth [47,48].

Neurologic Conditions

Evidence from uncontrolled clinical trials and studies in animal models suggest that the ketogenic diet can provide symptomatic and disease-modifying activity in a broad range of neurodegenerative disorders [48]. Anecdotal and uncontrolled studies have suggested that the ketogenic diet may have beneficial effects on Alzheimer disease [48,49], Parkinson disease, and amyotrophic lateral sclerosis. Some experts have suggested that the diet may be protective after traumatic brain injury [50,51] and stroke [52], and perhaps hypoxic-ischemic injuries in the newborn and adult. The diet may be useful in the management of autism [53] and severe hyperactivity [54]. Further studies of each of these areas will be interesting.

Nonneurologic Conditions

Some experts have also suggested that the diet, or even its modifications, may be useful in nonneurologic conditions, such as diabetes [55,56] and perhaps inflammatory diseases and pain [57].

In summary, the authors agree with the 2009 position statement of the Charlie Foundation:

> "The ketogenic diet has consistently been documented to effectively treat epilepsy in thousands of children since 1924. In the last fifteen years over 750 peer-reviewed articles regarding its success, implementation, and scientific mechanisms have been published. Two major reports which included 44 reviews of over one thousand children who received ketogenic diet treatment confirmed that at least half benefited with a 50% or greater improvement in seizure control."

A 2008 consensus report from 26 worldwide experts concluded that the ketogenic diet "should be offered to a child after two anticonvulsants (medications) are used unsuccessfully" [37].

SUMMARY

Interest in the ketogenic diet has come a long way since 1994. Its anticonvulsant and perhaps antiepileptic effectiveness have been accepted, although the mechanisms through which these are achieved are unknown. The effects of the diet on conditions such as tumors deserve more study. Its use in diabetes is promising. The use of ketones after brain trauma and strokes and in treating hyperactivity and other disorders will be interesting.

Acknowledgments

The authors would like to thank Dr Adam Hartman for his thoughtful suggestions and Elaine Freeman for her careful editing.

References

(These references represent many of the most recent references on the subject. They are intended to lead into the far more extensive literature using the references found within each. A more complete list of recently published articles is available on The Charlie Foundation Web site at www.charliefoundation.org.)

[1] Swink TD, Vining EP, Freeman JM. The ketogenic diet 1996. Adv Pediatr 1997;44: 297–329.

[2] Freeman JM. What every Pediatrician should know about the ketogenic diet. Contemp Pediatr 2003;20:113–27.

[3] Kossoff EH, Freeman JM, Turner Z, et al. The ketogenic diet: treatment for epilepsy and other disorders. 5th edition. New York: Demos Medical Publishers; 2011, in press.

[4] Phinney SD. Ketogenic diets and physical performance. Nutr Metab (Lond) 2004;1:2.

[5] Veech RL, Chance B, Kashiwaya Y, et al. Ketone bodies, potential therapeutic uses. IUBMB Life 2001;51:241–7.

[6] Veech RL. The therapeutic implications of ketone bodies: the effects of ketone bodies in pathological conditions: ketosis, ketogenic diet, redox states, insulin resistance, and mitochondrial metabolism. Prostaglandins Leukot Essent Fatty Acids 2004;70:309–19.

[7] Vining EP, Pyzik P, McGrogan J, et al. Growth of children on the ketogenic diet. Dev Med Child Neurol 2002;43:375–8.

[8] Nizamuddin J, Turner Z, Rubenstein JE, et al. Management and risk factors for dyslipidemia with the ketogenic diet. J Child Neurol 2008;23:758–61.

[9] Rubenstein JE. Use of the ketogenic diet in neonates and infants. Epilepsia 2008;49(Suppl 8): 30–2.

[10] Taubes G. What if it's all been a big fat lie? Available at: http://www.nytimes.com/2002/07/07/magazine/what-if-it-s-all-been-a-big-fat-lie.html. Accessed August 26, 2010.

[11] Yancy WS Jr, Olsen MK, Guyton JR. A low-carbohydrate, ketogenic diet versus a low-fat diet to treat obesity and hyperlipidemia: a randomized, controlled trial. Ann Intern Med 2004;40:769–77.

[12] Kwiterovitch PO, Vining EP, Pyzik P, et al. The effect of a high fat, ketogenic diet on the plasma levels of lipids, lipoproteins and apolipoproteins in children. JAMA 2003;290: 912–20.

[13] Patel A, Pyzik PL, Turner Z, et al. Long-term outcomes of children treated with the ketogenic diet in the past. Epilepsia 2010;51(7):1277–82.

[14] Kossoff EH, Pyzik PL, McGrogan JR, et al. Efficacy of the ketogenic diet for infantile spasms. Pediatrics 2002;109:780–3.

[15] Kossoff EH, Hedderick EF, Turner Z, et al. A case-control evaluation of the ketogenic diet versus ACTH for new-onset infantile spasms. Epilepsia 2008;49:1504–9.

[16] Kilaru S, Berqvist AG. Current treatment of myoclonic astatic epilepsy: clinical experience at the Children's Hospital of Philadelphia. Epilepsia 2007;48(9):1703–7.

[17] Wheless J. The history of the ketogenic diet. Epilepsia 2008;49(Suppl 8):3–5.

[18] A list of physicians world-wide who use the ketogenic diet. Available at: www.epilepsy.com/ketonews. Accessed August 13, 2010.

[19] Kossoff EH, Dorward JL, Molinero MR, et al. The modified Atkins diet: a potential treatment for developing countries. Epilepsia 2008;49:1646–7.

[20] Kossoff EH, Zupec-Kania BA, Amark PE, et al. Optimal clinical management of children receiving the ketogenic diet: recommendations of the International Ketogenic Diet Study Group. Epilepsia 2009;50(2):304–17.

[21] Kossoff EH, Laux LC, Blackford R, et al. When do seizures usually improve with the ketogenic diet? Epilepsia 2008;49(2):329–33.

[22] Villeneuve N, Pinton F, Bahi-Buisson N, et al. The ketogenic diet improves recently worsened epilepsy. Dev Med Child Neurol 2009;51:276–81.

[23] Prins M. Cerebral metabolic adaptation and ketone metabolism after brain injury. J Cereb Blood Flow Metab 2008;28(1):1–16.

[24] Hemingway C, Freeman JM, Pillas DJ, et al. The ketogenic diet: a 3–6 year follow-up of 150 children prospectively enrolled. Pediatrics 2001;108:898–905.

[25] Cross H, Neal EG. The ketogenic diet- update on recent clinical trials. Epilepsia 2008;49 (Suppl 8):6–10.

[26] Neal EG, Chaffe HM, Schwartz R, et al. The ketogenic diet for the treatment of childhood epilepsy: a randomized controlled trial. Lancet Neurol 2008;7(6):500–6.

[27] Freeman JM, Vining EP, Kossoff EH, et al. A blinded, crossover study of the ketogenic diet. Epilepsia 2009;50(2):322–5.

[28] Freeman J. The ketogenic diet: additional information from a crossover study. J Child Neurol 2009;24:509–12.

[29] Kossoff EH, Dorward JL. The modified Atkins diet. Epilepsia 2009;49(Suppl 8):37–41.

[30] Liu YC. Medium-chain triglyceride (MCT) ketogenic therapy. Epilepsia 2008;49(Suppl 8): 33–6.

[31] Neal EG, Chaffe HM, Schwartz RH, et al. A randomized trial of the classical and medium chain triglyceride diets in the treatment of childhood epilepsy. Epilepsia 2009;50: 1109–17.

[32] Pfeifer HH, Lyczkowski DA, Thiele EA. Low glycemic index treatment: Implementation and new insights into efficacy. Epilepsia 2008;49(Suppl 8):42–5.

[33] Muzykewicz DA, Lyczkowski DA, Memon N, et al. Efficacy, safety, and tolerability of the low glycemic index treatment in pediatric epilepsy. Epilepsia 2009;50:1118–26.

[34] Zupec-Kania B, Zupeck-Kania M. Long-term management of the ketogenic diet: seizure monitoring, nutrition, and supplementation. Epilepsia 2008;49(Suppl 8):23–36.

[35] Sampath A, Kossoff EH, Furth SL, et al. Kidney stones and the ketogenic diet: risk factors and prevention. J Child Neurol 2007;22:375–8.

[36] McNally MA, Pyzik PL, Rubenstein JE, et al. Empiric use of potassium citrate reduces kidney-stone incidence with the ketogenic diet. Pediatrics 2009;124:e300–4.

[37] Kossoff EH. International consensus statement on clinical Implementation of the ketogenic diet: agreement, flexibility and controversy. Epilepsia 2008;49(Suppl 8):11–3.

[38] Wirrell EC. Ketogenic ratio, calories and fluids: do they matter? Epilepsia 2008;49(Suppl 8): 17–9.

[39] Jung DE, Kang HC, Kim HD. Long-term outcome of the ketogenic diet for childhood intractable epilepsy due to focal malformation of cortical development. Pediatrics 2008;122:330.

[40] Freeman JM, Vining EP, Cost SS, et al. Does carnitine administration improve the symptoms attributed to anticonvulsant medications? A double-blinded, crossover study. Pediatrics 1994;93:893–5.

[41] Hartman AL. Does the effectiveness of the ketogenic diet yield insights into its mechanisms? Epilepsia 2008;49(Suppl 8):53–6.

[42] Rho JM, Sankar R. The ketogenic diet in a pill: is it possible? Epilepsia 2008;49(Suppl 8): 127–33.

[43] Baranano KW, Hartman AL. The ketogenic diet: uses in epilepsy and other neurologic illnesses. Curr Treat Options Neurol 2008;10:410–9.

[44] Nebeling LC, Miraldi F, Shurin SB, et al. Effects of a ketogenic diet on tumor metabolism and nutritional status in pediatric oncology patients: two case reports. J Am Coll Nutr 1995;14: 202–8.

[45] Seyfried TN, Kiebish M, Marsh J, et al. Targeting energy metabolism in brain cancer through caloric restriction and the ketogenic diet. J Cancer Res Ther 2009;5(Suppl 1):S7–15.

[46] Zuccoli G, Marcello N, Pisanello A. Metabolic management of glioblastoma multiforme using standard therapy together with a restricted ketogenic diet: case report. Nutr Metab (Lond) 2010;7:33.

[47] Yun J, Rago C, Cheong R, et al. Glucose deprivation contributes to the development of KRAS pathway mutations in tumor cells. Science 2009;325:1555–9.

[48] Gasior M, Rogawski MA, Hartman AL. Neuroprotective and disease-modifying effects of the ketogenic diet. Behav Pharmacol 2006;17(5–6):431–9.

[49] Henderson ST. Ketone bodies as a therapeutic for Alzheimer's disease. Neurotherapeutics 2008;5:470–80.

[50] Prins ML. Diet, ketones, and neurotrauma. Epilepsia 2008;49(Suppl 8):111–3.

[51] Appelberg KS, Hovda DA, Prins ML. The effects of a ketogenic diet on behavioral outcome after controlled cortical impact injury in the juvenile and adult rat. J Neurotrauma 2009;26(4):497–506.

[52] Tai KK, Nguyen N, Pham L, et al. Ketogenic diet prevents cardiac arrest-induced cerebral ischemic neurodegeneration. J Neural Transm 2008;115:1011–7.

[53] Evangeliou A, Vlachonikolis I, Mihailidou H, et al. Application of a ketogenic diet in children with autistic behavior: pilot study. J Child Neurol 2003;18(2):113–8.

[54] Murphy P, Burnham WM. The ketogenic diet causes a reversible decrease in activity level in Long-Evans rats. Exp Neurol 2006;201(1):84–9.

[55] Yancy WS Jr, Foy M, Chalecki AM, et al. A low-carbohydrate, ketogenic diet to treat type 2 diabetes. Nutr Metab (Lond) 2005;2:34.

[56] Westman EC, Yancy WS Jr, Mavropoulos JC, et al. The effect of a low-carbohydrate, ketogenic diet versus a low-glycemic index diet on glycemic control in type 2 diabetes mellitus. Nutr Metab (Lond) 2008;5:36.

[57] Ruskin DN, Kawamura M, Masino SA. Reduced pain and inflammation in juvenile and adult rats fed a ketogenic diet. PLoS One 2009;4(12):e8349.

Advances in Pediatrics 57 (2010) 331–351

ADVANCES IN PEDIATRICS

The GH/IGF-1 Axis in Growth and Development: New Insights Derived from Animal Models

Dara Cannata, MD, Archana Vijayakumar, BS,
Yvonne Fierz, MD, Derek LeRoith, MD, PhD*

Division of Endocrinology, Diabetes and Bone Diseases, The Samuel Bronfman Department of
Medicine, Mount Sinai School of Medicine, One Gustave L. Levy Place, Atran 4th Floor-36, PO
Box 1055, New York, NY 10029-6574, USA

L ongitudinal growth in humans follows a unique pattern that is characterized by rapid fetal growth, deceleration immediately after birth, a prolonged childhood growth phase, an additional deceleration prepubertally,
and a dramatic adolescent growth spurt leading ultimately to stagnancy in
adulthood [1]. Linear bone growth, which accompanies longitudinal body
growth, occurs during development and the childhood years until epiphyseal
fusion occurs after puberty [2]. Growth is dynamic in nature and is influenced
by nutritional, neuronal, and hormonal factors [3].

Growth hormone (GH), a hormone secreted from the anterior pituitary
gland, is a major regulator of somatic growth. The mammalian GH gene
(also known as GH-normal or GH-N) belongs to a family of genes that includes
the genes for GH, prolactin (PRL), and the placental lactogens [4]. The human
GH-N heterogeneous nuclear RNA transcript undergoes alternative splicing,
which leads to the creation of 2 mature mRNA transcripts, which then encode
2 polypeptides with molecular weights of 22 kDa and 20 kDa. In the circulation, the majority of human GH protein is the 22 kDa isoform; whereas, a small
amount is the 20 kDa isoform [4]. GH is secreted from the anterior pituitary
gland in a pulsatile fashion [5]. GH secretion exhibits sexual dimorphism in humans and rats. In humans, women exhibit more irregularity in GH secretion
than men [6]. Two hypothalamic factors regulate and maintain the pulsatile
secretion of GH from pituitary somatotrophs [7,8]. Growth hormone releasing
hormone (GHRH) stimulates GH release; whereas, somatostatin release-inhib-
iting factor (SRIF, or somatostatin) inhibits GH release [7,8]. In the circulation,
GH binds to the growth hormone binding protein (GHBP), a truncated form of
the growth hormone receptor (GHR). GHBP contains the extracellular portion
of the GHR [9–12]. In humans, the GHBP has been suggested to be formed by

*Corresponding author. E-mail address: derek.leroith@mssm.edu

0065-3101/10/$ – see front matter
doi:10.1016/j.yapd.2010.09.003

proteolytic cleavage of the extracellular domain of the GH receptor [13]; whereas, in rodents, the GHBP is produced by alternate mRNA splicing [10,11]. It has been proposed that up to 60% of circulating GH is bound to GHBP [14]. GHBP is thought to decrease the rate of clearance and degradation of GH, thereby increasing its half-life in the serum [14]. The main function of GH is to promote postnatal longitudinal growth. In fact, animals and humans with GH deficiency have been shown to have retarded body growth. Conversely, excess GH has been shown to cause gigantism and acromegaly in humans, which has also been reproduced in animals [15–18].

The growth-promoting effects of GH are brought about by the actions of GH on cellular metabolism and differentiation. Many of the effects of GH on somatic growth are mediated by its stimulatory effects on the secretion of the insulin-like growth factor-I (IGF-I) from the liver [19]. IGF-I, along with IGF-II, is a growth factor that shares a high degree of homology with the precursor form of insulin (proinsulin) [20]. In the circulation, the majority of IGFs are bound in a 150 kDa ternary complex with the IGF binding protein-3 (IGFBP-3) or IGF binding protein-5 (IGFBP-5) and the acid labile subunit (ALS). A smaller portion of IGFs are associated within 50 kDa binary complexes with the other IGFPBPs, such as IGFBP-1, IGFBP-2, IGFBP-4, and IGFBP-6, and less than 5% of the IGFs are found in their free 7.5 kDa form [3,21]. The major roles of the IGFBPs are to transport the IGFs in the circulation and across capillary barriers, to distribute them in the extravascular space and to mediate their access to receptors [22]. The IGFBPs prolong the half-lives of the IGFs by protecting them from proteolytic degradation [19]. During the postnatal period, circulating IGF-I levels are regulated mainly by GH [23–26]. However, IGF-I also negatively regulates GH secretion through feedback mechanisms [27,28]. Thus, the relationship between GH and IGF-I is complex and the effects of one cannot be considered mutually exclusive of the other. Given this complicated relationship, GH and IGF-I are often referred to as the GH/IGF-I axis.

Over the years, a large body of data on the mechanisms by which the GH/IGF-I axis regulates body growth has been compiled by genetically manipulating this axis in mice and other animal models Table 1. This review summarizes the findings of these studies and discusses their clinical implications.

SKELETAL DEVELOPMENT AND LONGITUDINAL GROWTH

Ossification, the process by which bone is formed, occurs by 2 mechanisms: intramembranous ossification and endochondral ossification. Intramembranous ossification is the formation of bone directly from connective tissue with no preliminary cartilage stage. Endochondral ossification entails the formation of osseous tissue by the replacement of cartilage anlagen. Thus, membranous bone originates from the mesenchyme: whereas, endochondral bone formation occurs within a cartilage template. Bone is a dynamic tissue. Old tissue is constantly replaced with new tissue, a process called bone remodeling. Bone remodeling occurs because of the synergistic actions of 2 classes of cells: the

Table 1
Transgenic and knockout models affecting the GH-IGF axis

Model	GH	IGF-I	Phenotype	References
GHKO mice	↓	↓	Large adipose stores, 2/3 size of control mice, reduced femoral bone mineral density	[84,88,90]
GHRKO mice	↓	↓	Postnatal growth retardation, dwarfism	[16,51]
Transgenic bGH mice	↑	↑	Larger size than control mice, increased femoral bone mineral density	[111–114]
IGF-I KO mice	↑	↓	Growth retardation in utero and postnatally, high rate of mortality after birth	[130,131]
IGF-IR KO mice	?	↑	Fetal growth deficiencies, delayed epiphyseal maturation	[127]
Bone IGF-I overexpression	↑	↓	Increased bone mineral density and bone remodeling	[134]

Abbreviations: GHKO, growth hormone knockout; GHRKO, growth hormone receptor knockout; IGF-I KO, insulin-like growth factor- I knockout; IGF-IR KO, insulin-like growth factor- I receptor knockout.

osteoclasts that remove the old, damaged tissue and the osteoblasts that form the new bone matrix. Childhood and adolescent linear (longitudinal) bone growth occurs via endochondral ossification at the epiphyseal (growth) plate at the end of long bones. Long bones, which include the femur, tibia, fibula, humerus, radius, ulna, metacarpals, metatarsals, and phalanges, typically contain an outer shell of cortical (compact bone) and a deeper layer of trabecular (cancellous) bone. Epiphyseal plates are present in growing bones; they are found in children throughout puberty and early adulthood. The growth plate has 3 main layers: the resting zone, the proliferative zone, and the hypertrophic zone [29]. Chondrogenesis, the formation of cartilage, results from chondrocyte (connective tissue cells that occupy lacuna within the cartilage matrix) proliferation, hypertrophy, and extracellular matrix secretion. Once cartilage is formed, new blood vessels and bone precursors are recruited and the cartilage is replaced by bone. As new bone is added at the bottom of the growth plate, bone elongation occurs [29]. Chondrocytes at different stages of differentiation occupy the 3 main layers of the growth plate. Resting zone chondrocytes replicate slowly and mainly function as stemlike cells for proliferative zone chondrocytes [30,31]. Proliferative zone chondrocytes replicate at a fast rate [30]. The hypertrophic process results in terminally differentiated chondrocytes. During this process, the zone of hypertrophic chondrocytes significantly increases in height, thereby greatly contributing to longitudinal growth [30,32]. When growth plate cartilage is completely replaced by bone, it is termed *epiphyseal fusion*. In humans, this typically occurs by the time of sexual maturation. It has been proposed that epiphyseal fusion is triggered when the proliferative potential of growth plate chondrocytes is finally exhausted [33]. Longitudinal bone growth is regulated by endocrine factors, such as GH, IGF-I, glucocorticoid, thyroid hormone, estrogen, androgen, vitamin D, and leptin [29]. The GH/IGF-I axis, in particular, leads to longitudinal growth by stimulating chondrocyte proliferation and hypertrophy [29,34].

The GH/IGF-I axis also affects the skeletal system by mediating achievement of peak bone mineral density [35]. The acquisition of peak bone mass, occurring at the end of skeletal maturation, is an important determinant of later development of osteoporosis and subsequent fracture risk [36].

Although it is clear that the GH/IGF-I axis plays a role in longitudinal growth, the exact mechanisms by which GH and IGF-I regulate somatic growth remains the subject of research and revision as new discoveries continue to be made.

THE SOMATOMEDIN HYPOTHESIS AND ITS EFFECT ON BONE GROWTH

In 1957, Salmon and Daughaday [37] found that GH (then called somatotropin) stimulated the incorporation of radioactive inorganic sulfate into cartilage. Further studies showed that this effect was lost when rats were hypophysectomized and was restored when rats were given exogenous bovine GH (bGH) injections, but this effect was not observed when cartilage slices were incubated with GH in vitro [38–40]. This finding suggested that GH did not mediate its effects directly but rather stimulated the expression of an intermediate factor that was responsible for the effects of GH. This intermediary factor was first named somatomedin C and later called insulin-like growth factor-I (IGF-I) to represent its structural and biologic similarities to insulin [41,42]. The original somatomedin hypothesis thereby postulated that somatic growth was a result of GH stimulating hepatic IGF-I production with IGF-I acting on peripheral tissues in an endocrine manner.

This hypothesis was questioned in 1980, when D'Ercole and colleagues [43] reported that multiple tissues of the fetal mouse synthesized IGF-I suggesting that IGF-I had local (autocrine/paracrine) effects. Moreover, Isaksson and colleagues [44] injected human growth hormone into the cartilage growth plate of the hind limbs of hypophysectomized rats and noted a significant increase in longitudinal bone growth. The contralateral limbs that did not receive an injection had no significant increase in growth rate, thereby demonstrating a local effect of GH. These investigators hypothesized that GH itself had local effects on somatic growth, independent of circulating IGF-I and suggested an alternative to the original somatomedin hypothesis.

In 1985, Green and colleagues [45] introduced the "dual effector hypothesis," which suggested that GH directly stimulates specific differentiation of preadipocytes into adipocytes, while it indirectly stimulates the clonal expansion of these newly differentiated cells via stimulating local IGF-I production for autocrine/paracrine action. Although the direct effect of GH on growth has been confirmed in other studies [32,46,47], questions have been posed regarding GH induction of IGF-I synthesis in proliferative chondrocytes. Multiple groups of researchers concluded that IGF-I is not needed for growth plate chondrocyte clonal expansion [47–49]. For example, Ohlsson and colleagues [47] found that injections of GH stimulated the multiplication of cells in the germinal layer of the epiphyseal plate; whereas, injections of IGF-I did not. The cells of the germinal layer are slow-cycling cells that are thought to function as progenitor cells of the growth plate. The investigators suggested that GH has a direct action on these cells; whereas, IGF-I acts only on the proliferation of chondrocytes. Wang and colleagues [50] reported that the IGF-I null mice had normal chondrocyte numbers and proliferation and suggested that IGF-I promotes longitudinal bone growth by augmenting chondrocyte hypertrophy through "insulin-like anabolic actions." Lupu and colleagues [51] formed a different conclusion when they studied the body length of mice with a null mutation of the GHR gene (GHRKO), mice with a null mutation of the IGF-I gene (IGF-I KO), and IGF-I/GHR double knock-out mice (IGF-I + GHR DKO). The investigators found that the IGF-I + GHR DKO mice demonstrated more severe growth retardation than the IGF-I KO or GHRKO mice, suggesting that GH and IGF-I promote growth by both common and independent functions (Fig. 1). In addition, the investigators demonstrated

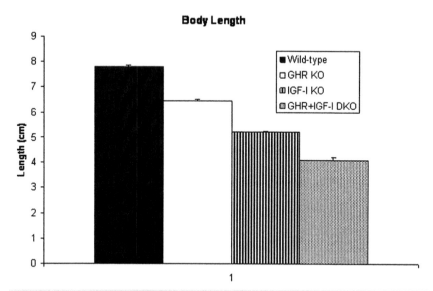

Fig. 1. Lupu and colleagues studied the body length of mice with a null mutation of the GHR gene (GHRKO), mice with a null mutation of the IGF-I gene (IGF-I KO), and IGF-I/GHR double knock-out mice (IGF-I + GHR DKO). As demonstrated, the IGF-I + GHR DKO mice demonstrate smaller size than did the IGF-I KO or GHR KO mice suggesting that GH and IGF-I promote growth by both common and independent functions. (*Data from* Lupu F, Terwilliger JD, Lee K, et al. Roles of growth hormone and insulin-like growth factor 1 in mouse postnatal growth. Dev Biol 2001;229:141–62.)

that GHR and IGF-IR were both expressed in the zone of proliferative chondrocytes, suggesting that IGF-I and GH are both involved in chondrocyte proliferation. Other groups found a greater reduction in longitudinal tibial growth rate in GHRKO mice as compared with IGF-I KO mice [52,53]. On the other hand, Hutchison and colleagues [54] reported that systemic IGF-I was a profound mediator of bovine epiphysial chondrocyte proliferation. Studies in IGF-I deficient mice demonstrate that IGF-I is a major stimulator of skeletal development in mice by promoting chondrocyte proliferation and hypertrophy while inhibiting apoptosis [53]. Thus, currently much controversy exists regarding the exact nature of the actions of GH and IGF-I on linear bone growth [55]. In addition, much study has been dedicated to elucidate the role of circulating and local IGF-I (subsequently discussed).

The roles of IGF-I and GH in somatic growth are constantly being reevaluated and have been the subject of much debate and discovery. The original somatomedin hypothesis was the first attempt to explain the effects of the GH/IGF-I axis on growth and has been revised continuously to reflect the most up-to-date findings. Studies have revealed that the GH/IGF-I system is more complex than it was originally thought to be. Currently, the thought is that both the endocrine and local effects of GH and IGF-I play a role in somatic growth. Further study is likely to continue to refine the somatomedin hypothesis and the understanding of the GH/IGF-I axis.

GROWTH HORMONE

As stated previously, GH is a major mediator of postnatal growth in mammals. Most of the GH in circulation is secreted by the somatotrope cells of the anterior pituitary [5]. However, extrapituitary production of GH has been reported in the brain, immune system, placenta, mammary gland, and testicles [56–60]. Synthesis of GH also occurs in prolactin- and gonadotropin-secreting cells of the anterior pituitary [61]. The secretion of GH from pituitary somatotrophs is regulated by the balance between GHRH and SRIF [7,8]. Several of the additional factors that have been shown to influence GH include IGF-I, which regulates GH secretion by feedback mechanisms; ghrelin, a peptide produced mainly by the stomach that stimulates GH release [62]; leptin, a cytokine hormone secreted by adipose tissue that stimulates spontaneous pulsatile GH secretion and the GH response to GHRH activity [63]; and free fatty acids, which inhibit GH release through a feedback mechanism, as GH is involved in lipid mobilization [64].

GH functions as a promoter of skeletal growth. Hypersecretion of GH leads to gigantism in children and acromegaly in adults. Individuals with these conditions develop enlarged bones and organomegaly [18]. Hyposecretion of GH leads to short stature and reduced height velocity [65]. In addition, GH has other important functions involving metabolism, reproduction, and aging that are beyond the scope of this article [66].

THE GROWTH HORMONE RECEPTOR AND SIGNAL TRANSDUCTION

GH mediates its effects on somatic growth by binding to the GHR on target tissues [67]. The GHR is a member of the cytokine receptor superfamily; other members of this class of receptors include receptors for prolactin; erythropoietin; thrombopoietin; leptin; interleukins 3, 5 and 6; granulocyte/macrophage colony stimulating factor; and interferons [68]. The GHR consists of 3 domains: an extracellular GH binding domain, a transmembrane domain, and an intracellular domain. The traditional view of GHR signaling was that 1 molecule of GH binds 2 GHR monomers and induces their dimerization. However, recent studies have demonstrated that the GHR exists as a preformed dimer that binds GH [69–71]. Upon binding GH, the GHR undergoes conformational changes that result in transphosphorylation and activation of the adjacent Janus kinase 2 (Jak2) molecules, which are cytoplasmic tyrosine kinases associated with the GHR [72]. Once activated, Jak2 phosphorylates tyrosine residues on the GHR, creating a binding site for Src homology 2 (SHC2) domain-containing proteins. The SHC2 domain-containing proteins include the signal transducers and activators of transcription (STAT) proteins, which are subsequently phosphorylated by Jak2. Once phosphorylated, the STATs homodimerize or heterodimerize and are translocated to the nucleus where they regulate gene expression of target genes, such as IGF-1, ALS, and suppressor of cytokine signaling (SOCS) proteins. SOCS proteins function as negative regulators of the JAK/STAT signaling pathways and act to terminate the GH signal cascade [68,73]. GH has been shown to activate STAT 1, 3, 5a, and 5b; however, STAT5b has been shown to be the major mediator of GH action [68]. Studies in rodents originally demonstrated that the one or both of the STAT 5 proteins were important for GH-induced IGF-I expression and skeletal growth [74,75]. Recent studies in rats have shown that the IGF-I gene contains response elements that bind STAT5b in a GH-dependent manner [76]. In humans, it has also been suggested that STAT5b is responsible for GH-mediated IGF-I stimulation as individuals with homozygous mutations of the STAT5b gene demonstrate severe growth retardation and reduced serum IGF-I, IGFBP, and ALS concentrations [77,78]. These individuals do demonstrate normal concentration of STAT5a, thus supporting the role of STAT5b as the sole mediator of GH-mediated IGF-I stimulation. GHR has also been shown to activate the phosphatidylinositol-triphosphate kinase (PI3K) and mitogen-activated protein kinase (MAPK) pathways, which both play critical roles in mediating the metabolic and mitogenic effects of insulin and IGF-I [79].

To study the importance of GH in linear growth, animal models have been employed. In mice, several recessive mutant genes have been identified that cause dwarfism as a result of decreased GH production or action [80,81]. Three of these mutant mouse models are the little mouse (*lit/lit*), Snell dwarf (dw), and Ames dwarf (df). The *lit/lit* mice exhibit isolated GH deficiency; whereas, the Snell and Ames dwarf mice have deficiencies in GH along with other anterior pituitary hormones [82–85]. Ames and Snell dwarf mice have mutations in transcription factors that regulate the expression of genes that encode for the embryonic development of the pituitary gland, and therefore they are deficient in GH, thyroid stimulating hormone (TSH), and PRL [86,87]. Phenotypically, the Ames and Snell dwarf mice exhibit small size, stunted growth, and infertility [86,87]. On the other hand, the *lit/lit* mouse has a mutation in the growth hormone releasing hormone receptor (GHRHR) gene, which leads to decreased GH production and GHRH resistance [84,88]. The pituitary glands of these mice have decreased secretory granules within somatotropes and decreased pituitary GH production as compared with control mice [80,89]. Because only the GH axis is affected, these mice have normal TSH and PRL levels and are fertile [88]. The *lit/lit* mice have abnormal body composition (with large adipose stores and decreased body water, protein, and minerals), and decreased serum IGF-I levels and IGFBP-3 levels [90]. They also achieve only two-thirds the size of wild-type litter mates [88] and exhibit reduced volumetric femoral bone density and reduced cortical bone volume with normal trabecular bone volume [84]. As the *lit/lit* mice have an isolated deficiency in GH, as compared with Snell and Ames dwarf mice which have deficiencies in all anterior pituitary hormones, the *lit/lit* mice provide a desirable mouse model to study the effects of GH on growth. Given the decreased size and abnormalities in bone development, the *lit/lit* mice demonstrate the importance of GH in skeletal development, linear growth, and bone mineral density.

Another mouse model was created by Zhou and colleagues, [16] the growth hormone receptor/binding protein (GHR/BP) knockout (GHRKO), which is a mouse model of GH resistance. Homozygous GHRKO mice are characterized by severe postnatal growth retardation, proportionate dwarfism, greatly decreased serum IGF-I concentration, and elevated serum GH concentration. Heterozygous GHRKO mice show only minimal growth impairment but demonstrate decreased GHR and GHBP expression and minimally decreased IGF-I levels. Similar to the *lit/lit* mice, GHRKO mice have decreased bone growth, bone mineral density, and bone turnover [51], which suggests that despite elevated GH levels, the GH resistance of GHRKO makes the mice phenotypically appear GH deficient. The GHRKO mouse model provides an in vivo model of Laron syndrome, a syndrome of growth hormone resistance (discussed later), and has been used to further explore clinical findings seen in humans with this disease [16,91].

Although much of the understanding of the effects of the GH/IGF-I axis on growth come from mouse models, much has also been learned from studying the clinical conditions affecting children with growth hormone deficiency (GHD) and growth hormone resistance. Prenatal growth is not dependent on GH because infants with GH and GHR deletions are born near-normal size [15]. GH does have important postnatal effects on growth because patients with congenital GHD or insensitivity demonstrate profound postnatal growth retardation [15].

GHD in children can be congenital or acquired. Regardless of which form of GHD a child has, clinically, patients demonstrate growth failure. Patients with congenital GHD are more likely to present breech and with perinatal asphyxia than non-GHD infants [92]. They often present with hypoglycemia, prolonged jaundice, microgenitalia in boys, and failure to thrive [65]. Many children with congenital GHD have multiple pituitary hormone deficiencies, such as adrenocorticotropic hormone and TSH [65]. Growth failure often presents in the first months of the infant's life [93–95]. Children with acquired GHD commonly present with short stature or a reduced height velocity [65]. In addition, children with GHD have lower bone mineral density [96,97], which can be increased with GH treatment [96]. Patients who are suboptimally treated have reduced bone mineral density upon reaching their final height [96]. Children with GHD demonstrate the importance of GH on bone growth and achieving peak bone mineral density. In particular, patients with congenital GHD highlight the importance of GH in the postnatal period, as these children are born of normal size and exhibit decreased growth in the first months of life.

Although children with Laron syndrome are technically resistant to and not deficient of GH, they clinically resemble patients with GHD. Laron syndrome was first described in Israeli patients in 1966 and since that time many independent populations of patients with Laron syndrome have been identified [15,98,99]. Laron syndrome is defined as hereditary dwarfism that results from a mutation in the GHR gene, resulting in resistance to GH. In most cases, the mutation is located in the extracellular domain of the GHR, thus affected patients often have absent or low levels of GHBP, as this is a truncated form of the GHR [100–104]. Laron syndrome phenotypically resembles GHD as patients demonstrate severe growth retardation and low serum IGF-I. However, unlike with GHD, in Laron syndrome, GH levels are elevated. Patients with Laron syndrome also metabolically resemble patients who are GH-deficient (much like the GHRKO mice resemble *lit/lit* mice) as they exhibit truncal obesity, delayed puberty, and hypoglycemia [105]. They are born near normal size but exhibit rapid postnatal decline with a reduced growth velocity. In addition, they do not experience a pubertal growth spurt [105]. Patients also traditionally have dysmorphic faces with a protruding forehead, saddle nose, underdeveloped facial bones, small chin, and sparse facial hair [105,106]. The long bones are thin and degenerative spinal changes are seen in young adults [107]. Decreased bone mineral density has been observed in young adults with Laron syndrome [108]. Further study showed that patients with Laron syndrome have less lean body mass and a higher percentage of body adiposity. However, when bone mineral density is normalized to overall body size, it is not reduced. In addition, markers of bone formation are not increased [109]. Patients with Laron syndrome are responsive to the growth-promoting effects of exogenous IGF-I but not to exogenous GH, implying that the defect lies at the level of the GHR and that IGF-I most likely mediates the GH effects on the bone [15,110]. Thus, Laron syndrome highlights the importance of the GH/IGF-1 axis in skeletal development and bone growth and maintenance.

Although the effects of a hormone can be demonstrated by studying deficiency states, much can be gleaned by studying states of excess. Mice with ubiquitous overexpression of the rat *GH* or *bGH* gene grow significantly larger than their control littermates [111–113]. Female GH-transgenic mice have higher femoral bone density than control mice. However, male GH-transgenic mice show no significant difference in bone mineral density as compared with control mice [114]. This gender difference likely reflects the interaction of female and male sex steroids and the bone [115]. Thus, although, further study is necessary to evaluate the effects of excessive GH on bone mineral density, animal models have confirmed the stimulatory effect of GH on growth.

In humans, gigantism and acromegaly are conditions of GH excess that result from GH-secreting adenomas [116]. Gigantism occurs when GH-secreting adenomas occur in young patients before epiphyseal fusion, resulting in the subsequent accelerated linear growth. When the GH-secreting adenoma occurs after epiphyseal fusion, acromegaly develops. Patients who are acromegalic demonstrate local overgrowth of bone, especially of the skull and mandible. As epiphyseal fusion has already occurred, linear growth is not affected [117]. In both conditions, elevated levels of GH and IGF-I are observed. In acromegaly, patients have an increase in body water and lean body mass and a decrease in body adiposity [118]. In general, bone mineral density is increased; however, often the effects of elevated GH are overshadowed by the effects of the hypogonadism (which can lead to a reduction in bone mineral density) that is often seen in this condition [119,120]. Cortical bone density appears to be less dependent on hypogonadism than trabecular bone density [119,120]. There is a paucity of data on fracture risk in patients who ae acromegalic; however, one small study did report a reduction in fracture risk [121]. Thus, data from patients with GH excess supports the conclusions formed from studying patients with GHD, as it suggests that GH may promote acquisition of ideal bone mineral density in addition to promoting linear bone growth. Moreover, observation of the phenotype of patients with gigantism and acromegaly demonstrates the importance of GH in linear body growth during the growth spurt seen in adolescence.

Taken together, GH plays an important role in skeletal development, linear growth, and bone mineral density. GH exerts its effects on somatic growth through signaling cascades. Animal models of GH deficiency and resistance highlight the importance of GH on linear growth, skeletal development, and the achievement of peak bone mineral density. Human syndromes of these conditions confirm GH as a mediator of somatic growth. The effects of GH on somatic growth has also been elucidated through the study of animal and human models of GH excess in which increased somatic and bone overgrowth are observed. Although the relative role of direct GH action versus IGF-I-mediated GH action is not quite clear at this time, animal models provide a means of addressing this complex question. Hence, further study using animal models is likely to continue to further delineate the complicated relationship between GH and IGF-I and their contributions to somatic and bone growth. Taken together,

GH is an important mediator of skeletal development, linear growth, and bone mineral density.

IGF-I

The IGF family consists of the ligands, IGF-I, IGF-II and insulin, the IGF binding proteins, IGFBP 1-6 and cell surface receptors, IGF-I receptor (IGF-IR), and insulin receptor (IR), that mediate the actions of the ligands. IGF-I and IGF-II share a high degree of homology with the precursor form of insulin (proinsulin) [20]. The IGF-IR and IR mediate the cellular responses of IGF-I and insulin, respectively. Similar to their ligands, the IGF-IR and IR demonstrate a high degree of homology and can thus exist as homodimers or heterodimers [122]. Both receptors have an extracellular α-subunit and an intracellular β-subunit with a transmembrane region [123]. Ligands bind the receptors at the α-subunit; whereas, the intracellular domains of the β-subunit contain the tyrosine kinase activity [124]. Ligand binding induces receptor activation, by transphosphorylation of tyrosine residues in the β-subunit, which in turn activates several downstream signaling pathways, predominantly the PI3K and MAPK pathways. These pathways are responsible for the metabolic and mitogenic effects of insulin and IGF-I [79].

IGF-I is a primary mediator of bone growth. IGF-I stimulates endochondral bone formation and rapidly activates bone turnover [125,126]. Unlike GH, which appears to have only postnatal effects on growth, the IGF system has been shown to have an important role in embryonic, fetal, and postnatal growth. Prenatally, IGF-I appears to have GH-independent effects on growth; however, these effects become GH-dependent around the time of birth [68]. For example, mice with deletions of the IGF-IR demonstrate decreased birth weight and postnatal growth failure [127]. Human studies also demonstrate reduced intrauterine and postnatal growth in individuals with mutations of the IGF-IR [128,129].

Animal studies have been used to define the role of IGF-I in skeletal growth. IGF-I null mice are born at 60% of the body weight of control mice [130,131]. Although most IGF-I null mice die shortly after birth, those that survive have deficits in postnatal growth and development, reaching only 30% of the body weight of control mice [130,131]. These mice show a reduction in femoral length, size, and bone mineral density as compared with control mice [52]. In fact, mice that are heterozygous for knock-out of the IGF-I gene also demonstrate a decrease in femoral bone content and bone mineral density [132]. Mice with deletions of the IGF-IR also demonstrate profound fetal growth deficiencies and delayed epiphyseal maturation postnatally [127,133]. Mice with genetic perturbation of both IGF-I and IGF-IR phenotypically resemble IGF-IR KO mice, suggesting that IGF-IR is responsible of the actions of IGF-I [127]. Thus, although animal models demonstrate that IGF-I plays an important role in prenatal and postnatal growth, IGF-I also seems to be required for the maintenance of bone mineral density.

Animal models of IGF-I excess also highlight a relationship between IGF-I and bone mineral density. Mouse models in which there is local IGF-I overexpression at the level of the bone demonstrate an increase in bone remodeling and bone mineral density as compared with control mice [132,134]. These findings of an association between bone mineral density and IGF-I have been replicated in human studies. Several groups have studied adolescent females and found a correlation between serum IGF-I levels and bone mineral density [135–136]. Thus, it is possible that exogenous IGF-I treatment might increase bone mineral density in children with IGF-I deficiency. However, because a clinical syndrome with primary IGF-I deficiency is rare, such a study is difficult to conduct. However, when recombinant human IGF-I was administered to healthy, postmenopausal women no change in bone mineral density was not seen [137–138]. Therefore, although it is clear that IGF-I plays a role in the achievement of peak bone mineral density, it is not yet clear if IGF-I administration can increase bone mineral density in older adults.

Human syndromes involving IGF-I-deficiency, IGF-I resistance, and ALS deficiency have been identified. For example, Woods and colleagues [128] first described a case of a patient with a homozygous partial deletion of the IGF-I gene. The manifestations of this patient's genetic disorder included severe prenatal and postnatal growth failure, sensorineural deafness, and mental retardation. Walenkamp and colleagues [139] presented a case of a patient with an inactivating mutation of IGF-I who presented with severe intrauterine and postnatal growth retardation, microcephaly, and sensorineural deafness. Bonapace and colleagues [140] reported a patient with a mutation in the E-domain of the IGF-I precursor, leading to low serum IGF-I levels, short stature, sensorineural deafness, and delayed psychomotor development. Patients with mutations in the IGF-IR exhibit both intrauterine growth retardation and poor postnatal growth [129,141].Cases of patients with mutations in the ALS gene have also been reported [142]. Patients with ALS deficiency present with reduced postnatal growth, short stature, and delayed puberty [142]. These patients demonstrate a marked reduction in bone mineral density and the development of fractures with minimal trauma [143]. Human genetic disorders involving IGF-I, IGF-IR, and ALS have been identified and the clinical presentations of the patients with these disorders, much like the aforementioned mouse models, demonstrate the importance of IGF-I in prenatal and postnatal growth and development.

Although it is clear that IGF-I has important functions on skeletal development and growth, the relative contributions of circulating (endocrine) and local IGF-I has been the subject of much investigation. D'Ercole and colleagues [43] reported IGF-I synthesis by multiple tissues of the fetal mouse, suggesting a local effect (autocrine/paracrine) of IGF-I. These findings were corroborated by the findings of other groups who reported IGF-I mRNA expression in many peripheral tissues [144–146]. As stated previously, these findings led to a revision of the original somatomedin hypothesis and questioned the relative contribution of circulating and autocrine/paracrine IGF-I to postnatal growth. The authors' earlier studies addressed whether circulating or autocrine/paracrine IGF-I was critical in postnatal growth. The Cre/LoxP system was used to create a mouse model with liver-specific deletion of the IGF-I gene (LID). The LID mice showed normal levels of IGF-I mRNA in nonhepatic tissues but no hepatic IGF-I mRNA. Total circulating IGF-I levels were only 25% of the levels found in control mice and GH levels were 4 times higher than levels in control mice. However, despite this dramatic reduction in circulating IGF-I, body and femoral lengths did not differ between control and LID mice [147]. Genetic deletion of the acid labile subunit in mice (ALSKO) resulted in a 62% decrease in levels of IGF-I as compared with control mice. Growth was only mildly affected with a growth deficit of 13% by 10 weeks of age [148]. Double trans-genic LID + ALSKO mice, on the other hand, showed an 85% to 90% reduc-tion in circulating IGF-I levels and a 30% reduction in linear growth as compared with control mice. Proximal growth plates of the LID + ALSKO mice were smaller as were the proliferative and hypertrophic zones of chondro-cytes as compared with control mice. Bone density, periosteal circumference, and cortical thickness were also decreased in the LID + ALSKO mice [3]. These studies using LID + ALSKO mice suggested that circulating IGF-I is critical for bone growth and that a threshold level of IGF-I is necessary for peak bone mass achievement Table 2.

To further explore the contributions of circulating and local IGF-I to devel-opment and maintenance of the bone, mouse models in which only the endo-crine form of IGF-I is active have been developed [149,150]. The authors have recently generated the KO-HIT mouse, a model in which the endogenous *Igf-1* gene was genetically ablated in all tissues and a rat *Igf-1* transgene was overex-pressed specifically in the liver. KO-HIT mice had serum IGF-I levels that were 2.5-fold higher than controls, but were born smaller. However, catch-up growth was seen at pubertal age such that adult KO-HIT mice exhibited normal body weight and body length. This finding suggests that tissue IGF-I is important for early neonatal growth, but in its absence, postnatal linear growth can be compensated for by increased circulating IGF-I [150]. Further study is necessary to better define if hepatic-derived endocrine IGF-I, in the absence of local IGF-I, is sufficient for normal bone acquisition.

Thus, IGF-I is a prominent mediator of prenatal and postnatal growth and skeletal development. The absence of IGF-I results in decreased bone length

Table 2
LID, ALSKO, LID+ ALSKO mice

Model	GH	IGF-I	Phenotype	References
LID	↑ by 4.5 fold	↓ by 75%	No difference in body or femoral length as compared to controls	[3,147]
ALSKO	—	↓ by 65%	Growth decreased by 13%	[3,148]
LID + ALSKO	↑ by 15 fold	↓ by 85%–90%	Growth decreased by 30%	[3]

Abbreviations: LID, liver IGF-I deficient knockout; ALSKO, acid labile subunit knockout; LID+ ALSKO, liver IGF-I deficient/ acid labile subunit knockout.

and bone mineral density. However, there may also be differential effects of local and circulating IGF-I as demonstrated by animal models. Moreover, it seems that there exists a threshold level for circulating IGF-I below which changes in bone parameters can be seen, suggesting that local IGF-I may not be able to compensate for the loss of circulating IGF-I; whereas, the latter seems feasible as seen with the KO-HIT mouse. As more data is collected, it is likely that answers to these questions will be provided and the understanding of the effects IGF-I on skeletal development, linear growth, and bone mineral density will be furthered.

SUMMARY

The GH/IGF-I axis plays an important role in skeletal development, linear growth, and the achievement of peak bone mineral density. The original somatomedin hypothesis stated that GH mediates its effect through an intermediate factor, later found to be IGF-I. Further study suggested that the GH/IGF-I axis was much more complicated than it was originally thought to be. Studies in human and animal models have highlighted the integral effects of GH and IGF-I on skeletal development, linear growth, and the achievement of peak bone mineral density. GH and IGF-I promote growth by both common and independent functions. Questions regarding the relative role of direct GH action versus IGF-I-mediated GH action and the precise role of circulating versus local IGF-I still remain. However, it is clear that the GH/IGF-I axis is a pivotal mediator of somatic growth and bone growth and maintenance.

References

[1] Rosenfeld RG. Insulin-like growth factors and the basis of growth. N Engl J Med 2003;349: 2184–6.

[2] Robson H, Siebler T, Shalet SM, et al. Interactions between GH, IGF-I, glucocorticoids, and thyroid hormones during skeletal growth. Pediatr Res 2002;52:137–47.

[3] Yakar S, Rosen CJ, Beamer WG, et al. Circulating levels of IGF-1 directly regulate bone growth and density. J Clin Invest 2002;110:771–81.

[4] Tuggle CK, Trenkle A. Control of growth hormone synthesis. Domest Anim Endocrinol 1996;13:1–33.

[5] Gahete MD, Duran-Prado M, Luque RM, et al. Understanding the multifactorial control of growth hormone release by somatotropes: lessons from comparative endocrinology. Ann N Y Acad Sci 2009;1163:137–53.

[6] Pincus SM, Gevers EF, Robinson IC, et al. Females secrete growth hormone with more process irregularity than males in both humans and rats. Am J Physiol 1996;270:E107–15.

[7] Brazeau P, Vale W, Burgus R, et al. Hypothalamic polypeptide that inhibits the secretion of immunoreactive pituitary growth hormone. Science 1973;179:77–9.

[8] Spiess J, Rivier J, Vale W. Characterization of rat hypothalamic growth hormone-releasing factor. Nature 1983;303:532–5.

[9] Spencer SA, Hammonds RG, Henzel WJ, et al. Rabbit liver growth hormone receptor and serum binding protein. Purification, characterization, and sequence. J Biol Chem 1988;263:7862–7.

[10] Baumbach WR, Horner DL, Logan JS. The growth hormone-binding protein in rat serum is an alternatively spliced form of the rat growth hormone receptor. Genes Dev 1989;3: 1199–205.

[11] Smith WC, Kuniyoshi J, Talamantes F. Mouse serum growth hormone (GH) binding protein has GH receptor extracellular and substituted transmembrane domains. Mol Endocrinol 1989;3:984–90.

[12] Barnard R, Waters MJ. Serum and liver cytosolic growth-hormone-binding proteins are antigenically identical with liver membrane 'receptor' types 1 and 2. Biochem J 1986;237:885–92.

[13] Trivedi B, Daughaday WH. Release of growth hormone binding protein from IM-9 lymphocytes by endopeptidase is dependent on sulfhydryl group inactivation. Endocrinology 1988;123:2201–6.

[14] Baumann G, Amburn K, Shaw MA. The circulating growth hormone (GH)-binding protein complex: a major constituent of plasma GH in man. Endocrinology 1988;122:976–84.

[15] Rosenfeld RG, Rosenbloom AL, Guevara-Aguirre J. Growth hormone (GH) insensitivity due to primary GH receptor deficiency. Endocr Rev 1994;15:369–90.

[16]. Zhou Y, Xu BC, Maheshwari HG, et al. A mammalian model for Laron syndrome produced by targeted disruption of the mouse growth hormone receptor/binding protein gene (the Laron mouse). Proc Natl Acad Sci U S A 1997;94:13215–20.

[17] Costa C, Solanes G, Visa J, et al. Transgenic rabbits overexpressing growth hormone develop acromegaly and diabetes mellitus. FASEB J 1998;12:1455–60.

[18] Colao A, Merola B, Ferone D, et al. Acromegaly. J Clin Endocrinol Metab 1997;82: 2777–81.

[19] Le Roith D, Bondy C, Yakar S, et al. The somatomedin hypothesis: 2001. Endocr Rev 2001;22:53–74.

[20] LeRoith D, Roberts CT Jr. Insulin-like growth factors. Ann N Y Acad Sci 1993;692:1–9.

[21] LeRoith D. Insulin-like growth factor receptors and binding proteins. Baillieres Clin Endocrinol Metab 1996;10:49–73.

[22] Clemmons DR, Busby W, Clarke JB, et al. Modifications of insulin-like growth factor binding proteins and their role in controlling IGF actions. Endocr J 1998;45(Suppl):S1–8.

[23] Hall LJ, Kajimoto Y, Bichell D, et al. Functional analysis of the rat insulin-like growth factor I gene and identification of an IGF-I gene promoter. DNA Cell Biol 1992;11:301–13.

[24] Bichell DP, Kikuchi K, Rotwein P. Growth hormone rapidly activates insulin-like growth factor I gene transcription in vivo. Mol Endocrinol 1992;6:1899–908.

[25] Mathews LS, Norstedt G, Palmiter RD. Regulation of insulin-like growth factor I gene expression by growth hormone. Proc Natl Acad Sci U S A 1986;83:9343–7.

[26] Pell JM, Saunders JC, Gilmour RS. Differential regulation of transcription initiation from insulin-like growth factor-I (IGF-I) leader exons and of tissue IGF-I expression in response to changed growth hormone and nutritional status in sheep. Endocrinology 1993;132:1797–807.

[27] Yamashita S, Melmed S. Insulinlike growth factor I regulation of growth hormone gene transcription in primary rat pituitary cells. J Clin Invest 1987;79:449–52.

[28] Yamashita S, Ong J, Melmed S. Regulation of human growth hormone gene expression by insulin-like growth factor I in transfected cells. J Biol Chem 1987;262:13254–7.

[29] Nilsson O, Marino R, De Luca F, et al. Endocrine regulation of the growth plate. Horm Res 2005;64:157–65.

[30] Kember NF. Cell population kinetics of bone growth: the first ten years of autoradiographic studies with tritiated thymidine. Clin Orthop Relat Res 1971;76:213–30.

[31]. Abad V, Meyers JL, Weise M, et al. The role of the resting zone in growth plate chondrogenesis. Endocrinology 2002;143:1851–7.

[32] Hunziker EB, Wagner J, Zapf J. Differential effects of insulin-like growth factor I and growth hormone on developmental stages of rat growth plate chondrocytes in vivo. J Clin Invest 1994;93:1078–86.

[33] Weise M, De-Levi S, Barnes KM, et al. Effects of estrogen on growth plate senescence and epiphyseal fusion. Proc Natl Acad Sci U S A 2001;98:6871–6.

[34] Wang Q, Seeman E. Skeletal growth and peak bone strength. Best Pract Res Clin Endocrinol Metab 2008;22:687–700.

[35] Tritos NA, Biller BM. Growth hormone and bone. Curr Opin Endocrinol Diabetes Obes 2009;16:415–22.

[36] Bonjour JP, Theintz G, Law F, et al. Peak bone mass. Osteoporos Int 1994;4(Suppl 1): 7–13.

[37] Salmon WD Jr, Daughaday WH. A hormonally controlled serum factor which stimulates sulfate incorporation by cartilage in vitro. J Lab Clin Med 1957;49:825–36.

[38] Murphy WR, Daughaday WH, Hartnett C. The effect of hypophysectomy and growth hormone on the incorporation of labeled sulfate into tibial epiphyseal and nasal cartilage of the rat. J Lab Clin Med 1956;47:715–22.

[39] Denko CW, Bergenstal DM. The effect of hypophysectomy and growth hormone on S35 fixation in cartilage. Endocrinology 1955;57:76–86.

[40] Daughaday WH, Reeder C. Synchronous activation of DNA synthesis in hypophysectomized rat cartilage by growth hormone. J Lab Clin Med 1966;68:357–68.

[41] Daughaday WH, Hall K, Raben MS, et al. Somatomedin: proposed designation for sulphation factor. Nature 1972;235:107.

[42] Rinderknecht E, Humbel RE. The amino acid sequence of human insulin-like growth factor I and its structural homology with proinsulin. J Biol Chem 1978;253:2769–76.

[43] D'Ercole AJ, Applewhite GT, Underwood LE. Evidence that somatomedin is synthesized by multiple tissues in the fetus. Dev Biol 1980;75:315–28.

[44] Isaksson OG, Jansson JO, Gause IA. Growth hormone stimulates longitudinal bone growth directly. Science 1982;216:1237–9.

[45] Green H, Morikawa M, Nixon T. A dual effector theory of growth-hormone action. Differentiation 1985;29:195–8.

[46] Isaksson OG, Lindahl A, Nilsson A, et al. Mechanism of the stimulatory effect of growth hormone on longitudinal bone growth. Endocr Rev 1987;8:426–38.

[47] Ohlsson C, Nilsson A, Isaksson O, et al. Growth hormone induces multiplication of the slowly cycling germinal cells of the rat tibial growth plate. Proc Natl Acad Sci U S A 1992;89:9826–30.

[48] Shinar DM, Endo N, Halperin D, et al. Differential expression of insulin-like growth factor-I (IGF-I) and IGF-II messenger ribonucleic acid in growing rat bone. Endocrinology 1993;132:1158–67.

[49] Wang E, Wang J, Chin E, et al. Cellular patterns of insulin-like growth factor system gene expression in murine chondrogenesis and osteogenesis. Endocrinology 1995;136:2741–51.

[50] Wang J, Zhou J, Bondy CA. Igf1 promotes longitudinal bone growth by insulin-like actions augmenting chondrocyte hypertrophy. FASEB J 1999;13:1985–90.

[51] Lupu F, Terwilliger JD, Lee K, et al. Roles of growth hormone and insulin-like growth factor 1 in mouse postnatal growth. Dev Biol 2001;229:141–62.

[52] Mohan S, Richman C, Guo R, et al. Insulin-like growth factor regulates peak bone mineral density in mice by both growth hormone-dependent and -independent mechanisms. Endocrinology 2003;144:929–36.

[53] Wang Y, Nishida S, Sakata T, et al. Insulin-like growth factor-I is essential for embryonic bone development. Endocrinology 2006;147:4753–61.

[54] Hutchison MR, Bassett MH, White PC. Insulin-like growth factor-I and fibroblast growth factor, but not growth hormone, affect growth plate chondrocyte proliferation. Endocrinology 2007;148:3122–30.

[55] Kaplan SA, Cohen P. The somatomedin hypothesis 2007: 50 years later. J Clin Endocrinol Metab 2007;92:4529–35.

[56] Boguszewski CL, Svensson PA, Jansson T, et al. Cloning of two novel growth hormone transcripts expressed in human placenta. J Clin Endocrinol Metab 1998;83:2878–85.

[57] Mol JA, Henzen-Logmans SC, Hageman P, et al. Expression of the gene encoding growth hormone in the human mammary gland. J Clin Endocrinol Metab 1995;80:3094–6.

[58] de Mello-Coelho V, Gagnerault MC, Souberbielle JC, et al. Growth hormone and its receptor are expressed in human thymic cells. Endocrinology 1998;139:3837–42.

[59] Kooijman R, Berus D, Malur A, et al. Human neutrophils express GH-N gene transcripts and the pituitary transcription factor Pit-1b. Endocrinology 1997;138:4481–4.

[60] Berry SA, Srivastava CH, Rubin LR, et al. Growth hormone-releasing hormone-like messenger ribonucleic acid and immunoreactive peptide are present in human testis and placenta. J Clin Endocrinol Metab 1992;75:281–4.

[61] Mertani HC, Waters MJ, Jambou R, et al. Growth hormone receptor binding protein in rat anterior pituitary. Neuroendocrinology 1994;59:483–94.

[62] Kojima M, Hosoda H, Date Y, et al. Ghrelin is a growth-hormone-releasing acylated peptide from stomach. Nature 1999;402:656–60.

[63] Tannenbaum GS, Gurd W, Lapointe M. Leptin is a potent stimulator of spontaneous pulsatile growth hormone (GH) secretion and the GH response to GH-releasing hormone. Endocrinology 1998;139:3871–5.

[64] Imaki T, Shibasaki T, Shizume K, et al. The effect of free fatty acids on growth hormone (GH)-releasing hormone-mediated GH secretion in man. J Clin Endocrinol Metab 1985;60:290–3.

[65] Herber SM, Milner RD. Growth hormone deficiency presenting under age 2 years. Arch Dis Child 1984;59:557–60.

[66] Lichanska AM, Waters MJ. How growth hormone controls growth, obesity and sexual dimorphism. Trends Genet 2008;24:41–7.

[67] Kopchick JJ, Andry JM. Growth hormone (GH), GH receptor, and signal transduction. Mol Genet Metab 2000;71:293–314.

[68] Rosenfeld RG, Hwa V. The growth hormone cascade and its role in mammalian growth. Horm Res 2009;71(Suppl 2):36–40.

[69] Gent J, van Kerkhof P, Roza M, et al. Ligand-independent growth hormone receptor dimerization occurs in the endoplasmic reticulum and is required for ubiquitin system-dependent endocytosis. Proc Natl Acad Sci U S A 2002;99:9858–63.

[70] Goffin V, Kelly PA. The prolactin/growth hormone receptor family: structure/function relationships. J Mammary Gland Biol Neoplasia 1997;2:7–17.

[71] Yang N, Wang X, Jiang J, et al. Role of the growth hormone (GH) receptor transmembrane domain in receptor predimerization and GH-induced activation. Mol Endocrinol 2007;21:1642–55.

[72] Argetsinger LS, Campbell GS, Yang X, et al. Identification of JAK2 as a growth hormone receptor-associated tyrosine kinase. Cell 1993;74:237–44.

[73] Hansen JA, Lindberg K, Hilton DJ, et al. Mechanism of inhibition of growth hormone receptor signaling by suppressor of cytokine signaling proteins. Mol Endocrinol 1999;13:1832–43.

[74] Udy GB, Towers RP, Snell RG, et al. Requirement of STAT5b for sexual dimorphism of body growth rates and liver gene expression. Proc Natl Acad Sci U S A 1997;94:7239–44.

[75] Teglund S, McKay C, Schuetz E, et al. Stat5a and Stat5b proteins have essential and nonessential, or redundant, roles in cytokine responses. Cell 1998;93:841–50.

[76] Chia DJ, Ono M, Woelfle J, et al. Characterization of distinct Stat5b binding sites that mediate growth hormone-stimulated IGF-I gene transcription. J Biol Chem 2006;281:3190–7.

[77] Rosenfeld RG, Belgorosky A, Camacho-Hubner C, et al. Defects in growth hormone receptor signaling. Trends Endocrinol Metab 2007;18:134–41.

[78] Kofoed EM, Hwa V, Little B, et al. Growth hormone insensitivity associated with a STAT5b mutation. N Engl J Med 2003;349:1139–47.

[79] Saltiel AR, Kahn CR. Insulin signaling and the regulation of glucose and lipid metabolism. Nature 2001;414:799–806.

[80] Eicher EM, Beamer WG. Inherited ateliotic dwarfism in mice. Characteristics of the mutation, little, on chromosome 6. J Hered 1976;67:87–91.

[81] Eicher EM, Beamer WG. New mouse dw allele: genetic location and effects on lifespan and growth hormone levels. J Hered 1980;71:187–90.

[82] Bartke A. Histology of the anterior hypophysis, thyroid and gonads of two types of dwarf mice. Anat Rec 1964;149:225–35.

[83] Bartke A. The response of two types of dwarf mice to growth hormone, thyrotropin, and thyroxine. Gen Comp Endocrinol 1965;5:418–26.

[84] Beamer WH, Eicher EM. Stimulation of growth in the little mouse. J Endocrinol 1976;71: 37–45.

[85] Bartke A, Goldman BD, Bex F, et al. Effects of prolactin (PRL) on pituitary and testicular function in mice with hereditary PRL deficiency. Endocrinology 1977;101:1760–6.

[86] Brown-Borg HM, Borg KE, Meliska CJ, et al. Dwarf mice and the ageing process. Nature 1996;384:33.

[87] Flurkey K, Papaconstantinou J, Miller RA, et al. Lifespan extension and delayed immune and collagen aging in mutant mice with defects in growth hormone production. Proc Natl Acad Sci U S A 2001;98:6736–41.

[88] Lin SC, Lin CR, Gukovsky I, et al. Molecular basis of the little mouse phenotype and implications for cell type-specific growth. Nature 1993;364:208–13.

[89] Cheng TC, Beamer WG, Phillips JA 3rd, et al. Etiology of growth hormone deficiency in little, Ames, and Snell dwarf mice. Endocrinology 1983;113:1669–78.

[90] Donahue LR, Beamer WG. Growth hormone deficiency in 'little' mice results in aberrant body composition, reduced insulin-like growth factor-I and insulin-like growth factor-binding protein-3 (IGFBP-3), but does not affect IGFBP-2, -1 or -4. J Endocrinol 1993;136:91–104.

[91] Kopchick JJ, Laron Z. Is the Laron mouse an accurate model of Laron syndrome? Mol Genet Metab 1999;68:232–6.

[92] Craft WH, Underwood LE, Van Wyk JJ. High incidence of perinatal insult in children with idiopathic hypopituitarism. J Pediatr 1980;96:397–402.

[93] Gluckman PD, Gunn AJ, Wray A, et al. Congenital idiopathic growth hormone deficiency associated with prenatal and early postnatal growth failure. The International Board of the Kabi Pharmacia International Growth Study. J Pediatr 1992;121:920–3.

[94] De Luca F, Bernasconi S, Blandino A, et al. Auxological, clinical and neuroradiological findings in infants with early onset growth hormone deficiency. Acta Paediatr 1995;84: 561–5.

[95] Pena-Almazan S, Buchlis J, Miller S, et al. Linear growth characteristics of congenitally GH-deficient infants from birth to one year of age. J Clin Endocrinol Metab 2001;86:5691–4.

[96] Saggese G, Baroncelli GI, Bertelloni S, et al. The effect of long-term growth hormone (GH) treatment on bone mineral density in children with GH deficiency. Role of GH in the attainment of peak bone mass. J Clin Endocrinol Metab 1996;81:3077–83.

[97] Saggese G, Baroncelli GI, Bertelloni S, et al. Effects of long-term treatment with growth hormone on bone and mineral metabolism in children with growth hormone deficiency. J Pediatr 1993;122:37–45.

[98] Laron Z, Pertzelan A, Mannheimer S. Genetic pituitary dwarfism with high serum concentration of growth hormone—a new inborn error of metabolism? Isr J Med Sci 1966;2: 152–5.

[99] Woods KA, Savage MO. Laron syndrome: typical and atypical forms. Baillieres Clin Endocrinol Metab 1996;10:371–87.

[100] Baumann G, Shaw MA, Winter RJ. Absence of the plasma growth hormone-binding protein in Laron-type dwarfism. J Clin Endocrinol Metab 1987;65:814–6.

[101] Daughaday WH, Trivedi B. Absence of serum growth hormone binding protein in patients with growth hormone receptor deficiency (Laron dwarfism). Proc Natl Acad Sci U S A 1987;84:4636–40.

[102] Laron Z, Klinger B, Erster B, et al. Serum GH binding protein activities identifies the heterozygous carriers for Laron type dwarfism. Acta Endocrinol (Copenh) 1989;121: 603–8.

[103] Amselem S, Duquesnoy P, Duriez B, et al. Spectrum of growth hormone receptor mutations and associated haplotypes in Laron syndrome. Hum Mol Genet 1993;2:355–9.

[104] Rosenbloom AL, Guevara Aguirre J, Rosenfeld RG, et al. The little women of Loja–growth hormone-receptor deficiency in an inbred population of southern Ecuador. N Engl J Med 1990;323:1367–74.

[105] Rosenbloom AL, Guevara-Aguirre J, Rosenfeld RG, et al. Growth hormone receptor deficiency in Ecuador. J Clin Endocrinol Metab 1999;84:4436–43.

[106] Laron Z. Laron syndrome (primary growth hormone resistance or insensitivity): the personal experience 1958–2003. J Clin Endocrinol Metab 2004;89:1031–44.

[107] Kornreich L, Horev G, Schwarz M, et al. Laron syndrome abnormalities: spinal stenosis, os odontoideum, degenerative changes of the atlanto-odontoid joint, and small oropharynx. AJNR Am J Neuroradiol 2002;23:625–31.

[108] Laron Z, Klinger B. IGF-I treatment of adult patients with Laron syndrome: preliminary results. Clin Endocrinol (Oxf) 1994;41:631–8.

[109] Bachrach LK, Marcus R, Ott SM, et al. Bone mineral, histomorphometry, and body composition in adults with growth hormone receptor deficiency. J Bone Miner Res 1998;13:415–21.

[110] Carel JC, Chaussain JL, Chatelain P, et al. Growth hormone insensitivity syndrome (Laron syndrome): main characteristics and effects of IGF1 treatment. Diabetes Metab 1996;22: 251–6.

[111] Palmiter RD, Brinster RL, Hammer RE, et al. Dramatic growth of mice that develop from eggs microinjected with metallothionein-growth hormone fusion genes. Nature 1982;300: 611–5.

[112] Knapp JR, Chen WY, Turner ND, et al. Growth patterns and body composition of transgenic mice expressing mutated bovine somatotropin genes. J Anim Sci 1994;72:2812–9.

[113] McGrane MM, de Vente J, Yun J, et al. Tissue-specific expression and dietary regulation of a chimeric phosphoenolpyruvate carboxykinase/bovine growth hormone gene in transgenic mice. J Biol Chem 1988;263:11443–51.

[114] Eckstein F, Lochmuller EM, Koller B, et al. Body composition, bone mass and microstructural analysis in GH-transgenic mice reveals that skeletal changes are specific to bone compartment and gender. Growth Horm IGF Res 2002;12:116–25.

[115] Callewaert F, Venken K, Kopchick JJ, et al. Sexual dimorphism in cortical bone size and strength but not density is determined by independent and time-specific actions of sex steroids and IGF-I: evidence from pubertal mouse models. J Bone Miner Res 2010;25: 617–26.

[116] Melmed S. Medical progress: acromegaly. N Engl J Med 2006;355:2558–73.

[117] Keil MF, Stratakis CA. Pituitary tumors in childhood: update of diagnosis, treatment and molecular genetics. Expert Rev Neurother 2008;8:563–74.

[118] Katznelson L. Alterations in body composition in acromegaly. Pituitary 2009;12:136–42.

[119] Diamond T, Nery L, Posen S. Spinal and peripheral bone mineral densities in acromegaly: the effects of excess growth hormone and hypogonadism. Ann Intern Med 1989;111: 567–73.

[120] Colao A, Pivonello R, Scarpa R, et al. The acromegalic arthropathy. J Endocrinol Invest 2005;28:24–31.

[121] Vestergaard P, Mosekilde L. Fracture risk is decreased in acromegaly–a potential beneficial effect of growth hormone. Osteoporos Int 2004;15:155–9.

[122] Ullrich A, Gray A, Tam AW, et al. Insulin-like growth factor I receptor primary structure: comparison with insulin receptor suggests structural determinants that define functional specificity. EMBO J 1986;5:2503–12.

[123] Steele-Perkins G, Turner J, Edman JC, et al. Expression and characterization of a functional human insulin-like growth factor I receptor. J Biol Chem 1988;263:11486–92.

[124] Sasaki N, Rees-Jones RW, Zick Y, et al. Characterization of insulin-like growth factor I-stimulated tyrosine kinase activity associated with the beta-subunit of type I insulin-like growth factor receptors of rat liver cells. J Biol Chem 1985;260:9793–804.

[125] Bianda T, Hussain MA, Glatz Y, et al. Effects of short-term insulin-like growth factor-I or growth hormone treatment on bone turnover, renal phosphate reabsorption and 1,25 di-hydroxyvitamin D3 production in healthy man. J Intern Med 1997;241:143–50.

[126] Mauras N, Doi SQ, Shapiro JR. Recombinant human insulin-like growth factor I, recombinant human growth hormone, and sex steroids: effects on markers of bone turnover in humans. J Clin Endocrinol Metab 1996;81:2222–6.

[127] Liu JP, Baker J, Perkins AS, et al. Mice carrying null mutations of the genes encoding insulin-like growth factor I (Igf-1) and type 1 IGF receptor (Igf1r). Cell 1993;75:59–72.

[128] Woods KA, Camacho-Hubner C, Savage MO, et al. Intrauterine growth retardation and postnatal growth failure associated with deletion of the insulin-like growth factor I gene. N Engl J Med 1996;335:1363–7.

[129] Abuzzahab MJ, Schneider A, Goddard A, et al. IGF-I receptor mutations resulting in intra-uterine and postnatal growth retardation. N Engl J Med 2003;349:2211–22.

[130] Baker J, Liu JP, Robertson EJ, et al. Role of insulin-like growth factors in embryonic and post-natal growth. Cell 1993;75:73–82.

[131] Liu JL, Grinberg A, Westphal H, et al. Insulin-like growth factor-I affects perinatal lethality and postnatal development in a gene dosage-dependent manner: manipulation using the Cre/loxP system in transgenic mice. Mol Endocrinol 1998;12:1452–62.

[132] Mohan S, Baylink DJ. Impaired skeletal growth in mice with haploinsufficiency of IGF-I: genetic evidence that differences in IGF-I expression could contribute to peak bone mineral density differences. J Endocrinol 2005;185:415–20.

[133] DeChiara TM, Efstratiadis A, Robertson EJ. A growth-deficiency phenotype in heterozy-gous mice carrying an insulin-like growth factor II gene disrupted by targeting. Nature 1990;345:78–80.

[134] Zhao G, Monier-Faugere MC, Langub MC, et al. Targeted overexpression of insulin-like growth factor I to osteoblasts of transgenic mice: increased trabecular bone volume without increased osteoblast proliferation. Endocrinology 2000;141:2674–82.

[135] Baylink D, Lau KH, Mohan S. The role of IGF system in the rise and fall in bone density with age. J Musculoskelet Neuronal Interact 2007;7:304–5.

[136] Adami S, Zivelonghi A, Braga V, et al. Insulin-like growth factor-1 is associated with bone formation markers, PTH and bone mineral density in healthy premenopausal women. Bone 2010;46:244–7.

[137] Thompson JL, Butterfield GE, Gylfadottir UK, et al. Effects of human growth hormone, insulin-like growth factor I, and diet and exercise on body composition of obese postmen-opausal women. J Clin Endocrinol Metab 1998;83:1477–84.

[138] Butterfield GE, Thompson J, Rennie MJ, et al. Effect of rhGH and rhIGF-I treatment on protein utilization in elderly women. Am J Physiol 1997;272:E94–9.

[139] Walenkamp MJ, Karperien M, Pereira AM, et al. Homozygous and heterozygous expression of a novel insulin-like growth factor-I mutation. J Clin Endocrinol Metab 2005;90:2855–64.

[140] Bonapace G, Concolino D, Formicola S, et al. A novel mutation in a patient with insulin-like growth factor 1 (IGF1) deficiency. J Med Genet 2003;40:913–7.

[141] Kawashima Y, Kanzaki S, Yang F, et al. Mutation at cleavage site of insulin-like growth factor receptor in a short-stature child born with intrauterine growth retardation. J Clin Endocrinol Metab 2005;90:4679–87.

[142] Domene HM, Hwa V, Argente J, et al. Human acid-labile subunit deficiency: clinical, endocrine and metabolic consequences. Horm Res 2009;72:129–41.

[143] van Duyvenvoorde HA, Kempers MJ, Twickler TB, et al. Homozygous and heterozygous expression of a novel mutation of the acid-labile subunit. Eur J Endocrinol 2008;159:113–20.

[144] Lowe WL Jr, Roberts CT Jr, Lasky SR, et al. Differential expression of alternative 5′ untranslated regions in mRNAs encoding rat insulin-like growth factor I. Proc Natl Acad Sci U S A 1987;84:8946–50.

[145] Lowe WL Jr, Lasky SR, LeRoith D, et al. Distribution and regulation of rat insulin-like growth factor I messenger ribonucleic acids encoding alternative carboxy terminal E-peptides: evidence for differential processing and regulation in liver. Mol Endocrinol 1988;2: 528–35.

[146] Murphy LJ, Bell GI, Friesen HG. Tissue distribution of insulin-like growth factor I and II messenger ribonucleic acid in the adult rat. Endocrinology 1987;120:1279–82.

[147] Yakar S, Liu JL, Stannard B, et al. Normal growth and development in the absence of hepatic insulin-like growth factor I. Proc Natl Acad Sci U S A 1999;96:7324–9.

[148] Ueki I, Ooi GT, Tremblay ML, et al. Inactivation of the acid labile subunit gene in mice results in mild retardation of postnatal growth despite profound disruptions in the circulating insulin-like growth factor system. Proc Natl Acad Sci U S A 2000;97:6868–73.

[149] Stratikopoulos E, Szabolcs M, Dragatsis I, et al. The hormonal action of IGF1 in postnatal mouse growth. Proc Natl Acad Sci U S A 2008;105:19378–83.

[150] Wu Y, Sun H, Yakar S, et al. Elevated levels of insulin-like growth factor (IGF)-I in serum rescue the severe growth retardation of IGF-I null mice. Endocrinology 2009;150: 4395–403.

Advances in Pediatrics 57 (2010) 353–372

ADVANCES IN PEDIATRICS

ELSEVIER
MOSBY

Fetal Surgery: Progress and Perspectives

Miho Watanabe, MD[a,b], Alan W. Flake, MD[a,b],*

[a]Center for Fetal Diagnosis and Treatment and The Children's Center for Fetal Research, Children's Hospital of Philadelphia, 34th Street and Civic Center Boulevard, Philadelphia, PA 19104, USA
[b]Department of Surgery, University of Pennsylvania School of Medicine, 3600 Spruce Street, Philadelphia, PA 19104, USA

The first description of open maternal fetal surgery for correction of an anatomic anomaly by Harrison and colleagues [1] was published nearly 30 years ago. At that time, the diagnostic and surgical tools for prenatal treatment of the fetus were just being developed and the concept of the fetus as a patient was the subject of philosophic and ethical debate [2]. Over the past 3 decades, great progress has been made in our ability to diagnose fetal abnormalities, predict their outcome, and to perform surgical interventions when appropriate. The concept of the fetus as a patient has become a standard of care and the ethical framework for maternal fetal intervention is well developed [3]. Although application of open fetal surgery has remained limited to a relatively small number of highly selected fetuses and is practiced in only a few centers, the development of this field has accelerated technological progress in prenatal diagnosis and intervention, led to improved understanding of the pathophysiology and natural history of candidate disorders, allowed comprehensive counseling of prospective parents in centers with focused expertise in fetal anomalies, and driven the evolution of less invasive therapeutic approaches. The purpose of this review was to describe the current status of fetal surgical intervention and to speculate regarding future developments in this rapidly evolving field.

RATIONALE AND GENERAL PRINCIPALS OF FETAL SURGICAL INTERVENTION

Fetal surgery was born of clinical necessity. Observations by pediatric surgeons and neonatologists of neonates who were born with irreversible organ damage led to the compelling rationale that the only way to prevent this alteration of normal development was to correct the defect before birth. This led to

*Corresponding author. Department of Surgery, Abramson Research Center, Room 1116B, 3615 Civic Center Boulevard, Philadelphia, PA 19104-4318. E-mail address: flake@email.chop.edu

0065-3101/10/$ – see front matter
doi:10.1016/j.yapd.2010.08.011

experimental validation of the pathophysiology of specific fetal defects in the fetal lamb model and to the development of techniques for their prenatal surgical correction [4–6]. Subsequent studies in the primate model defined the anesthetic, tocolytic, and technical methods and devices [7] essential for clinical translation [8–10]. Ultimately, these efforts supported the first systematic clinical application of fetal surgery at the University of California, San Francisco (UCSF), in the early 1980s [11].

During this formative period, prerequisites for fetal surgery were formulated that with slight modification still apply today (Fig. 1). Although the prerequisites have not changed significantly, our ability to satisfy them for specific anomalies has improved dramatically. For instance, the requirement for an accurate prenatal diagnosis and the exclusion of associated anomalies is now practically taken for granted. The armamentarium for examining the fetus in the womb, including high-resolution ultrasound (2D, 3D, and 4D), haste MRI, and fetal echocardiography, when expertly applied, are capable of detecting essentially any significant fetal structural anomaly. When combined with maternal serum screening, karyotype analysis, and molecular screening techniques, the likelihood of missing an associated anomaly or performing an intervention on an unrecognized syndromic fetus has been dramatically reduced. In addition, with accumulated experience and normograms for many fetal parameters, the limits of normality and abnormality have been clarified, allowing appropriate interpretation of normal variation (for instance, minimal renal pelviectasis). There has also been tremendous progress in our ability to safely

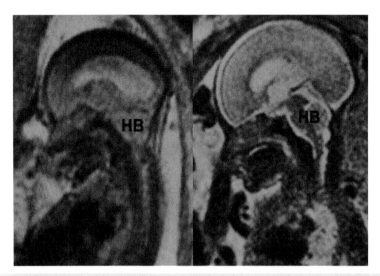

Fig. 1. Example of reversal of hindbrain herniation 3 weeks after fetal repair of myelomeningocele. Note the restoration of fluid spaces in the cisterna magna, a uniform finding after fetal repair.

operate on a mother and her fetus and correct specific anatomic defects. Advances in technical aspects of fetal intervention, maternal anesthesia, tocolysis, and the accumulation of clinical experience have evolved to the point where open fetal surgery can be performed with a minimum of maternal morbidity, and to this date no maternal mortality in a few experienced centers [12]. Having said that, fetal surgical interventions have until recently been limited to fetal anomalies perceived to be lethal because of the potential risk of this major surgical procedure to the usually young, healthy mother. The fetal surgical treatment of myelomeningocele (MMC), a nonlethal disorder, has extended the original prerequisites for fetal surgery to disorders causing irreversible organ damage with associated quality-of-life–impacting morbidities before birth [13]. If proven efficacious, this may open the door for other nonlethal fetal anomalies for which there is an appropriate rationale for prenatal treatment.

Despite this progress, fetal surgery remains controversial. The controversies primarily relate to our understanding of the "natural history" of specific anomalies, and whether we can accurately select fetuses that will benefit from fetal intervention. Our knowledge of the natural history of many disorders without fetal treatment has improved allowing accurate selection of fetuses that might benefit from fetal intervention. The natural history of congenital cystic adenomatoid malformation (CCAM), fetal sacrococcygeal teratoma (SCT), MMC, and lower urinary tract obstruction (LUTO) for instance, are relatively well understood. However, the natural history remains controversial for congenital diaphragmatic hernia (CDH) and cardiac outflow tract anomalies [14], making interpretation of the results of fetal therapy more difficult. The importance of randomized controlled trials to resolve these controversies cannot be overemphasized and the design and implementation of such trials is a current focus for fetal treatment centers [13,15].

Currently, there are a relatively limited number of fetal anomalies for which a compelling rationale exists for fetal intervention. The anomalies discussed in this article and their associated pathophysiology are shown in Table 1. These anomalies were chosen because they represent the spectrum of fetal surgery, both from a technical perspective (open fetal surgery, fetoscopy, and ultrasound-guided shunt placements), and from the perspective of proven efficacy. In some cases (CCAM, SCT, twin-to-twin transfusion syndrome), fetal intervention has clearly improved upon the natural history of the disease. For MMC, the efficacy of fetal surgery is being appropriately evaluated by a well-designed prospective randomized trial. For CDH and LUTO, fetal intervention is of unproven benefit and remains controversial.

ANATOMIC ANOMALIES CURRENTLY TREATED BY FETAL SURGERY
Fetal Lung Lesions
Fetal intervention for CCAM is one of the few unequivocal success stories of fetal surgery. CCAM is a hamartomatous tumor that is thought to arise

Table 1
Anatomic anomalies currently treated by fetal surgery

Anomaly	Pathophysiologic consequence	Fetal treatment
Cystic adenomatoid malformation	Hydrops Lung hypoplasia	Open surgery lobectomy
Sacrococcygeal teratoma	High-output cardiac failure	Open surgery Tumor debulking
Myelomeningocele	Spinal chord damage Brain stem compression Hydrocephalus	Open surgery Defect closure
Posterior urethral valves	Renal dysplasia Pulmonary hypoplasia	Vesicoamniotic shunt or cystoscopic valve ablation
Diaphragmatic hernia	Pulmonary hypoplasia	Fetoscopic balloon Tracheal occlusion
Twin-twin transfusion syndrome	Hypervolemia and hypovolemia Cardiac failure, organ damage	Fetoscopic laser photocoagulation

from aberrant events during lung branching morphogenesis [16]. Grossly, CCAMs appear as discrete intraparenchymal masses that derive their blood supply from the pulmonary circulation and can contain cysts of any size ranging from the visually imperceptible (microcystic CCAM) to the predominantly cystic (macrocystic CCAM). Histologically, CCAM is characterized by an overgrowth of one or several components of lung tissue with typically bronchial and epithelial elements. Bronchopulmonary sequestration (BPS) consists of a mass of nonfunctional lung tissue that arises as an aberrant outpouching from the developing foregut. Characteristic features include the absence of a communicating bronchus and aberrant systemic blood supply. Intralobar sequestration shares a visceral pleural lining with usually a lower pulmonary lobe and may be aerated by intra-alveolar communications. The combination of systemic vascular inflow with pulmonary venous outflow in these lesions often results in a high-flow, low-resistance circuit leading to cardiac failure in childhood. In reality, all of these lesions are part of a spectrum of pulmonary maldevelopment. CCAMs may have systemic blood supply (hybrid lesions) or BPS may contain CCAM histology. In addition, lobar or segmental bronchial stenosis or atresia may be present, suggesting an etiologic link with obstruction.

Pathophysiology and natural history
The natural history of postnatally recognized CCAM includes recurrent pulmonary infection that is resistant to antibiotic treatment, pneumothorax, and ultimately a propensity for malignant degeneration [17–19]. For these reasons, we recommend resection of all CCAMS even when asymptomatic.

The postnatal natural history of BPS is dependent upon whether they are intra-lobar or extralobar. Intralobar BPS should always be resected because of likely events of infection or high-output cardiac failure. Extralobar BPS should be re-sected if there appears to be risk for cardiac failure, there is significant mass effect, or lymphatic congestion results in associated pleural effusion. In contrast, the natural history of prenatal cystic lung lesions is relatively unpre-dictable. Approximately 15% to 20% of fetal CCAM lesions will decrease in size and two-thirds of BPS lesions shrink considerably before birth [20,21]. Despite a relative or absolute decrease in size and a tendency to become iso-echogenic with lung tissue by ultrasound examination in the third trimester, few if any of these lesions truly disappear and postnatal CT scan will confirm the persistence of the lesion after birth. Other CCAMs will grow dramatically during gestation with secondary compression of the surrounding lung and mediastinal structures. This may result in heart failure (hydrops) in the fetus or the presence of a large mass preventing ventilation at term. In addition, there is a low incidence of significant pulmonary hypoplasia that may affect survival after birth. The evolution of hydrops associated with CCAM is nearly uniformly fatal without intervention and is the sole indication for fetal surgery [20]. Given the uncertain natural history of these lesions, and the requirement for early intervention when hydrops develops, it was important to develop predictive parameters for the development of hydrops. One such parameter is the CCAM volume (using the formula for a prolate ellipse – length × height × width × 0.52) divided by the head circumference (to control for gestational age) ratio, called the CVR [22]. By serial measurement of the CVR, we have determined that most CCAMs follow a predictable growth profile, increasing in size until they plateau at about 28 weeks of gestation. A CVR on presenta-tion of 1.6 or higher predicts an 80% likelihood of the development of hydrops, and these fetuses require very close sonographic surveillance (2 to 3 times per week) to monitor for signs of hydrops. A CVR lower than 1.6 portends a low likelihood of hydrops and we recommend initial weekly surveillance with decreasing frequency after 28 weeks. CCAMs with a predominant macrocystic component must be observed frequently throughout pregnancy, as their growth is less predictable than microcystic CCAMs and we have observed rapid growth after 28 weeks in a few cases.

Fetal intervention for lung lesions

Most lung lesions require no fetal intervention and can be managed postnatally as described previously with excellent outcomes [23]. CCAMs that present with CVRs of 1.6 or higher are a high-risk category and require close surveil-lance. We [24] and others [25,26] have observed growth arrest of these tumors with steroid therapy but this is an experimental treatment that needs assess-ment by a randomized trials. At the present time, we empirically treat CCAMs at risk for evolution of hydrops, or in early stages of hydrops, with steroids before fetal intervention. If signs of hydrops persist or progress in the fetus of less than 32 weeks' gestation, fetal surgery is indicated, either open resection for microcystic lesions (see Fig. 1), or thoracoamniotic shunt placement for macrocystic lesions with a single dominant cyst. If hydrops develops in a fetus after 32 weeks of gestation, or if there is persistence of major mediastinal shift closer to term, we recommend delivery and resection by the Ex Utero Intrapartum Treatment (EXIT) procedure [27]. The results of fetal therapy for hydrops induced by fetal lung lesions have significantly improved upon the natural history. Of 24 fetuses undergoing open fetal surgery at the Children's Hospital of Philadelphia (CHOP) between 21 and 31 weeks of gestation, there are 13 healthy survivors with 1 to 16 years of follow-up. Resections involved a single lobectomy in 18 cases, right middle and lower lobectomies in 4 cases, extralobar BPS resection in 1 case, and 1 left pneumonectomy for CCAM. In survivors, resection resulted in resolution of hydrops within 1 to 2 weeks after resection and impressive compensatory lung growth before delivery. Follow-up developmental testing has been normal in all survivors. The results of thoracoamniotic shunt placement for hydrops attributable to CCAMs with a predominant cyst are even better with good quality-of-life survival of approximately 75% of shunted patients.

Sacrococcygeal Teratoma

A particularly challenging fetal anomaly requiring expertise in its pre- and perinatal management is sacrococcygeal teratoma (SCT) [28]. SCT is a teratoma arising from the presacral area that occurs in 1 of 30,000 to 1 of 40,000 live births. SCTs have malignant potential but are predominantly benign at birth. By definition they are composed of elements from all 3 germ layers on microscopic examination and usually contain cystic and solid elements. Fetal karyotype is usually normal and there are usually no associated anomalies. SCTs have been classified (American Academy of Pediatrics Surgical Section Classification) based on the anatomic distribution of the tumor [29]. Type I SCT is predominantly external with a minimal presacral component. Type IV SCT is predominantly presacral with extension into the pelvis and abdomen and Types II and III are intermediate between these extremes. Most SCTs are Types I or II. Type IV is of significance because it can be missed after birth if not detected prenatally with subsequent presentation with pelvic outlet obstruction or malignancy.

Pathophysiology and natural history
The natural history of prenatally diagnosed SCT is considerably worse than that after delivery [30]. After birth, most patients with SCT do well after early surgical resection, which must include the coccyx to prevent recurrence of the tumor. In contrast, the mortality associated with prenatally diagnosed SCT ranges from 30% to 50%. The high mortality rate of fetal SCT can be attributed to a variety of mechanisms, all of which relate to the size or blood flow of the tumor. Mass effect can result in preterm labor and/or dystocia and these were common mechanisms of fetal demise before the advent of prenatal diagnosis. SCTs can hemorrhage internally resulting in rapid enlargement of the tumor and fetal anemia, or rupture and bleed into the amniotic fluid resulting in fetal

anemia or sudden death. Finally, predominantly solid SCTs have high associated blood flow with arteriovenous shunting. This represents a low-resistance vascular steal from the fetus and placenta and can ultimately result in high-output cardiac failure [31]. Serial echocardiographic assessment can document the evolution of high-output failure with increasing combined cardiac outputs and descending aortic blood flow, increasing left and right ventricular end diastolic diameters, increasing inferior vena caval diameter, and increasing placental thickness [32]. Fetal hydrops and placentomegaly may subsequently occur with the end result of fetal demise and often the maternal mirror syndrome. The evolution of hydrops secondary to high-output cardiac failure in the immature fetus with SCT is associated with near 100% mortality and is the sole indication for fetal resection of these tumors.

Fetal intervention for SCT

The fetus presenting with a large predominantly solid SCT is at high risk for progression to hydrops [33]. We recommend frequent surveillance by sonography and echocardiography with measurement of the cardiovascular parameters noted previously. This may be as often as 3 times per week in the fetus verging on hydrops as the fetus can decompensate rapidly and success of fetal treatment is dependent on intervention before progression of hydrops. Fetal debulking of the tumor to remove the vascular steal is recommended when the evolution of high-output cardiac failure is recognized before 28 weeks of gestation in a fetus with Type I SCT. Timing of intervention is critical and should be recommended when the first overt evidence of hydrops occurs. The presence of advanced hydrops and/or the presence of placentomegaly are contraindications for fetal intervention. If hydrops occurs after 28 weeks, the fetus should be delivered and debulked by the EXIT procedure. In either case, once the cardiac failure has resolved and the infant has been stabilized after birth, a formal resection of the residual tumor and coccyx can be performed. After fetal resection of the SCT, hydrops will generally resolve within 2 to 3 weeks. Since 1995, we have operated on 5 anatomically appropriate fetuses with SCT and associated high-output failure with 4 survivors. One survivor has required postnatal treatment of pulmonary metastases of germ cell tumor but at 11 years of age has no evidence of disease. Another survivor had significant morbidity likely related to emboli at the time of tumor resection. The other 2 survivors remain healthy. These cases demonstrate that fetal resection of a large tumor can reverse the pathophysiology of high-output cardiac failure in carefully selected cases and that early intervention offers the best hope of survival once high-output failure is documented. However, SCT remains one of the most difficult and challenging fetal anomalies to manage and parents should be counseled appropriately.

Fetal Myelomeningocele

Myelomeningocele (MMC), or open spina bifida, is a common and devastating congenital anomaly for which there is no satisfactory postnatal treatment. It is the first nonfatal anomaly considered for fetal surgical intervention necessitating a careful analysis of risks and benefit. It is characterized by protrusion of meninges and neural elements through a defect in the vertebral arches with secondary complications of lifelong paralysis and varying degrees of mental retardation, bowel and bladder dysfunction, and orthopedic disabilities [34]. MMC has been determined to have both genetic and micronutrient causes. Although substantial progress could be made in preventing this disorder through folic acid supplementation, MMC still affects approximately 1 of 2000 live births and this figure does not include the 23% of MMC pregnancies in which the fetus is aborted [35–37].

Pathophysiology and natural history
There is experimental and clinical evidence implicating the "2-hit hypothesis" in the pathophysiology of MMC recently reviewed by Adzick. [13] The first "hit" is failure of neurulation resulting in an open spinal defect. Interestingly, there is minimal evidence for primary neural injury during this phase of the pathogenesis. The second "hit" results from exposure of the neural elements to the amniotic fluid and mechanical effects within the intrauterine environment. This is where evidence suggests the neural damage occurs and this evidence constitutes the rationale for fetal coverage of the MMC defect. A secondary result of the open spinal defect is the Arnold-Chiari malformation, which is responsible for a significant component of the morbidity and mortality of MMC. Loss of cerebral spinal fluid through the defect results in a sump effect that causes descent of the hindbrain into the posterior fossa with secondary brainstem compression. With current postnatal treatment, nearly 14% of all MMC neonates do not survive past 5 years of age, with the mortality rising to 35% of those with symptoms of brainstem compression from the Arnold-Chiari malformation. Whereas 70% of patients have an IQ higher than 80, only half are able to live independently as adults, even with adapted accommodations. [38,39] In addition to the motor and sensory deficits caused by the spinal cord lesion, patients with MMC have significant complications from hydrocephalus, the Arnold-Chiari II malformation, and tethering of the cord at the site of surgical repair. Hydrocephalus occurs in more than 85% of patients with MMC and at least 80% require placement of shunts to prevent neurologic and intellectual compromise associated with hydrocephalus. The rate of shunt-related complications and morbidity is high contributing significantly to the overall morbidity of MMC. Thus, it is clear that improvements in treatment are desperately needed.

Fetal intervention for MMC
Fetal intervention for MMC was first reported in 1997 by Bruner and colleagues at Vanderbilt University Medical Center who reported endoscopic coverage of 2 MMC defects with a maternal split-thickness skin graft [40]. This unsuccessful experience was followed by several reports from Vanderbilt and CHOP describing the first early results of open prenatal repair of MMC [41–43]. As the selection criteria for fetal intervention differed between the 2 institutions, the results also differed and only the CHOP results are reviewed

here. Between 1998 and 2003 we performed MMC repairs on 58 fetuses [44]. The selection criteria required that the fetus be less than 25 weeks of gestation, with a thoracic or lumbosacral MMC, associated Arnold-Chiari malformation, mild to moderate ventriculomegaly, normal leg movements without evidence of club foot, and normal karyotype without evidence of other abnormalities. Of the 58 fetuses, 4 died because of premature delivery with an average age at delivery of 34 weeks, 4 days. There was resolution of hindbrain herniation in 100% of operated fetuses by 3 weeks after surgery (see Fig. 1). Comprehensive follow-up examinations were performed at 1, 2, 3, and 5 years of age. The vast majority of children demonstrated no or minimal symptoms related to brainstem dysfunction. The ventriculoperitoneal shunt rate was 46%, which is much lower than the expected shunt rate of 84% based on 297 historical controls followed at the CHOP Spina Bifida Clinic between 1983 and 2000. As a group, these patients had better than expected lower extremity function at birth with 66% of patients being independent walkers on long-term follow-up. However, these children continue to exhibit deficits in movement coordination and balance that are characteristic of children with MMC [45]. Most importantly, 28 of the children have undergone neurodevelopmental evaluation at 5 years of age. Most (83%) have overall cognitive function in the average or high range. There was a pattern of consistently higher scores in the verbal areas compared with scores for visual-motor or nonverbal reasoning suggesting the possibility of later learning difficulties. These results were promising and have led to a carefully designed National Institutes of Health (NIH)-sponsored multicenter, prospective, randomized trial of fetal myelomeningocele repair (MOMS Trial) that began in 2003. The surgical centers for the trial are CHOP, Vanderbilt University Medical Center, and UCSF, with an independent Data and Study Coordinating Center at George Washington University Biostatistics Center. By early 2009, more than three-fourths of the proposed number of patients had been randomized. The results of this trial will determine whether fetal repair of MMC is more or less effective than postnatal management and will have major influence on the future of fetal intervention for MMC.

Lower Urinary Tract Obstruction

Fetuses with some form of obstructive uropathy are frequently diagnosed by prenatal ultrasound. In this article, the discussion is limited to potential candidates for fetal intervention that are a subset of fetuses with lower urinary tract obstruction (LUTO). LUTO refers to distal obstruction of the urinary tract caused by a variety of anatomic anomalies. In females, it is often associated with cloacal anomalies that independently complicate the outcome of these fetuses. In males, the most common anomalies are posterior urethral valves (PUV), urethral atresia (UA), and prune belly syndrome (PBS).

Pathophysiology and natural history

The pathophysiology of LUTO is related to the effects of urinary obstruction during development on the kidneys, and the secondary effects of oligohydramnios. LUTO results in bladder dilation and hypertrophy, megaureters, and hydronephrosis. If the obstruction is high grade and develops early in development it causes fibrocystic dysplasia of the kidneys, an irreversible condition leading to renal failure. The associated oligohydramnios gives rise to Potter's sequence, manifest by pulmonary hypoplasia and physical deformations. The extent of pathophysiology related to LUTO is dependent on the degree and duration of obstruction. Early, high-grade obstruction results in severe renal fibrocystic dysplasia, oligohydramnios, and the Potter's sequence. Minimal obstruction may result in only dilation without associated dysplasia. Unfortunately, the natural history of this disorder when diagnosed prenatally is poor. The untreated mortality of prenatally diagnosed LUTO is 45%. When LUTO is associated with mid-trimester oligohydramnios, the untreated mortality is 95%. Survivors have a more than 50% incidence of renal failure and even in circumstances where normal amniotic fluid is maintained throughout gestation, approximately one-third of patients will develop renal failure [46].

Fetal intervention for LUTO
It is important to appreciate that most fetuses evaluated for LUTO will not be candidates for fetal intervention. Female fetuses with LUTO are not candidates because of the complicating issues related to the associated cloacal anomalies. Karyotypic abnormalities are present in 8% to 25% of LUTO fetuses, excluding them as candidates [47,48]. Fetuses that maintain normal amniotic fluid into the third trimester are not candidates because most will have normal renal function and will not benefit from fetal intervention. Most fetuses presenting with oligohydramnios will already have evidence of fibrocystic dysplasia with renal parenchymal cysts by ultrasound examination. We consider the minimal requirements for fetal intervention to be (1) an ultrasound examination consistent with LUTO with associated oligohydramnios; (2) a normal male karyotype; and (3) urinary electrolytes on serial analysis consistent with preserved renal function. Although controversial, in our hands the use of 3 bladder taps at 24-hour intervals for urinary electrolyte analysis has been highly predictive of renal function [49–51]. The rationale is that the first tap represents stagnant urine in the bladder that has partially equilibrated with serum, the second tap represents run down from the megaureters, and the third tap represents relatively "fresh" urine from the kidneys. A profile that trends toward less salt and protein in the urine with normalization of values supports preserved renal function. Decompression of LUTO has evolved over the years and is still in evolution. It is of historical interest that the first open fetal surgical procedures for the treatment of anatomic anomalies were performed for obstructive uropathy [1]. Since the early 1980s, open fetal surgery has been replaced by ultrasound-guided placement of vesicoamniotic shunts and, more recently, ultrasound-guided vesicoscopy has been used to confirm the diagnosis of PUV and in some cases treat the obstruction by laser ablation or mechanical disruption of the PUVs [52,53]. The outcome of fetal treatment of LUTO has

been highly variable and in most series poor with survivals of less than 50% and renal failure in as high as 40% of survivors [54]. In addition, 25% of survivors require bladder augmentation. In addition to the baseline poor natural history of this disease, the results are in part because of poor case selection and technical issues related to shunt placement. With the application of the selection criteria stated previously and experienced shunt placement, 31 of 49 good urinary prognosis patients survived of which 84% had good renal function. In long-term assessment of survivors, 45% have normal renal function and 61% had normal bladder function. Patients with PUV had a better outcome than those with PBS or UA with only 14% requiring transplantation and 72% having normal bladder function [55,56]. In summary, it appears that in appropriately selected patients fetal intervention for LUTO can improve on the natural history of the disease and result in good quality-of-life outcomes in a subset of patients. It is likely that in the future, improved instrumentation will allow vesicoscopic selection of patients with PUV with preserved renal function for valve ablation. Restoration of urethral patency will allow normal bladder cycling and will potentially improve bladder outcomes as well.

Fetal Congenital Diaphragmatic Hernia

Congenital diaphragmatic hernia (CDH) affects 1 in 2500 to 1 in 4000 liveborn infants. It is a simple anatomic defect that results in a devastating physiologic consequence, ie, pulmonary hypoplasia. There is a long history of fetal surgical treatment for CDH, which is beyond the scope of this article but has recently been reviewed elsewhere [57]. The approach has evolved from open surgical repair of the defect to open tracheal occlusion to induce lung growth to the most recent technique of minimally invasive fetoscopic balloon tracheal occlusion [58]. Although the rationale for fetal treatment of CDH remains compelling, the controversy relates to the natural history of this anomaly, selection of patients with CDH who are most likely to benefit, and whether fetal treatment improves upon the natural history [59].

Pathophysiology and natural history of fetal CDH

CDH results from failure of closure of the foramen of Bochdalek between 8 and 10 weeks of gestation. The cause of that failure is the subject of active debate and will not be resolved here [60,61]. The pathophysiology of CDH is composed of both fixed and reversible components. The fixed component is pulmonary hypoplasia, which arises from interference with branching morphogenesis during lung development. A lung with severe hypoplasia has fewer branch points and therefore fewer airways, arteries, veins, and alveolar structures than a normal lung [62]. This results in fixed increased vascular resistance, and decreased surface area for gas exchange [62,63]. In addition to the relatively fixed deficit from pulmonary hypoplasia, lungs in severe CDH also have markedly abnormal pulmonary vasculature. The peripheral pulmonary arteries are hypermuscular, with a thickened medial muscular layer that extends further distal on the arterioles than normal. The clinical correlate of this anatomic observation is increased pulmonary vasoreactivity accounting for the marked clinical lability of patients with severe CDH. The resultant pulmonary hypertension results in persistence of the fetal circulation with shunting through the patent ductus arteriosus, or foramen ovale with secondary hypoxemia and acidosis. As hypoxemia and acidosis stimulate further pulmonary vasospasm a "vicious cycle" is initiated with rapid clinical deterioration of the patient and inability to ventilate using conventional techniques [64]. Thus, a combination of pulmonary hypoplasia and pulmonary vascular abnormality results in the still considerable mortality and morbidity of CDH. Nevertheless, views of the natural history of CDH have evolved considerably over the past 2 decades. Where is was once felt that a lethal degree of pulmonary hypoplasia was present in as high as 40% of patients with CDH [65], the number is now considered to be closer to 10%. With improvements in neonatal management including lung-sparing ventilatory strategies, delayed surgery, and extracorporeal membrane oxygenation (ECMO), survival of CDH has improved [66]. Nevertheless, severe CDH remains a disease with significant mortality and quality-of-life–impacting morbidity. As the damage is done before birth, there remains a compelling rationale for fetal intervention.

Fetal intervention for CDH

The controversy over fetal intervention for CDH, whether by open surgery or by fetoscopic balloon tracheal occlusion, revolves around the natural history, whether we can identify fetuses that will benefit from fetal intervention, and whether fetal intervention can improve upon the natural history. As stated previously, the natural history has been a moving target with improvement in most centers over the years. Therefore, selection criteria that once selected a population of fetuses with greater than 90% mortality in any given institution probably are no longer as predictive. This is best exemplified by the randomized trial of prenatal tracheal occlusion performed at UCSF [67]. In that trial, the control group that was predicted based on historical prognostic factors to have a mortality of 63%, had a survival of 75%. Thus, any trial of prenatal treatment of CDH must have contemporaneous controls from the same institution, and the patients must be stratified for severity.

Prenatal prognostic parameters that have proven helpful in predicting severity of fetal CDH include liver position and lung volume measurements. Liver position is the most significant and reproducible independent determinant of outcome with liver herniation predictive of poor outcome [68–70]. Lung volume measurements, whether indirect lung area to head circumference ratio (LHR) or direct (MRI or 3-dimensional ultrasound), do not provide additional independent predictive value for mortality over liver herniation, but do provide confirmatory evidence of severity. In our most recent series, fetuses with liver up have a mortality of approximately 55% [69]. Thus, our ability to predict mortality for an individual fetus with CDH, even with our best prognostic test is little better than 50/50, hardly adequate for selection of fetuses for fetal intervention. The ability to predict morbidity for an individual fetus is even less well defined. So, at the present time, we cannot predict a "most severe subset" of fetuses with CDH that are destined to die or have quality-of-life–impacting morbidity without fetal intervention. The question of whether prenatal treatment (now balloon tracheal occlusion) will improve the natural history of CDH is also controversial. Although tracheal occlusion in animal models has been shown to induce lung growth, it has not been shown to create structurally and functionally normal lungs [71,72]. The human experience suggests that even when lung growth occurs, many of the neonates have severe respiratory compromise resulting in death or significant morbidity [73–75]. The only randomized trial of prenatal tracheal occlusion completed thus far has shown no benefit [67]. Since the early 2000s there have been a series of optimistic publications from the Eurofetus group describing improved survival in non-randomized series of CDH patients using single-port balloon tracheal occlusion (TO) with and without release [58,76–78]. The investigators have demonstrated that they can perform the technical maneuvers with remarkable finesse. They have demonstrated that an approximately 50% survival can be achieved in patients with CDH selected by historical criteria to have a less than 10% survival. Although these results appear impressive, the studies have cited historical control LHR data accrued from multiple institutions, including UCSF. More recently, they have stated results for contemporaneous controls but provide no data describing their control group. In summary, they have performed more than 200 of these procedures and have not defined the contemporaneous natural history for the population of patients that they are treating and they have not tested their approach by a randomized controlled clinical trial. Until these basic standards are met, it is critical that the community at large maintain a healthy skepticism regarding TO for CDH. It is important that European and US centers maintain their equipoise and cooperate to combine data and perform well-designed, randomized, controlled studies examining both morbidity and mortality end points before widespread application of TO in patients with severe CDH can be condoned.

Twin-to-Twin Transfusion Syndrome

Monozygotic (MZ) twin pregnancies account for about 30% of spontaneously conceived twins and that incidence is rising owing to the increased prevalence of MZ twins after assisted reproductive technology. Approximately 70% to 75% of MZ twins are monochorionic, diamniotic (MCDA), and 1% to 2% are monochorionic, monoamniotic (MCMA). It is the monochorionic twins that are susceptible to twin-to-twin transfusion syndrome (TTTS) because of their placental architecture and shared circulation. Because of the high frequency of this disorder, and its potential to be fetoscopically treated, it is now the most common fetal surgical intervention in most fetal treatment centers [79].

Pathophysiology and natural history
TTTS is a heterogeneous disorder comprising a spectrum of presentations and severity. It develops because of vascular communications between the

placentas of monochorionic twins. Although all MC twins have these communications, normally the exchange of circulation between the twins is balanced, but in about 15% of cases the flow becomes unbalanced and this creates the potential for TTTS. TTTS can be rapidly progressive or indolent in presentation and course. It can occur early or late in gestation and at the present time the clinical progression of TTTS in any pair of twins is unpredictable. Commonly, MC placentas have anastomoses between pairs of arteries (AA) and less commonly between pairs of veins (VV). These connections lie on the surface of the placenta and allow bidirectional flow dependent on the pressure dynamics between the 2 circulations at any given time. The unilateral transfer of blood is mediated in most circumstances by arteriovenous (AV) communications within the placenta. The presence of an AV anastomosis without a compensating AA anastomosis is associated with a higher rate of TTTS [80,81]. When unbalanced blood flow occurs, the donor twin becomes hypovolemic and oliguric while the recipient twin becomes hypervolemic and polyuric. Activation of the renin-angiotensin system in the donor to conserve intravascular volume results in hypertension, with paradoxic reduction in placental perfusion and growth retardation. Opposite hormonal influences act in the recipient, which increases renal perfusion and urine output. The volume overload results in myocardial hypertrophy, AV valve regurgitation, and increased pulmonary outflow and aortic outflow velocities. However, other cardiac findings are more difficult to explain. The development of pulmonic stenosis and right ventricular outflow tract obstruction cannot be explained on the basis of volume loading alone and suggest an increase in cardiac afterload owing to systemic hypertension, which is likely mediated by Endothelin 1, a potent vasoconstrictor. The end result of TTTS is a cascade of metabolic events in both fetuses that result in a mortality approaching 90% if left untreated [79].

Fetal intervention for TTTS

Accurate diagnosis of TTTS is crucial and dependent upon specific sonographic features. There must be evidence of monochorionicity, ie, a single placenta, a thin inter-twin membrane usually measuring less than 2 mm, and the absence of a twin peak sign. This is best established at the earliest ultrasound evaluation. There must be a discrepancy in amniotic fluid between the 2 fetuses (poly/oli). Other features include a size discrepancy between the cotwins of more than 20%, concordant fetal gender, and Doppler changes within the fetal vasculature or frank hydrops or twin demise. Current clinical staging (Table 2) follows that described by Quintero and colleagues [82], which has been very useful but does not incorporate cardiovascular indices that are important in the pathophysiology of the disease. Therefore, we also use a cardiovascular scoring system described by Rychik and colleagues [83] in assessing severity of the physiology of TTTS and in selection of cotwins for fetal treatment. Although many treatments have been proposed over the past few decades for TTTS, since publication of the Eurofetus randomized trial [84]

Table 2
Staging of twin-to-twin transfusion syndrome

Stage	Findings
1.	Polyhydramnios in recipient sac (MVP >8 cm) and oligohydramnios in the donor sac (MVP <2 cm).
2.	No visible bladder in the donor twin.
3.	Doppler abnormality consisting of absent or reverse flow in the umbilical artery, reverse flow in the ductus venosus, or pulsatile flow in the umbilical vein.
4.	Ascites or hydrops in either fetus.
5.	Demise of either fetus.

Abbreviation: MVP, maximum vertical pocket of amniotic fluid.

comparing amnioreduction with selective laser photocoagulation, the treatment of choice has been fetoscopic laser therapy. This therapy directly interrupts the vascular connections on the chorionic plate that are responsible for development of the syndrome and, therefore, if applied at a suitable stage of progression, should prevent further pathophysiology. The procedure is now performed percutaneously using ultrasound guidance to appropriately position the fetoscope, usually under local anesthesia or conscious sedation. The current technique has evolved from ablation of all vessels crossing the intertwin membrane to a selective approach identifying and obliterating each anastomotic site. This has resulted in an improvement in survival of at least one fetus from 61% in the nonselective group to 83% in the selective group [85]. As many Quintero Stage 1 patients do not progress, laser therapy is reserved for Stage 2 or above by most fetal centers including ours. However, the best management for Stage 1 disease remains controversial. Overall, laser therapy has dramatically improved the natural history of this devastating condition. Although significant mortality and morbidity persist, it is predominantly related to preexisting damage or premature delivery. The largest study of long-term follow-up of surviving twins treated by laser therapy before 26 weeks of gestation showed normal development in 83% and minor neurologic abnormality in 7% of survivors at 3 years of age [86].

THE FUTURE OF FETAL SURGERY

The past 3 decades have seen dramatic progress in our ability to diagnose, appropriately select, and treat fetuses with life-threatening or quality-of-life–impacting disease. Despite this success, application of fetal intervention remains fairly limited. There are a number of keys that can be envisioned for the future success and expansion of fetal surgery [87]. In the short term, the single most important requirement is accountability. For fetal surgery to become permanently established, the benefit to patients must be clearly established by randomized clinical trials when applicable. The second area of required progress is reduction of maternal and fetal risk. The 2 areas that are most pressing are improvement in maternal tocolysis to control the inevitable preterm delivery that occurs after fetal surgery, and the development of technologic solutions specifically designed to address fetal surgical obstacles that would allow truly "minimally invasive" fetal surgery. The third area is the development of improved imaging technology. The holy grail of fetal imaging is the realization of real-time, 3-dimensional, ultra–high resolution imaging. There has been rapid progress in ultrasound and MRI technology that is likely to realize this goal in the foreseeable future. High-frequency transducers (40–50 MHz) can already clearly visualize fetal mouse cardiac anatomy at 9.5 days' gestation with resolution approaching 30 μm. In combination with advances in 3-dimensional rendering of ultrasound images, this technology could provide real-time 3-dimensional imaging of early gestational fetuses. Perhaps even more powerful is the promise of MRI. MRI is now a highly useful modality in fetal treatment centers providing confirmation and at times enhanced detail compared with ultrasound alone for some anatomic diagnoses. If rapid multiplanar acquisition can be achieved simultaneously eliminating movement artifact, than each point in the fetus becomes a pixel, allowing the ability to 3-dimensionally render the fetus and view the fetus from any angle. Add to that the ability of different MRI modes to provide internal contrast between organs and you obtain a 3-dimensional representation of the fetus that would allow "fly-through" capabilities. If this technology can be upscaled for real-time imaging of early gestational human fetuses, then the capacity for image-guided intervention will exist at any gestational age at a level of precision that is far beyond what is currently available. Precise delivery of needles, shunts, ablative probes, micromachines with specific tasks, or site-specific cellular or gene delivery could all potentially be achieved. In the long term it is likely that fetal surgery, as currently practiced, will become obsolete. Large uterine incisions with their attendant risk and morbidity will no longer be necessary. Whereas there will always be a niche for anatomic correction of fetal abnormalities, it will be filled by less invasive approaches performed using vastly superior imaging, instrumentation, and technology. In addition, a more developmental approach will be required to fully correct specific defects, with earlier and more discrete interventions.

References

[1] Harrison MR, Golbus MS, Filly RA, et al. Fetal surgery for congenital hydronephrosis. N Engl J Med 1982;306:591–3.

[2] Harrison MR. Unborn: historical perspective of the fetus as a patient. Pharos Alpha Omega Alpha Honor Med Soc 1982;45:19–24.

[3] Flake AW. Prenatal intervention: ethical considerations for life-threatening and non-life-threatening anomalies. Semin Pediatr Surg 2001;10:212–21.

[4] Glick PL, Harrison MR, Adzick NS, et al. Correction of congenital hydronephrosis in utero IV: in utero decompression prevents renal dysplasia. J Pediatr Surg 1984;19:649–57.

[5] Harrison MR, Ross NA, de Lorimier AA. Correction of congenital diaphragmatic hernia in utero. III. Development of a successful surgical technique using abdominoplasty to avoid compromise of umbilical blood flow. J Pediatr Surg 1981;16:934–42.

[6] Adzick NS, Harrison MR, Glick PL, et al. Fetal urinary tract obstruction: experimental pathophysiology. Semin Perinatol 1985;9:79–90.

[7] Adzick N, Harrison M, Flake A, et al. Automatic uterine stapling devices in fetal surgery: experience in a primate model. Surg Forum 1985;36:479–81.

[8] Adzick NS, Harrison MR, Glick PL, et al. Fetal surgery in the primate. III. Maternal outcome after fetal surgery. J Pediatr Surg 1986;21:477–80.

[9] Harrison MR, Anderson J, Rosen MA, et al. Fetal surgery in the primate I. Anesthetic, surgical, and tocolytic management to maximize fetal-neonatal survival. J Pediatr Surg 1982;17:115–22.

[10] Nakayama DK, Harrison MR, Seron-Ferre M, et al. Fetal surgery in the primate II. Uterine electromyographic response to operative procedures and pharmacologic agents. J Pediatr Surg 1984;19:333–9.

[11] Harrison MR. Fetal surgery. West J Med 1993;159:341–9.

[12] Adzick NS. Open fetal surgery for life-threatening fetal anomalies. Semin Fetal Neonatal Med 2010;15:1–8.

[13] Adzick NS. Fetal myelomeningocele: natural history, pathophysiology, and in-utero intervention. Semin Fetal Neonatal Med 2010;15:9–14.

[14] McElhinney DB, Marshall AC, Wilkins-Haug LE, et al. Predictors of technical success and postnatal biventricular outcome after in utero aortic valvuloplasty for aortic stenosis with evolving hypoplastic left heart syndrome. Circulation 2009;120:1482–90.

[15] Johnson MP. The North American Fetal Therapy Network (NAFTNet): a new approach to collaborative research in fetal diagnosis and therapy. Semin Fetal Neonatal Med 2010;15:52–7.

[16] Gonzaga S, Henriques-Coelho T, Davey M, et al. Cystic adenomatoid malformations are induced by localized FGF10 overexpression in fetal rat lung. Am J Respir Cell Mol Biol 2008;39:346–55.

[17] d'Agostino S, Bonoldi E, Dante S, et al. Embryonal rhabdomyosarcoma of the lung arising in cystic adenomatoid malformation: case report and review of the literature. J Pediatr Surg 1997;32:1381–3.

[18] Granata C, Gambini C, Balducci T, et al. Bronchioloalveolar carcinoma arising in congenital cystic adenomatoid malformation in a child: a case report and review on malignancies originating in congenital cystic adenomatoid malformation. Pediatr Pulmonol 1998;25:62–6.

[19] Sudou M, Sugi K, Murakami T. Bronchioloalveolar carcinoma arising from a congenital cystic adenomatoid malformation in an adolescent: the first case report from the Orient. J Thorac Cardiovasc Surg 2003;126:902–3.

[20] Adzick NS, Harrison MR, Crombleholme TM, et al. Fetal lung lesions: management and outcome. Am J Obstet Gynecol 1998;179:884–9.

[21] MacGillivray TE, Harrison MR, Goldstein RB, et al. Disappearing fetal lung lesions. J Pediatr Surg 1993;28:1321–4.

[22] Crombleholme TM, Coleman B, Hedrick H, et al. Cystic adenomatoid malformation volume ratio predicts outcome in prenatally diagnosed cystic adenomatoid malformation of the lung. J Pediatr Surg 2002;37:331–8.

[23] Tsai AY, Liechty KW, Hedrick HL, et al. Outcomes after postnatal resection of prenatally diagnosed asymptomatic cystic lung lesions. J Pediatr Surg 2008;43:513–7.

[24] Peranteau WH, Wilson RD, Liechty KW, et al. Effect of maternal betamethasone administration on prenatal congenital cystic adenomatoid malformation growth and fetal survival. Fetal Diagn Ther 2007;22:365–71.

[25] Morris LM, Lim FY, Livingston JC, et al. High-risk fetal congenital pulmonary airway malformations have a variable response to steroids. J Pediatr Surg 2009;44:60–5.

[26] Curran PF, Jelin EB, Rand L, et al. Prenatal steroids for microcystic congenital cystic adenomatoid malformations. J Pediatr Surg 2010;45:145–50.

[27] Hedrick HL, Flake AW, Crombleholme TM, et al. The ex utero intrapartum therapy procedure for high-risk fetal lung lesions. J Pediatr Surg 2005;40:1038–43.

[28] Flake AW. Fetal sacrococcygeal teratoma. Eur J Med 1993;2:113–20.

[29] Altman RP, Randolph JG, Lilly JR. Sacrococcygeal teratoma: American Academy of Pediatrics Surgical Section Survey-1973. J Pediatr Surg 1974;9:389–98.

[30] Flake AW, Harrison MR, Adzick NS, et al. Fetal sacrococcygeal teratoma. J Pediatr Surg 1986;21:563–6.

[31] Bond SJ, Harrison MR, Schmidt KG, et al. Death due to high-output cardiac failure in fetal sacrococcygeal teratoma. J Pediatr Surg 1990;25:1287–91.

[32] Schmidt KG, Silverman NH, Harison MR, et al. High-output cardiac failure in fetuses with large sacrococcygeal teratoma: diagnosis by echocardiography and Doppler ultrasound. J Pediatr 1989;114:1023–8.

[33] Hedrick HL, Flake AW, Crombleholme TM, et al. Sacrococcygeal teratoma: prenatal assessment, fetal intervention, and outcome. J Pediatr Surg 2004;39:430–8.

[34] Mitchell LE, Adzick NS, Melchionne J, et al. Spina bifida. Lancet 2004;364:1885–95.

[35] Botto LD, Moore CA, Khoury MJ, et al. Neural-tube defects. N Engl J Med 1999;341:1509–19.

[36] Velie EM, Shaw GM. Impact of prenatal diagnosis and elective termination on prevalence and risk estimates of neural tube defects in California, 1989–1991. Am J Epidemiol 1996;144:473–9.

[37] Edmonds LD, James LM. Temporal trends in the prevalence of congenital malformations at birth based on the birth defects monitoring program, United States, 1979–1987. MMWR CDC Surveill Summ 1990;39:19–23.

[38] Oakeshott P, Hunt GM. Long-term outcome in open spina bifida. Br J Gen Pract 2003;53:632–6.

[39] Hunt GM. Open spina bifida: outcome for a complete cohort treated unselectively and followed into adulthood. Dev Med Child Neurol 1990;32:108–18.

[40] Bruner JP, Tulipan NE, Richards WO. Endoscopic coverage of fetal open myelomeningocele in utero. Am J Obstet Gynecol 1997;176:256–7.

[41] Tulipan N, Hernanz-Schulman M, Bruner JP. Reduced hindbrain herniation after intrauterine myelomeningocele repair: a report of four cases. Pediatr Neurosurg 1998;29:274–8.

[42] Adzick NS, Sutton LN, Crombleholme TM, et al. Successful fetal surgery for spina bifida. Lancet 1998;352:1675–6.

[43] Sutton LN, Adzick NS, Bilaniuk LT, et al. Improvement in hindbrain herniation demonstrated by serial fetal magnetic resonance imaging following fetal surgery for myelomeningocele. JAMA 1999;282:1826–31.

[44] Johnson MP, Sutton LN, Rintoul N, et al. Fetal myelomeningocele repair: short-term clinical outcomes. Am J Obstet Gynecol 2003;189:482–7.

[45] Danzer E, Gerdes M, Bebbington MW, et al. Lower extremity neuromotor function and short-term ambulatory potential following in utero myelomeningocele surgery. Fetal Diagn Ther 2009;25:47–53.

[46] Wu S, Johnson MP. Fetal lower urinary tract obstruction. Clin Perinatol 2009;36:377–90, x.

[47] Brumfield CG, Davis RO, Joseph DB, et al. Fetal obstructive uropathies. Importance of chromosomal abnormalities and associated anomalies to perinatal outcome. J Reprod Med 1991;36:662–6.

[48] Donnenfeld AE, Lockwood D, Custer T, et al. Prenatal diagnosis from fetal urine in bladder outlet obstruction: success rates for traditional cytogenetic evaluation and interphase fluorescence in situ hybridization. Genet Med 2002;4:444–7.

[49] Johnson MP, Bukowski TP, Reitleman C, et al. In utero surgical treatment of fetal obstructive uropathy: a new comprehensive approach to identify appropriate candidates for vesicoamniotic shunt therapy. Am J Obstet Gynecol 1994;170:1770–6.

[50] Freedman AL, Johnson MP, Gonzalez R. Fetal therapy for obstructive uropathy: past, present, future? Pediatr Nephrol 2000;14:167–76.

[51] Johnson MP, Corsi P, Bradfield W, et al. Sequential urinalysis improves evaluation of fetal renal function in obstructive uropathy. Am J Obstet Gynecol 1995;173:59–65.

[52] Quintero RA, Hume R, Smith C, et al. Percutaneous fetal cystoscopy and endoscopic fulguration of posterior urethral valves. Am J Obstet Gynecol 1995;172:206–9.

[53] Ruano R, Duarte S, Bunduki V, et al. Fetal cystoscopy for severe lower urinary tract obstruction—initial experience of a single center. Prenat Diagn 2010;30:30–9.

[54] Coplen DE. Prenatal intervention for hydronephrosis. J Urol 1997;157:2270–7.

[55] Freedman AL, Johnson MP, Smith CA, et al. Long-term outcome in children after antenatal intervention for obstructive uropathies. Lancet 1999;354:374–7.

[56] Biard JM, Johnson MP, Carr MC, et al. Long-term outcomes in children treated by prenatal vesicoamniotic shunting for lower urinary tract obstruction. Obstet Gynecol 2005;106:503–8.

[57] Grethel EJ, Nobuhara KK. Fetal surgery for congenital diaphragmatic hernia. J Paediatr Child Health 2006;42:79–85.

[58] Jani JC, Nicolaides KH, Gratacos E, et al. Severe diaphragmatic hernia treated by fetal endoscopic tracheal occlusion. Ultrasound Obstet Gynecol 2009;34:304–10.

[59] Flake A. Fetal surgery for congenital diaphragmatic hernia. Semin Pediatr Surg 1996;5:266–74.

[60] Clugston RD, Greer JJ. Diaphragm development and congenital diaphragmatic hernia. Semin Pediatr Surg 2007;16:94–100.

[61] Rottier R, Tibboel D. Fetal lung and diaphragm development in congenital diaphragmatic hernia. Semin Perinatol 2005;29:86–93.

[62] Kitagawa M, Hislop A, Boyden EA, et al. Lung hypoplasia in congenital diaphragmatic hernia. A quantitative study of airway, artery, and alveolar development. Br J Surg 1971;58:342–6.

[63] Hislop A, Reid L. Persistent hypoplasia of the lung after repair of congenital diaphragmatic hernia. Thorax 1976;31:450–5.

[64] Mohseni-Bod H, Bohn D. Pulmonary hypertension in congenital diaphragmatic hernia. Semin Pediatr Surg 2007;16:126–33.

[65] Harrison MR, Adzick NS, Estes JM, et al. A prospective study of the outcome for fetuses with diaphragmatic hernia [see comments]. JAMA 1994;271:382–4.

[66] Deprest JA, Hyett JA, Flake AW, et al. Current controversies in prenatal diagnosis 4: Should fetal surgery be done in all cases of severe diaphragmatic hernia? Prenat Diagn 2009;29:15–9.

[67] Harrison MR, Keller RL, Hawgood SB, et al. A randomized trial of fetal endoscopic tracheal occlusion for severe fetal congenital diaphragmatic hernia. N Engl J Med 2003;349:1916–24.

[68] Albanese CT, Lopoo J, Goldstein RB, et al. Fetal liver position and perinatal outcome for congenital diaphragmatic hernia. Prenat Diagn 1998;18:1138–42.

[69] Hedrick HL, Danzer E, Merchant A, et al. Liver position and lung-to-head ratio for prediction of extracorporeal membrane oxygenation and survival in isolated left congenital diaphragmatic hernia. Am J Obstet Gynecol 2007;197:422, e1–4.

[70] Jani J, Keller RL, Benachi A, et al. Prenatal prediction of survival in isolated left-sided diaphragmatic hernia. Ultrasound Obstet Gynecol 2006;27:18–22.

[71] Davey MG, Hedrick HL, Bouchard S, et al. Temporary tracheal occlusion in fetal sheep with lung hypoplasia does not improve postnatal lung function. J Appl Physiol 2003;94:1054–62.

[72] Davey MG, Danzer E, Schwarz U, et al. Prenatal glucocorticoids and exogenous surfactant therapy improve respiratory function in lambs with severe diaphragmatic hernia following fetal tracheal occlusion. Pediatr Res 2006;60:131–5.

[73] Danzer E, Davey MG, Kreiger PA, et al. Fetal tracheal occlusion for severe congenital diaphragmatic hernia in humans: a morphometric study of lung parenchyma and muscularization of pulmonary arterioles. J Pediatr Surg 2008;43:1767–75.

[74] Flake AW, Crombleholme TM, Johnson MP, et al. Treatment of severe congenital diaphragmatic hernia by fetal tracheal occlusion: clinical experience with fifteen cases. Am J Obstet Gynecol 2000;183:1059–66.

[75] Heerema AE, Rabban JT, Sydorak RM, et al. Lung pathology in patients with congenital diaphragmatic hernia treated with fetal surgical intervention, including tracheal occlusion. Pediatr Dev Pathol 2003;6:536–46.

[76] Deprest J. Towards an endoscopic intra-uterine treatment for congenital diaphragmatic hernia. Verh K Acad Geneeskd Belg 2002;64:55–70.

[77] Deprest J, Gratacos E, Nicolaides KH. Fetoscopic tracheal occlusion (FETO) for severe congenital diaphragmatic hernia: evolution of a technique and preliminary results. Ultrasound Obstet Gynecol 2004;24:121–6.

[78] Deprest J, Jani J, Cannie M, et al. Prenatal intervention for isolated congenital diaphragmatic hernia. Curr Opin Obstet Gynecol 2006;18:355–67.

[79] Bebbington M. Twin-to-twin transfusion syndrome: current understanding of pathophysiology, in-utero therapy and impact for future development. Semin Fetal Neonatal Med 2010;15:15–20.

[80] Denbow ML, Cox P, Taylor M, et al. Placental angioarchitecture in monochorionic twin pregnancies: relationship to fetal growth, fetofetal transfusion syndrome, and pregnancy outcome. Am J Obstet Gynecol 2000;182:417–26.

[81] Denbow ML, Eckersley R, Welsh AW, et al. Ex vivo delineation of placental angioarchitecture with the microbubble contrast agent levovist. Am J Obstet Gynecol 2000;182:966–71.

[82] Quintero RA, Morales WJ, Allen MH, et al. Staging of twin-twin transfusion syndrome. J Perinatol 1999;19:550–5.

[83] Rychik J, Tian Z, Bebbington M, et al. The twin-twin transfusion syndrome: spectrum of cardiovascular abnormality and development of a cardiovascular score to assess severity of disease. Am J Obstet Gynecol 2007;197:392, e1–8.

[84] Senat MV, Deprest J, Boulvain M, et al. Endoscopic laser surgery versus serial amnioreduction for severe twin-to-twin transfusion syndrome. N Engl J Med 2004;351:136–44.

[85] Quintero RA, Comas C, Bornick PW, et al. Selective versus non-selective laser photocoagulation of placental vessels in twin-to-twin transfusion syndrome. Ultrasound Obstet Gynecol 2000;16:230–6.

[86] Graef C, Ellenrieder B, Hecher K, et al. Long-term neurodevelopmental outcome of 167 children after intrauterine laser treatment for severe twin-twin transfusion syndrome. Am J Obstet Gynecol 2006;194:303–8.

[87] Flake AW. Surgery in the human fetus: the future. J Physiol 2003;547:45–51.

Advances in Pediatrics 57 (2010) 373–389

ADVANCES IN PEDIATRICS

Advances in the Surgical Management of Gastroesophageal Reflux

John A. Sandoval, MD[a], David A. Partrick, MD[b],*

[a]St Jude Children's Research Hospital, Department of Surgery, 262 Danny Thomas Place, Mail Stop 332, Memphis, TN 38105, USA
[b]University of Colorado School of Medicine, Department of Pediatric Surgery, The Children's Hospital, 13123 East 16th Avenue, B323, Aurora, CO 80045, USA

Gastroesophageal reflux (GER) is common in infants and children. The functional process occurs daily in one-half of infants 0 to 3 months of age and two-thirds of infants 4 months of age [1] and is characterized by the involuntary passage of gastric contents into the lower esophagus. In general, most infants with GER eventually "outgrow" or spontaneously resolve their reflux with only 5% of infants having persistent symptoms after the age of 12 months [2,3]. The subsequent development of a pathologic condition associated with reflux is termed GER disease (GERD) and may include poor weight gain, irritability, esophagitis, esophageal stricture, stridor, reactive airway disease, recurrent pneumonia, bronchitis, laryngitis, and apparent life-threatening events (ALTEs) [4]. Over the past 5 decades, the understanding and treatment of reflux disease has grown, in part, owing to the development and use of flexible upper endoscopy and sophisticated approaches to the measurement of pathophysiologic factors leading to GER. Additionally, the increased utilization and improvements in antireflux surgical procedures have furthered our ability to help the subset of infants and children requiring operative intervention to control GERD symptoms. Gastric dissociation procedures, robot-assisted laparoscopic surgery, and single-site techniques are operations that have a role in selected cases. Lastly, developments in novel endoluminal therapies have extended the armamentarium for the management of GERD and may create the next generation of interventional options in the treatment of pediatric GERD.

HISTORY

An extensive body of literature has documented the historical perspective of GERD in children. For example, in 1828, GERD was first recorded at autopsy in children with repeated bouts of emesis [5]. The term peptic esophagitis was first mentioned in 1935 [6]. Allison [7] is generally credited for initiating the

*Corresponding author. E-mail address: partrick.david@tchden.org

0065-3101/10/$ – see front matter
doi:10.1016/j.yapd.2010.09.004

modern era of antireflux surgery. In his classic article published in 1951, he aimed to "emphasize the relation between the altered physiology at the cardia, and a common form of indigestion consisting mainly of heartburn, gastric flatulence and postural regurgitation." He attributed the occurrence of these symptoms to reflux esophagitis caused by incompetence of the gastroesophageal junction and stated that "the cause of the incompetence is a sliding hernia of the stomach through the esophageal hiatus of the diaphragm into the posterior mediastinum." Allison focused on the crural sling as the key factor in preventing reflux. He believed these crural fibers functioned as a pinchcock to prevent reflux. Barrett [8] focused on restoration of the cardioesophageal angle as the critical component in the prevention of GER, and his efforts stimulated surgeons to design procedures aimed at improving the function of the cardia. Following the description of "chalasia" by Berenberg and Neuhauser and of partial thoracic stomach by Carre and Astley [9], GERD was recognized as a pediatric clinical entity. Not until the 1950s did surgery become an option for childhood GERD because of the limited experience with antireflux operations in children. As advancements of the physiology of GER were made during the second half of the twentieth century, (Fig. 1) Nissen and Belsey developed their famous operations. In 1957, Collis published his innovative operation. Thal described his technique in 1965, and in 1967, Hill published his procedure. Many modifications of these procedures were published by

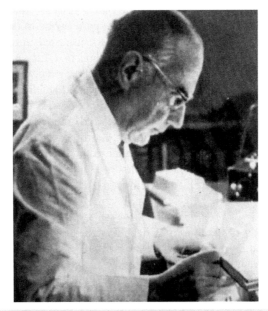

Fig. 1. Rudolf Nissen pictured during the time of development of the antireflux surgery. (*From* Liebermann-Meffer, Stein. Rudolf Nissen and the World Revolution of Fundoplication. St Louis, MI: Quality Medical Publishing Inc; 1999; with permission.)

Pearson and Henderson, Orringer and Sloan, and Rossetti et al. More recently, the widespread availability of physiologic and diagnostic testing with esophageal motility studies, 24-hour pH probe studies, endoscopy, and barium esophagography has greatly improved the identification of infants/children who are likely to benefit from surgery. These progressive innovations in the approaches to delineating GERD and the development of minimally invasive surgical techniques have led to a dramatic increase in the number of antireflux operations being performed by pediatric surgeons [10].

PATHOGENESIS

Understanding the mechanisms that result in GER as well as protect against GER are important in the effective management of GERD. Physiologic mechanisms protecting against GER are effective esophageal motility (facilitates esophageal clearance), antral contractions (promotes gastric emptying), and the production of mucus, prostaglandin, and epithelial growth factors (prevents esophageal mucosa damage). A number of important anatomic mechanisms are responsible for GER; these include the lower esophageal sphincter (LES; pressure >10–30 mm Hg), length of the intra-abdominal segment of the esophagus, acute angle of His, mucosal rosette in the distal esophagus, phrenoesophageal membrane, and the pinchcock effect of the diaphragmatic crura. Of the different components interacting at various levels, the most important in preventing reflux is the LES. The primary mechanism of GER in children is the transient lower esophageal sphincter relaxation (TLESR) [11]. Other mechanisms that account for a small fraction of reflux in patients with GERD include low resting LES pressure and increased intragastric pressure (stress reflux) [12,13]. TLESRs are physiologic relaxations of the LES to intragastric pressure that occur in the absence of a swallow. These relaxations are prolonged compared with swallow-induced relaxations, typically lasting longer than 10 seconds, and are associated with a characteristic pattern of pharyngeal and esophageal motility on manometric studies [14]. TLESR is the underlying mechanism for nearly all reflux episodes in healthy adults and in adults [12,13] and children [11] with GERD. Although there is conflicting evidence regarding whether TLESRs are more common in patients with GERD, it seems that GER occurs more frequently during TLESR in patients with reflux esophagitis [12,13]. TLESRs are activated by a vagally mediated pathway in response to fundal stretch [15]. There is evidence that several signaling molecules, both excitatory and inhibitory, play a role in this pathway, including acetylcholine, cholecystokinin, γ-aminobutyric acid (GABA), and nitric oxide [15]. These transmitters are potential targets for pharmacologic therapy, particularly agents that affect the GABA inhibitory pathway [16]. Other novel molecular biology work providing insight into the cause of GERD involves a connective tissue component (collagen type III α 1 [COL3A1]). Asling and coworkers [17] showed the expression of COL3A1 was associated with GERD in children and adults and with hiatal hernia in men, indicating that a tissue remodelling mechanism may be implicated in some cases. Derangement in the inherent balance of the gastroesophageal mechanism, driven by the interactions of biology, physiology, and anatomy, are responsible for contributing to pediatric GERD.

CLINICAL DIAGNOSIS

A diversity of clinical signs and symptoms attributed to GER can be appreciated in infants and children. Infants generally present with recurrent nonbilious emesis, but regurgitation of feedings are not exclusive to the diagnosis of GER. For these reasons, other extraesophageal features such as apnea, chronic lung disease (bronchopulmonary dysplasia), failure to thrive, and behavioral symptoms (irritability, facial grimacing, head arching, and frequent swallowing) may also indicate complications from GER (Box 1). In children, persistent nonbilious vomiting continues to be the prevalent symptom, but GER may also present with esophageal strictures, hypochromic microcytic anemia from ulcerative esophagitis, asthma, or frequent respiratory symptoms (silent refluxers). GER may also be present in special pediatric populations. These include infants and children with associated anatomic defects (insertion of gastrostomy tubes, esophageal atresia and/or tracheoesophageal fistula, antral dysmotility, or antral and pyloric webs), congenital diaphragmatic hernia and anterior abdominal defects, neurologic abnormalities, aspiration syndromes (ALTEs), and unusual presentations (Sandifer syndrome and protein-losing enteropathy). Furthermore, it is important to delineate vomiting caused by GER from other systemic disorders, such as infections (eg, sepsis, meningitis, urinary tract infection), obstruction (hypertrophic pyloric stenosis, malrotation, or intussusception), and neurologic (hydrocephalus, elevated intracranial pressure,

---

Box 1: Operative indications for GERD

Absolute indications

Apnea/near sudden infant death syndrome with GER

Pneumonitis with associated lung changes

Esophagitis with ulceration or stricture

Relative indications

Failure of medical management

Failure to thrive

Recurrent pneumonia

Atypical asthma

Chronic cough

Chronic vomiting

Adapted from Partrick DA. Gastroesophageal reflux in infants and children. In: Patterson GA, Cooper JD, Deslauriers J, et al, editors. Pearson's thoracic and esophageal surgery. Philadelphia: Churchill Livingstone Elsevier; 2008. p. 217–23.

migraines, or subdural hematoma), metabolic (diabetic ketoacidosis, galacto-semia, fructose intolerance, or urea cycle defects), or renal (obstructive urop-athy or renal insufficiency).

DIAGNOSIS

Several investigations are used to diagnose GER, including contrast esophagram, esophageal pH monitoring, and esophagoscopy. Barium esophagography is a noninvasive, inexpensive, and readily available test that can simultaneously evaluate swallowing function, esophageal motility, GER, and a host of structural abnormalities in the pharynx and esophagus. The purpose of barium studies in patients with reflux symptoms is not only to document the presence of a hiatal hernia or GER but also to detect the morphologic sequelae of reflux, including reflux esophagitis or peptic strictures. Additionally, this test can be valuable in the evaluation of the postoperative antireflux surgical patient. An esophogram can determine if the fundoplication is intact, or whether recurrent GER is present. It can also help define the main mechanism of failure after an antireflux procedure such as a herniated fundoplication through the hiatus, a disrupted fundoplication, a paraesophageal hernia, a tight fundoplication, or a tight esophageal hiatus. However, contrast esophogram is not a good study to quantitate the amount of GER occurring.

pH monitoring has long been considered the gold standard in the diagnosis of GERD. Acid reflux occurs when the measured pH falls below 4, and this can be continuously measured over time. Additional information regarding the number and duration of each reflux episode as well as symptom correlation are also recorded. Although widely accepted and available, pH monitoring has important limitations. Traditional pH probes do not measure nonacid re-flux (refluxed material that has a pH ≥ 4.0). Furthermore, pH probes require transnasal placement, which may cause discomfort, decrease appetite and activity, disrupt normal routines, and, thus, underestimate the true incidence of reflux.

Multichannel intraluminal impedance (MII) and the wireless pH capsule have been added to the repertoire of tests available to study esophageal path-ophysiology in children to address the shortcomings of pH monitoring. The main advantage of MII over traditional pH monitoring is its ability to detect both acid and nonacid GER and to discern liquid from gas GER. Although feasible with multiple pH sensors, the MII technique routinely detects the prox-imal extent of a GER episode. When a pH sensor is added to the MII catheter, important information about the acidity of a GER event can be obtained. The role of MII has also been investigated in esophageal function testing. Manom-etry classically reveals information about esophageal pressure patterns and sphincter function but not about bolus flow. MII not only detects the presence of esophageal flow but also adds information on the direction of flow, duration of bolus presence, completeness of bolus clearance, and composition of the bolus.

A wireless pH capsule is intended to be less uncomfortable and facilitates activity during the measuring period compared with the usual method with a nasoesophageal catheter. The pH radiotransmitted device is an oblong 6 × 5.5 × 25-mm capsule deployed from the end of an 80-cm, 6F catheter that is placed transorally. The capsule is attached to the esophageal mucosa and transmits pH data to a portable receiver, using radiotelemetry. The wireless system has mostly been studied in adults and causes less discomfort than traditional pH monitoring with a catheter [18].

Information on the use of the wireless system in children is limited, but the system has been recommended by those who have used it [19]. Most patients tolerate wireless pH monitoring without incident, and in a recent study comparing catheter-based pH monitoring and wireless monitoring in children aged 4 to 18 years, patients reported greater satisfaction with the wireless monitoring system [20]. Complications and drawbacks include failure of attachment, chest pain, foreign body sensation, early detachment (11% before 48 hours in original adult studies), failure to detach within 14 days, inability to measure nonacid reflux, and a need to place with endoscopy. Contraindications to capsule placement include bleeding diatheses, esophageal strictures, severe esophagitis, esophageal varices, gastrointestinal tract obstruction, and pacemakers [21].

Endoscopic evaluation of patients with GERD using standard endoscopy is specific for the diagnosis when esophageal erosions are present. Using standard white-light endoscopy, however, less than half of the patients with GERD have findings of erosive esophagitis. Endoscopy is more useful for excluding other conditions that mimic GERD, such as eosinophilic esophagitis, pill esophagitis, or Crohn disease, or in the assessment of reflux complications (esophagitis or stricture) as well as obtaining biopsies for the detection of microscopic disease (*Helicobacter pylori* infections or Barrett's esophagus).

The routine use of nuclear scintigraphy to assess for delayed gastric emptying and to measure reflux is controversial, and the authors think that this test offers no real advantage over the upper gastrointestinal contrast study. Another modality used in adults, yet limited in children, is esophageal manometry. The effectiveness of esophageal manometry for GERD has minimal clinical value except in children with suspected primary or secondary esophageal motility disorders. Manometry has identified abnormal distal esophageal motility in infants after repair of esophageal atresia.

Finally, bronchoscopy can be useful to assess vocal cord inflammation or edema in patients with pulmonary symptoms secondary to GER. The lipid-laden macrophage index (LLMI) obtained from bronchoalveolar lavage specimens has been reported to correspond with aspiration events related to GER, but recent data suggest that the LLMI has limited use in predicting reflux-related respiratory disease in children [22].

TREATMENT

Most infants with physiologic reflux generally require no intervention [23]. Nevertheless, the aim of therapy for the fraction of infants with GERD is to achieve symptomatic relief, promote normal growth, and prevent relapses and complications. The treatment of GER can be divided into traditional measures, pharmacologic treatments, and surgery.

Conservative measures include feeding modifications, positioning, and avoiding tobacco smoke exposure and medications that reduce LES tone (eg, caffeine, theophylline, anticholinergics). Although some of these techniques have little proven efficacy, a recent double-blind, randomized, placebo-controlled trial evaluated standard approaches (feeding changes, positioning, and tobacco smoke avoidance) to treat GER symptoms in infants [24]. Using a symptom-scoring instrument, the authors concluded that 2 weeks of conservative therapy taught to parents in a primary care setting caused improvement in 78% of infants with GERD; 59% had improvement by at least 5 points, and 24% normalized. The study reinforces that many GER symptoms improved or resolved in most infants within 2 weeks and underscores that the nonpharmacologic approach should be the first-line therapy. Level I and level III evidence also support feed thickening [23,25], thereby strengthening the evidence-based literature on these time-tested methods. Other alternative therapies include temporary placement of a transpyloric, nasoduodenal, or nasojejunal feeding tube. Transpyloric feedings have been shown to reduce episodes of apnea and bradycardia in preterm infants with suspected GER [26].

Pharmacologic Medical Therapy

Modern medical therapy allows the physician to heal the esophagitis and relieve the patients from troublesome GERD symptoms. Medical therapy is effective with H2 receptor antagonists and proton pump inhibitors and is supported by type I evidence [23]. These therapies have a low side-effect profile but have considerable side effects for chronic suppression of gastric acid consistent with diarrhea (especially *Clostridium difficile*, *Salmonella*, and *Campylobacter* infections), community-acquired pneumonia, and hip fractures [27–30]. Moreover, the widespread use of acid inhibitors in infants and children has been noted. Medco Health Solutions Inc, a pharmacy benefit manager, determined that the number of acid suppressant medications prescribed in children younger than 4 years increased by 56% between 2002 and 2006; it was estimated that 3% of all children in this age group are prescribed some form of acid-suppression medication [31]. When medical management is compared with surgery for GERD, cost-effective analysis shows surgery to be more cost-effective in adults [32]; there are no randomized controlled trials of fundoplication versus medical therapy in children [23].

Surgical Treatment

For selected patients, that is, children with severe and/or chronic, relapsing GERD or those who experience extraesophageal complications, there is an established role for the surgical treatment of reflux. Fundoplication is the standard surgical approach to GER in a child and currently recommended by type II-3 evidence. The laparoscopic Nissen fundoplication has largely replaced the open Nissen fundoplication as the preferred operative approach in children who have normal esophageal body peristalsis. These procedures are safe and have similar outcomes [33–35]. The main benefits of the laparoscopic approach in adults and children are shorter hospital stays and fewer perioperative problems, such as prolonged ileus and respiratory infections. The fundamental platform of the procedures (Figs. 2 and 3) (1) a limited circumferential dissection of the esophagus with a complete dissection of the esophageal hiatus and both crura, (2) mobilization of the gastric fundus by dividing the short gastric vessels, (3) closure of the associated hiatal defect, (4) creation of a tensionless floppy 360° gastric wrap at the distal esophagus around an appropriately sized intraesophageal dilator [36], (5) limiting the wrap to no more than 2 cm, and (6) stabilization of the wrap to the esophagus by partial-thickness bites of the esophagus during the creation of the wrap. The overall physiologic action of antireflux surgery is such that an elevation in the gastric volume causes the wrap to compress the lower esophagus/cardia, creating a pneumohydraulic valve. Additional aims are to reestablish intra-abdominal esophageal length and recreate a high-pressure zone in the distal esophagus by accentuating the angle of His; the intended surgical intervention seeks to establish or restore the antireflux barrier and correct other abnormalities contributing to a reflux.

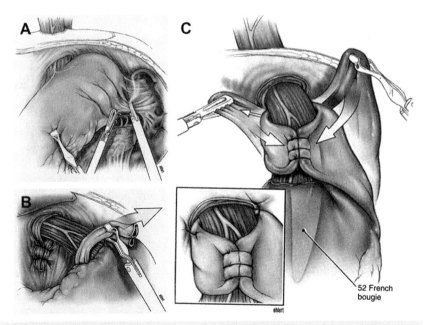

Fig. 2. Surgical sequence for Nissen fundoplication. (A) Left crus approach is followed by an incision in the phrenoesophageal membrane and dissection of the right crus; (B) posterior crural closure; (C) involvement of the esophagus with the gastric fundus. (Adapted from Townsend. Sabiston textbook of surgery. 16th edition. WB Saunders Company; 2001; with permission.)

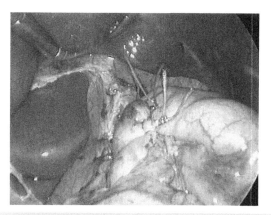

Fig. 3. Final appearance of Nissen fundoplication.

Postoperatively, depending on open or laparoscopic technique, the course may vary. In general, patients are allowed to drink after laparoscopic repair. Carbonated beverages are eschewed to avoid gastric distension, and patients are advanced to a soft mechanical diet the first postoperative day. In selected cases in which extensive paraesophageal hernial dissection occurs, redo surgery or concomitant gastric emptying procedure (pyloroplasty), feeds may be delayed 1–3 days. On average, children are discharged home 1 to 3 days after the procedure when tolerating a soft mechanical diet and reasonable pain control is achieved. Secondary to edema at the fundoplication, patients are maintained on a soft diet for 1 week and gradually advanced to a regular diet at home. A dietician consultation is obtained before discharge to underscore to parents/caretakers that children be instructed to chew food well and avoid swallowing large pieces of bread or dry foods that have the potential to become lodged at the fundoplication site. There are no limitations on activity and no long term dietary restrictions. In patients recovering from open surgery, neurologically impaired children, or those having a concomitant gastrostomy tube inserted, the time for feeds and discharge are potentially longer.

Most series indicate complications after antireflux surgery can be divided into intraoperative, early, and late postoperative events. Intraoperative complications, such as bleeding, bowel injury, pneumothorax, esophageal/gastric perforations, and vagal nerve injury, occur in 0.5% to 11.5% [37]. A high index of suspicion needs to be maintained to detect these intraoperative complications. Favorable recovery depends intraoperative recognition such that most of these events can be rectified laparoscopically, avoiding the need for a major laparotomy. Early complications are uncommon in the initial recovery period, but a minority has dysphagia (2%–12%) and gas bloat (4%–10%). While some transitory and mild dysphagia occurs in patients, most commonly after a circumferential wrap, this condition generally settles in most patients by 2 to 4 weeks. The causes of persistent postoperative dysphagia include inappropriate patient selection, lack of an adequate objective preoperative evaluation, type of antireflux procedure, and technical problem with how the fundoplication was formed. Various mechanisms may cause the gas bloat syndrome and, in some cases, interact to generate the syndrome; these mechanisms include abnormal motility, impaired gastric accommodation, gastric hypersensitivity, and dumping syndrome (30%) [38]. Other anatomic complications, such as disrupted (8%–12%) or slipped wrap, herniated wrap, too tight or too long fundoplication, twisted wrap, or the 2-compartment stomach [39], are related to technical failures and constitute unsuccessful surgery. Late events such as adhesional small-bowel obstruction (2%–10%) have lower incidence after laparoscopic fundoplication than after open fundoplication and are more common if patients undergo other concomitant procedures (eg, Ladd's procedure, gastrotomy, appendectomy, etc).

To offset the known adverse effects associated with a complete circumferential wrap, several different antireflux procedures with numerous modifications (Nissen-Rosseti, Toupet, and Thal procedures) have been reported. Some surgeons favor partial fundoplication because they argue that a partial fundoplication is more physiologic, allowing venting of air from the stomach, and therefore reduces the rate of adverse effects of a total fundoplication. In addition, a partial fundoplication may be more appropriate in patients with known esophageal dysmotility, such as after esophageal atresia repair. Regardless of the technique used, there are no randomized studies comparing partial or complete fundoplication, but reports show that the efficacy and complications of partial and complete fundoplication are similar [40]. The primary concern with the various partial fundoplications is an increased risk of recurrent GER compared to a Nissen fundoplication.

The recurrence of GERD after Nissen fundoplication represents a significant clinical problem. Recurrent GERD must be differentiated from transient symptoms because up to two-thirds of infants who undergo fundoplication can have persistent GERD-related sequelae requiring medical therapy for up to 2 months after the procedure [41]. Wrap disruption and/or transmigration are the most common reasons for recurrent reflux. In children younger than 6 years, preoperative hiatal hernia, postoperative retching, postoperative esophageal dilation, and neurologic impairment are risk factors that have been associated with fundoplication failure [42,43]. Revision of the fundoplication is a reasonable approach that can be accomplished laparoscopically the first time up to 89% of the time, but this decreases to 68% for second revisions [4]. Conversion to an open procedure was usually because of difficulties with dissection secondary to scarring or poor visualization. Laparoscopic failures requiring a redo laparoscopic procedure were associated with a failure rate of 4%, 7%, and 10% [44–46]. There is evidence that limiting the paraesophageal and hiatal dissection during the initial surgery can decrease the recurrence rate [47]. Other options for the child with a failed fundoplication include medical management, jejunal feeding using a percutaneous tube or a Roux-en-Y jejunostomy, total esophagogastric dissociation (TEGD), or laparoscopic Roux-en-Y gastrojejunal bypass (RYGB). TEGD is an alternative to the classic fundoplication procedure because this approach involves dividing the esophagus from the stomach at the gastroesophageal junction, forming an esophagojejunal anastomosis using a Roux-en-Y configuration, and placing feeding access through a gastrostomy. TEGD seeks to reduce GER recurrence and supraesophageal complications and thus avoid the need for reiterative procedures. Published series support effectiveness compared with a fundoplication with a lower failure rate [48,49]. The TEGD is a nonreversible procedure, with limited capabilities for jejunum-compatible oral feeds, meaning gastrostomy feeding alone. The laparoscopic RYGB procedure differs from the TEGD procedure in that it maintains normal viability through the stomach and the gastrojejunal diversion offers an 'escape valve' that may aid gastric emptying. Recent work by Mattioli and colleagues [50] offers preliminary proof of principal evidence on the RYGB to treat children with GERD. While recurrent operations for failed antireflux surgery can achieve good long-term results in most patients, focus should be on prevention. Evolving technology such as fundoplication and hiatal-area endoscopic ultrasound evaluation may be an applicable tool to assess the integrity and position of an existing fundoplication [51]. This will help inform surgeons regarding factors influencing re-do operations and potentially lead to individualized surgery.

Robot-Assisted Antireflux Surgery

Robotic surgery is a relatively new technology, which may expand the variety of operations a pediatric surgeon can perform with minimally invasive methods. Robot-assisted laparoscopic (RAL) surgery has been readily adopted by the adult urological, gynecologic, and general surgical community (Fig. 4). The literature on robotic surgery on adults contains publications regarding the technological applications and successes as well as the significant learning curve that is required to achieve proficiency. However, pediatric robotic surgery remains in its infancy, with only 2 institutions reporting their experiences with initiating a pediatric RAL program [52]. While most reports have

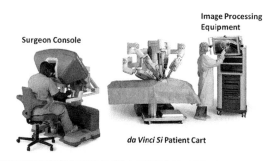

Fig. 4. Typical set up for robotic-assisted laparoscopic surgery. (*Courtesy of* Intuitive Surgical, Inc, Copyright 2010, How Stuff Works; with permission.)

addressed the feasibility and safety of RAL surgery, few reports compare robotic surgery with the laparoscopic approach. Albassam and colleagues [53] recently published a comparative study in 50 children undergoing either a RAL or traditional Nissen fundoplication. They reported no significant differences in outcomes between both groups, and no clear benefit was perceived given the high cost associated with robotic devices. Other reports echo these findings in addition to longer operating times and the lack of clinical advantage. To make RAL a reality, standard clinical protocols, established training programs, defined patient criteria, and favorable cost analyses are required to conclude the value of this important technology [54]. Nevertheless, the robotic interface is crucial for advancing surgical care, as the foundations in RAL have led to the development of miniature camera robots and microrobots [55]. These advances in the extension of the robotic platform promise to change the future of robotic technology for general surgery.

Laparoendoscopic Single-Site Surgery

One-port, single-incision laparoscopy is part of the natural development of minimally invasive surgery. The laparoscopic paradigm to place different ports according to ergonomic principles is presently challenged by laparoendoscopic single-site surgery (LESS). The objective is to perform a complex task with several instruments using only 1 access port (Fig. 5). However, this approach introduces distinct ergonomic problems and requires innovative technical solutions to allow for more complex surgical tasks. The LESS approach has been applied mainly in the adult population and has been used for a variety of laparoscopic operations, including tubal ligation, hysterectomy, fundoplication, appendectomy, cholecystectomy, sleeve gastrectomy, colectomy, and nephrectomy [56–61]. LESS in pediatric surgery is less extensive [62]. Using a modified single-site technique, Rothenberg et al [63] reported their laparoscopic experience with cholecystectomy (n = 10), appendectomy (n = 8), enterolysis (n = 2), ovarian cystectomy (n = 1), and inguinal hernial repair (n = 15). All procedures, except one, were completed using the modified single-port technique. As further refinements in instrumentation and operative techniques improve, the authors think that this technique will aptly be applied to pediatric fundoplications. The implementation of robotics may help ease the ergonomic difficulties associated with LESS. The advantages of combining both surgical disciplines are the improvements in articulated and rotating instruments with flexible sections and fine handling modalities. An experimental prospective report by Allemann and coworkers [64] compared laparoscopic and robot-assisted single-port access Nissen fundoplication in an animal model. All procedures were successfully completed, with the mean operative time and number of conflicts significantly lowered in the robot-assisted series. The co-use of both techniques may help open paths for these minimally invasive platforms. However, before use in the broader population, prospective, randomized studies are required to determine the true benefit and utility of this novel surgical approach compared with current alternatives.

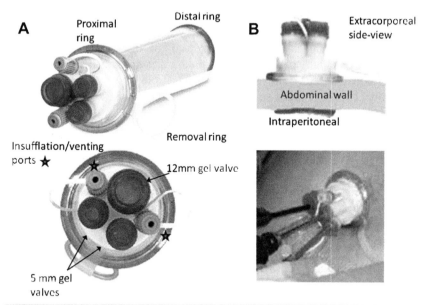

Fig. 5. Access for laparoendoscopic single site surgery (LESS). TriPortTM Disposable Multi-Instrument Port. (A) The TriPortTM device consists of a retractor component and a valve component. The valve component is made of a unique elastomeric material that allows passage of standard laparoscopic instruments and scopes simultaneously. The TriPort has one inlet for a 12 mm instrument and two for 5 mm instruments. Two separate insufflation/venting ports are used for feeding CO_2 gas and evacuating smoke from electrocautery and laser procedures to ensure the operating field remains clear. The high elasticity of the gel valve allows small specimens to be removed through this route, while larger specimens are withdrawn into the distal end of the port and removed simultaneously with the device at the end of the surgery. (B) The extracorporeal view of the TriPort with a bent modified instrument through the superior port. (*Courtesy of* Olympus America Incorporated; with permission.)

Endoscopic Antireflux Techniques

As the era of minimally invasive procedures in antireflux surgery has become prominent, new technologies that promise to be even less invasive has the potential to become the next-generation therapy for GERD. Three novel endoscopic techniques (Stretta, Curon Medical, EndoCinch, C.R. Bard Inc, and Enteryx procedures, Boston Scientific Corporation) are approved by the US Food and Drug Administration for the treatment of GERD. The procedures involve the injection or implantation of biopolymers into the LES as a bulking agent (Enteryx), the application of radiofrequency energy to the LES region (Stretta), and endoluminal suturing/plication of the gastric cardia (EndoCinch) [65,66]. Initial attempts to endoscopically control reflux have failed when compared with surgical partial fundoplication, and as a result, first-generation devices have been removed from further clinical application [67]. A fourth type of endoscopic approach has been described using a transoral anterior partial fundoplication (EsophyX, EndoGastric Solutions, Redmond, WA, USA), which attempts to attach the fundus of the stomach to a length of the intra-abdominal esophagus, thereby replicating the partial surgical fundoplication of up to 240° in extent. The first clinical use of the device was encouraging, as reflux control was touted in up to 80% of the patients at 6 months with little morbidity [68]. A current study by Repici and colleagues [69] enrolling 20 patients describes a 20% rate of early revision and poor objective outcomes; 17% improvement in 24 pH outcomes versus 67% worsening after treatment. Although the newer procedure is based on the principle of the surgical technique, they are limited to individuals with mild reflux and those with hiatal hernias less than 2 cm in length; therefore, these endoscopic approaches may be suitable for a subpopulation of patients. At present, endoscopic antireflux therapy is not recommended for routine use, but continued development and improvement in these devices is expected to have more effect in the future.

SUMMARY

Cornerstones for the optimal surgical management of pediatric GERD include careful patient selection, a complete and thorough preoperative workup, a meticulous operation in experienced hands, and well-informed parents/caretakers. Nissen fundoplication is the current standard of care in the majority of patients. As the panorama of newer approaches broadens for GERD, these contributions will open up new paradigms for treatment. In this constantly advancing field of surgical investigation, it will be paramount to understand how these developing procedures will fit in the spectrum of options for infants and children with GERD.

References

[1] Nelson SP, Chen EH, Syniar GM, et al. Prevalence of symptoms of gastroesophageal reflux during infancy. Arch Pediatr Adolesc Med 1997;151:569–72.

[2] Nelson SP, Chen EH, Syniar GM, et al. Prevalence of symptoms of gastroesophageal reflux during childhood. Arch Pediatr Adolesc Med 2000;154:150–4.

[3] Locke GR, Talley NJ, Fett SL, et al. Prevalence and clinical spectrum of gastroesophageal reflux: a population-based study in Olmsted County. Minnesota. Gastroenterology 1997;112:1448–56.

[4] Partrick DA. Gastroesophageal reflux in infants and children. In: Patterson GA, Cooper JD, Deslauriers J, et al, editors. Pearson's thoracic and esophageal surgery. Philadelphia: Churchill Livingstone Elsevier; 2008. p. 217–23.

[5] Billiard MC. Traite des maladies des enfans nouveaux-nes et a la mamelle. In: Billiard M, editor. Atlas d'anatomie pathologique pour servir a l'historie des maladies des enfants. Paris: Imprimerie se H Balzac; 1828. p. 271.

[6] Winkelstein A. Peptic esophagitis: a new clinical entity. JAMA 1935;104:906.

[7] Allison PR. Reflux esophagitis, sliding hiatal hernia, and the anatomy of repair. Surg Gynecol Obstet 1951;92:419–31.

[8] Barrett NR. Hiatus hernia. Br J Surg 1954;42:231–43.

[9] Carre IJ, Astley R. The fate of the partial thoracic stomach ('hiatus hernia') in children. Arch Dis Child 1960;35:484–6.

[10] Sydorak RM, Albanese CT. Laparoscopic antireflux procedures in children: evaluating the evidence. Semin Laparosc Surg 2002;9:133–8. Available at: http://www.ncbi.nlm.nih.gov/pubmed/12407520. Accessed September 2, 2010.

[11] Kawahara H, Dent J, Davidson G. Mechanisms responsible for gastroesophageal reflux in children. Gastroenterology 1997;113:399–408.

[12] Dodds WJ, Dent J, Hogan WJ, et al. Mechanisms of gastroesophageal reflux in patients with reflux esophagitis. N Engl J Med 1982;307:1547–52.

[13] Mittal RK, McCallum RW. Characteristics and frequency of transient relaxations of the lower esophageal sphincter in patients with reflux esophagitis. Gastroenterology 1988;95:593–9.

[14] Mittal RK, Holloway RH, Penagini R, et al. Transient lower esophageal sphincter relaxation. Gastroenterology 1995;109:601–10.

[15] Hirsch DP, Tytgat GNJ, Boeckxstaens GEE. Review article: transient lower oesophageal sphincter relaxations—a pharmacological target for gastrooesophageal reflux disease. Aliment Pharmacol Ther 2002;16:17–26.

[16] Lehmann A. Novel treatments of GERD: focus on the lower esophageal sphincter. Eur Rev Med Pharmacol Sci 2008;12:103–10.

[17] Asling B, Jirholt J, Hammond P, et al. Collagen type III alpha I is a gastro-oesophageal reflux disease susceptibility gene and a male risk factor for hiatus hernia. Gut 2009;58:1063–9.

[18] Wenner J, Johnsson F, Johansson J, et al. Wireless oesophageal pH monitoring: feasibility, safety and normal values in healthy subjects. Scand J Gastroenterol 2005;40:768–74.

[19] Bothwell M, Phillips J, Bauer S. Upper esophageal pH monitoring of children with the Bravo pH capsule. Laryngoscope 2004;114:786–8.

[20] Croffie JM, Fitzgerald JF, Molleston JP, et al. Accuracy and tolerability of the Bravo catheter-free pH capsule in patients between the ages of 4 and 18 years. J Pediatr Gastroenterol Nutr 2007;45:559–63.

[21] Dranove JE. Focus on diagnosis: new technologies for the diagnosis of gastroesophageal reflux disease. Pediatr Rev 2008;29:317–20.

[22] Rosen R, Fritz J, Nurko A, et al. Lipid-laden macrophage index is not an indicator of gastroesophageal reflux-related respiratory disease in children. Pediatrics 2008;121:e879–84.

[23] Rudolph CD, Mazur LJ, Liptak GS, et al. Guidelines for evaluation and treatment of gastroesophageal reflux in infants and children: recommendations of the North American Society for Pediatric Gastroenterology and Nutrition. J Pediatr Gastroenterol Nutr 2001;32:S1–31.

[24] Orenstein SR, Hassall E, Furmaga-Jablonska W, et al. Multicenter, double-blind, randomized, placebo-controlled trial assessing the efficacy and safety of proton pump inhibitor lansoprazole in infants with symptoms of gastroesophageal reflux disease. J Pediatr 2009;154:514–20.

[25] Wenzl TG, Schneider S, Scheele F, et al. Effects of thickened feeding on gastroesophageal reflux in infants: a placebo-controlled crossover study using intraluminal impedance. Pediatrics 2003;111:e355–9.

[26] Malcolm WF, Smith PB, Mears S, et al. Transpyloric tube feeding in very low birthweight infants with suspected gastroesophageal reflux: impact on apnea and bradycardia. J Perinatol 2009;29:372–5.

[27] Canani RB, Cirillo P, Roggero P, et al. Therapy with gastric acidity inhibitors increases the risk of acute gastroenteritis and community-acquired pneumonia in children. Pediatrics 2006;117:e817–20.

[28] Leonard J, Marshall JK, Moayyedi P. Systematic review of the risk of enteric infection in patients taking acid suppression. Am J Gastroenterol 2007;102:2047–56.

[29] Yang YX, Lewis JD, Epstein S, et al. Long-term proton pump inhibitor therapy and risk of hip fracture. J Am Med Assoc 2006;296:2947–53.

[30] O'Connell MB, Madden DM, Murray AM, et al. Effects of proton pump inhibitors on calcium carbonate absorption in women: a randomized crossover trial. Am J Med 2005;118:778–81.

[31] Medico Health Solutions, Inc. (NYSE: MHS) Children's aching stomachs: New research finds young children are increasingly using medications to treat gastrointestinal ailments. Infants and preschoolers show greatest increase in use, followed by elementary age children. Franklin Lakes, NJ, October 4, 2007.

[32] Epstein D, Bojke L, Sculpher MJ. REFLUX trial group. Laparoscopic fundoplication compared with medical management for gastro-oesophageal reflux disease: cost effectiveness study. BMJ 2009;339:b2576.

[33] Kane TD, Brown MF, Chen MK. Members of the APSA New Technology Committee. Position paper on laparoscopic antireflux operations in infants and children for gastroesophageal reflux disease. American Pediatric Surgery Association. J Pediatr Surg 2009;44:1034–40.

[34] Chung DH, Georgeson KE. Fundoplication and gastrostomy. Semin Pediatr Surg 1998;7: 213–9.

[35] Mattioli G, Sacco O, Gentilino V, et al. Outcome of laparoscopic Nissen-Rossetti fundoplication in children with gastroesophageal reflux disease and supraesophageal symptoms. Surg Endosc 2004;18:463–5.

[36] Ostlie DJ, Miller KA, Holcomb GW 3rd. Effective Nissen fundoplication length and bougie diameter size in young children undergoing laparoscopic Nissen fundoplication. J Pediatr Surg 2002;37:1664–6.

[37] Lobe TE. The current role of laparoscopic surgery for gastroesophageal reflux disease in infants and children. Surg Endosc 2007;21:167–74.

[38] Di Lorenzo C, Orenstein S. Fundoplication: friend or foe? J Pediatr Gastroenterol Nutr 2002;34:117–24.

[39] Hunter JG, Smith CD, Branum GD, et al. Laparoscopic fundoplication failures: patterns of failure and response to fundoplication revision. Ann Surg 1999;230:595–604.

[40] Esposito C, Montupet P, van Der Zee D, et al. Long-term outcome of laparoscopic Nissen, Toupet, and Thal antireflux procedures for neurologically normal children with gastroesophageal reflux disease. Surg Endosc 2006;20:855–8.

[41] Gilger MA, Yeh C, Chiang J, et al. Outcomes of surgical fundoplication in children. Clin Gastroenterol Hepatol 2004;2:978–84.

[42] Ngerncham M, Barnhart DC, Haricharan RN, et al. Risk factors for recurrent gastroesophageal reflux disease after fundoplication in pediatric patients: a case-control study. J Pediatr Surg 2007;42:1478–85.

[43] Pearl RH, Robie DK, Ein SH, et al. Complications of gastroesophageal antireflux surgery in neurologically impaired versus neurologically normal children. J Pediatr Surg 1990;25: 1169–73.

[44] Granderath FA, Kamolz T, Schweiger UM, et al. Is laparoscopic refundoplication feasible in patients with failed primary open antireflux surgery? Surg Endosc 2002;16:381–5.

[45] Graziano K, Teitelbaum DH, McLean K, et al. Recurrence after laparoscopic and open Nissen fundoplication: a comparison of the mechanism of failure. Surg Endosc 2003;17: 704–7.

[46] Rothenberg SS. Laparoscopic redo Nissen fundoplication in infant and children. Surg Endosc 2006;20:1518–20.

[47] St Peter SD, Valusek PA, Calkins CM, et al. Use of esophagocrural sutures and minimal esophageal dissection reduces the incidence of postoperative transmigration of laparoscopic Nissen fundoplication wrap. J Pediatr Surg 2007;42:25–9.

[48] Lall A, Morabito A, Bianchi A. "Total gastric dissociation (TGD)" in difficult clinical situations. Eur J Pediatr Surg 2006;16:396–8.

[49] Goyal A, Khalil B, Choo K, et al. Esophagogastric dissociation in the neurologically impaired: an alternative to fundoplication? J Pediatr Surg 2005;40:915–8.

[50] Mattioli G, Buffa P, Gandullia P, et al. Laparoscopic proximal Roux-en-Y gastrojejunal diversion in children: preliminary experience from a single center. J Laparoendosc Adv Surg Tech A 2009;19:807–13.

[51] Chang EY, Minjarez RC, Kim CY, et al. Endoscopic ultrasound for the evaluation of Nissen fundoplication integrity: a blinded comparison with conventional testing. Surg Endosc 2007;21:1719–25.

[52] Sorensen MD, Johnson MH, Delostrinos C, et al. Initiation of a pediatric robotic surgery program: institutional challenges and realistic outcomes. Surg Endosc 2010. [Epub ahead of print].

[53] Albassam AA, Mallick MS, Gado A, et al. Nissen fundoplication, robotic-assisted versus laparoscopic procedure: a comparative study in children. Eur J Pediatr Surg 2009;19:316–9.

[54] van Haasteren G, Levine S, Hayes W. Pediatric robotic surgery: early assessment. Pediatrics 2009;124:1642–9.

[55] Shah BC, Buettner SL, Lehman AC, et al. Miniature in vivo robotics and novel robotic surgical platforms. Urol Clin North Am 2009;36:251–63.

[56] Wheeless CR Jr. Outpatient laparoscope sterilization under local anesthesia. Obstet Gynecol 1972;39:767–70.

[57] Pelosi MA, Pelosi MA. Laparoscopic supracervical hysterectomy using a single-umbilical puncture (mini-laparoscopy). J Reprod Med 1992;37:777–84.

[58] Rispoli G, Armellino MF, Esposito C. One-trocar appendectomy: sense and nonsense. Surg Endosc 2002;16:833–5.

[59] Navarra G, Pozza E, Occhionorelli S, et al. One-wound laparoscopic cholecystectomy. Br J Surg 1997;84:695.

[60] Reavis KM, Hinojosa HW, Smith BR, et al. Single-laparoscopic incision transabdominal surgery sleeve gastrectomy. Obes Surg 2008;18:1492–4.

[61] Bucher P, Pugin F, Morel P. Single port access laparoscopic right hemicolectomy. Int J Colorectal Dis 2008;23:1013–6.

[62] Garey CL, Ostlie DJ, St Peter SD. A review of single site minimally invasive surgery in infants and children. Pediatr Surg Int 2010;26(5):451–6.

[63] Rothenberg SS, Shipman K, Yoder S. Experience with modified single-port laparoscopic procedures in children. J Laparoendosc Adv Surg Tech A 2009;19:695–8.

[64] Allemann P, Leroy J, Asakuma M, et al. Robotics may overcome technical limitations of single-trocar surgery: an experimental prospective study of Nissen fundoplication. Arch Surg 2010;145:267–71.

[65] Torquati A, Houston HL, Kaiser J, et al. Long-term follow-up study of the Stretta procedure for the treatment of gastroesophageal reflux disease. Surg Endosc 2004;18:1475–9.

[66] Johnson DA, Ganz R, Aisenberg J, et al. Endoscopic implantation of Enteryx for treatment of GERD: 12-month results of a prospective, multicenter trial. Am J Gastroenterol 2003;98:1921–30.

[67] Hogan WJ. Clinical trials evaluating endoscopic GERD treatments: is it time for a moratorium on the clinical use of these procedures? Am J Gastroenterol 2006;101:437–9.

[68] Cadière GB, Rajan A, Germay O, et al. Endoluminal fundoplication by a transoral device for the treatment of GERD: a feasibility study. Surg Endosc 2008;22:333–42.

[69] Repici A, Fumagalli U, Malesci A, et al. Endoluminal fundoplication (ELF) for GERD using EsophyX: a 12-month follow-up in a single-center experience. J Gastrointest Surg 2010;14:1–6.

Advances in Pediatrics 57 (2010) 391–397

ELSEVIER
MOSBY

ADVANCES IN PEDIATRICS

INDEX

Note: Page numbers of article titles are in **boldface** type.

0065-3101/10/$ – see front matter
doi:10.1016/S0065-3101(10)00027-7

Printed and bound by CPI Group (UK) Ltd, Croydon, CR0 4YY

08/05/2025

01864676-0002